Advances in Oral Administration

Advances in Oral Administration

Guest Editor

Guanyu Chen

MDPI

Basel • Beijing • Wuhan • Barcelona • Belgrade • Novi Sad • Cluj • Manchester

Guest Editor
Guanyu Chen
School of Pharmaceutical
Sciences (Shenzhen)
Shenzhen Campus of Sun
Yat-sen University
Shenzhen
China

Editorial Office
MDPI AG
Grosspeteranlage 5
4052 Basel, Switzerland

This is a reprint of the Special Issue, published open access by the journal *Pharmaceutics* (ISSN 1999-4923), freely accessible at: https://www.mdpi.com/journal/pharmaceutics/special_issues/T71C4OMV46.

For citation purposes, cite each article independently as indicated on the article page online and as indicated below:

Lastname, A.A.; Lastname, B.B. Article Title. *Journal Name* **Year**, *Volume Number*, Page Range.

ISBN 978-3-7258-6918-3 (Hbk)
ISBN 978-3-7258-6919-0 (PDF)
https://doi.org/10.3390/books978-3-7258-6919-0

Contents

pharmaceutics

MDPI

Editorial

Advances in the Oral Delivery of Protein and Peptide Drugs

Guanyu Chen

School of Pharmaceutical Sciences (Shenzhen), Shenzhen Campus, Sun Yat-sen University, Shenzhen 518107, China; chengy239@mail.sysu.edu.cn; Tel.: +86-020-84723750

Protein and peptide drugs (PPDs) are highly effective therapies for a wide range of diseases, including cancer, diabetes, and autoimmune disorders [1]. However, delivering these drugs orally presents significant challenges. PPDs face substantial barriers to attaining oral bioavailability, such as the rapid cleavage of PPDs by proteases in the gastrointestinal tract (GIT), and the low intestinal permeability of PPDs due to their hydrophilicity properties and high-molecular-weight structures [2]. Additionally, the denaturation of PPDs in acidic gastric environments due to their sensitivity to pH, as well as their short half-life with rapid systemic clearance, limits their therapeutic efficacy [3].

To overcome these barriers, advanced strategies for the delivery of innovative formulations are presented, such as nanocarriers. These include lipid-based carriers such as liposomes and polymeric nanoparticles; mucoadhesive systems including inorganic carriers, such as mesoporous silica, for enzymatic protection and controlled release [4]; enteric coatings such as chitosan or thiolated polymers to prolong intestinal residence [5]; absorption/permeation enhancement in the form of pH-responsive polymers (Eudragit®) for site-specific delivery to the small intestine [6]; targeted transport, such as SNAC (used in oral semaglutide), medium-chain fatty acids, or zonula occludens toxin, to transiently open tight junctions; chemical modification through receptor-mediated uptake (e.g., FcRn, vitamin B12 conjugation) [7]; enzyme inhibitors for PEGylation, cyclization, or D-amino acid substitution to resist proteolysis; the co-administration of protease inhibitors (e.g., aprotinin, soybean trypsin inhibitor) [8]; etc.

In the clinical translation of protein and peptide formulations, three major aspects should be considered: First, scalability, such as the manufacturing reproducibility of complex formulations (e.g., nanoparticle size uniformity). Secondly, safety, such as the long-term effects of permeation enhancers on intestinal integrity. Lastly, bioavailability, as even with advanced systems, achieving > 1% bioavailability remains a hurdle [9]. Therefore, more investigations and advanced formulation approaches are required for the oral delivery of protein and peptide drugs.

In this Special Issue on Advances in Oral Administration, twelve articles have been published, including eight research articles and four review articles. In the following sections, the highlights of these 12 articles will be summarized.

Csilla et al. conducted a study that successfully scaled up a wet grinding method using a planetary ball mill and ZrO_2 pearls, producing submicron meloxicam particles (~580 nm) with preserved crystallinity (70%) and enhanced dissolution (~100% in 5 min) without toxicity. The tenfold scale-up proved feasible by optimizing the milling parameters and excipient amounts, ensuring consistent drug quality for oral delivery (contribution 1).

Klervi et al. established a pharmacometric model which showed that CHILD-IVITAB, a child-friendly ivermectin formulation, exhibited faster and more consistent absorption than STROMECTOL®, enabling effective dosing for children under 15 kg, and their simulations demonstrated that a 250 μg/kg dose of CHILD-IVITAB provided an equivalent drug exposure in children < 15 kg to 200 μg/kg of STROMECTOL® in adults and heavier children, supporting its use in pediatric studies (contribution 2).

Ivan et al. developed Archaeosomes, which were made from archaeal lipids via microfluidics, exhibiting exceptional stability (100 nm size, low polydispersity) and retaining > 95% of encapsulated drugs (calcein/insulin) in harsh gastrointestinal conditions, with a 35% insulin encapsulation efficiency. Their resilience during freeze-/spray-drying and their strong adhesion to intestinal cells in co-culture models highlighted their potential as stable oral drug carriers, enabling solid dosage forms for biologics like insulin (contribution 3).

Guanyu et al. developed gemcitabine-loaded β-glucan nanoparticles using film-casting and freezer-milling, achieving sustained release, enhanced intestinal permeation, and greater oral bioavailability compared to a plain drug solution. Additionally, the nanomedicine showed excellent safety characteristics and potent tumor growth inhibition in 4T1 breast cancer models, demonstrating its potential as an effective chemotherapy platform for oral gemcitabine delivery (contribution 4).

Mengyang Liu et al. developed PEGylated niosomes which significantly improved thymopentin stability and cellular uptake via active endocytosis, though the transport rates remained similar to those of the free drug, with the mechanisms shifting to energy-dependent pathways (adsorptive/clathrin-mediated) instead of passive diffusion/MRP5 efflux. The formulation, enhanced further by permeation aids (EDTA/sodium taurocholate), demonstrated promise for oral peptide delivery by balancing uptake and transport while maintaining safety, offering a potential solution to thymopentin's metabolic instability (contribution 5).

Solene Masloh et al. introduced a novel oral delivery strategy for biotherapeutics using Nanofitin 1-F08, a robust affinity protein that targets the leptin receptor (LepR) without competing with leptin, enabling receptor-mediated transport across the intestinal barriers. Their approach demonstrated successful ex vivo transport in a porcine model, offering a promising pathway for the oral delivery of biologically active molecules while maintaining their efficacy, with the potential for future in vivo applications (contribution 6).

Else Holmfred et al. explored the compaction behavior of protein–excipient blends, revealing that lysozyme enhances the tablet strength in brittle excipients due to the improved particle bonding, while larger BSA particles reduce tensile strength, demonstrating non-linear effects with an increasing protein content. Additionally, the findings emphasized that the particulate properties of protein powders critically influence their compaction performance, showing that protein-based tablets can be designed using small-molecule pharmaceutical principles, supporting the development of oral protein formulations (contribution 7).

Clémence et al. reported that oral somatostatin receptor ligands (SRLs) like octreotide capsules (OOCs) and paltusotine show promise in acromegaly management, maintaining biochemical control in patients previously stabilized on injectable SRLs, as evidenced by recent trials (MPOWERED, PATHFNDR-1). While OOCs demonstrate long-term efficacy, gaps in the research remain—including direct drug comparisons and trials in SRL-naïve patients—highlighting the need for further research to optimize oral SRLs as a viable alternative to injections (contribution 8).

Xinxin et al.'s review article highlighted the potential for nano-formulations (liposomes, self-emulsifying systems, polymer particles) to enhance the oral delivery of antidiabetic peptides, offering promising solutions to improve gastrointestinal absorption and therapeutic efficacy (contribution 9).

Wanneng et al. introduced the gut microbiota, which plays a critical role in human health, and its regulation presents both therapeutic potential and challenges for treating disease. Additionally, they introduced the associated nanomaterials, with their protective, targeted, and biocompatible properties, demonstrated their significant promise in advancing the modulation of the gut microbiota, as highlighted by recent research and future development prospects (contribution 10).

Dan et al.'s review was focused on oxytocin, known for enhancing social cognition and reducing anxiety, and which is being explored as a therapy for social dysfunction disorders. While intranasal administration yielded a higher oxytocin bioavailability (11.1%) compared to oromucosal routes (4.4%), both methods showed similar peak concentration times (approximately 30 min) and comparable behavioral effects, highlighting the therapeutic potential of oromucosal delivery for oxytocin and other peptides in clinical and broader pharmaceutical applications (contribution 11).

Sílvio et al. discussed how inflammatory bowel disease (IBD) remains challenging to treat, but highlighted that probiotics show promise in managing symptoms, particularly for ulcerative colitis, though their stability and delivery need improvement. While the micro- and nanoencapsulation of probiotics and drugs enhances targeted colon delivery, overcoming gastrointestinal tract barriers and offering a novel therapeutic strategy for IBD, further clinical validation is needed for their long-term safety and efficacy (contribution 12).

Lastly, we would like to take this opportunity to thank all of the scientific researchers for their contributions to this Special Issue. While the oral delivery of protein/peptide drugs remains a formidable challenge, interdisciplinary advances in formulation science, nanotechnology, and molecular biology are driving progress in this field. Success in this area could revolutionize treatment by offering patients a more convenient and non-invasive alternative to injections, improving adherence and quality of life. Moreover, success hinges on balancing bioavailability, safety, and scalable manufacturing—a frontier requiring collaboration across pharmaceutics, biochemistry, and regulatory sciences. Continued research and collaboration are essential to bring these advanced therapies to the market.

Conflicts of Interest: The author declares no conflicts of interest.

List of Contributions

1. Bartos, C.; Motzwickler-Németh, A.; Kovács, D.; Burián, K.; Ambrus, R. Study on the Scale-Up Possibility of a Combined Wet Grinding Technique Intended for Oral Administration of Meloxicam Nanosuspension. *Pharmaceutics* **2024**, *16*, 1512.
2. Golhen, K.; Buettcher, M.; Huwyler, J.; van den Anker, J.; Gotta, V.; Dao, K.; Rothuizen, L.E.; Kobylinski, K.; Pfister, M. Pharmacometrics to Evaluate Dosing of the Patient-Friendly Ivermectin CHILD-IVITAB in Children ≥15 kg and <15 kg. *Pharmaceutics* **2024**, *16*, 1186.
3. Vidakovic, I.; Kornmueller, K.; Fiedler, D.; Khinast, J.; Fröhlich, E.; Leitinger, G.; Horn, C.; Quehenberger, J.; Spadiut, O.; Prassl, R. Archaeosomes for oral drug delivery: From continuous microfluidics production to powdered formulations. *Pharmaceutics* **2024**, *16*, 694.
4. Chen, G.; Liu, Y.; Svirskis, D.; Li, H.; Ying, M.; Lu, W.; Wen, J. Cryo-Milled β-Glucan Nanoparticles for Oral Drug Delivery. *Pharmaceutics* **2024**, *16*, 546.
5. Liu, M.; Svirskis, D.; Proft, T.; Loh, J.; Huang, Y.; Wen, J. Cellular Uptake and Transport Mechanism Investigations of PEGylated Niosomes for Improving the Oral Delivery of Thymopentin. *Pharmaceutics* **2024**, *16*, 397.
6. Masloh, S.; Chevrel, A.; Culot, M.; Perrocheau, A.; Kalia, Y.N.; Frehel, S.; Gaussin, R.; Gosselet, F.; Huet, S.; Zeisser Labouebe, M.; Scapozza, L. Enhancing Oral Delivery of Biologics: A Non-Competitive and Cross-Reactive Anti-Leptin Receptor Nanofitin Demonstrates a Gut-Crossing Capacity in an Ex Vivo Porcine Intestinal Model. *Pharmaceutics* **2024**, *16*, 116.
7. Holmfred, E.; Hirschberg, C.; Rantanen, J. Compaction Properties of Particulate Proteins in Binary Powder Mixtures with Common Excipients. *Pharmaceutics* **2023**, *16*, 19.

8. Reverdiau, C.; Denimal, D. Advances in the Oral Administration of Somatostatin Receptor Ligands in Acromegaly: A Systematic Review Focusing on Biochemical Response. *Pharmaceutics* **2024**, *16*, 1357.
9. Yang, X.; Lin, R.; Feng, C.; Kang, Q.; Yu, P.; Deng, Y.; Jin, Y. Research Progress on Peptide Drugs for Type 2 Diabetes and the Possibility of Oral Administration. *Pharmaceutics* **2024**, *16*, 1353.
10. Li, W.; Zhan, M.; Wen, Y.; Chen, Y.; Zhang, Z.; Wang, S.; Tian, D.; Tian, S. Recent Progress of Oral Functional Nanomaterials for Intestinal Microbiota Regulation. *Pharmaceutics* **2024**, *16*, 921.
11. Xu, D.; Lan, C.; Kou, J.; Yao, S.; Zhao, W.; Kendrick, K.M. Oromucosal administration of oxytocin: The development of 'Oxipops'. *Pharmaceutics* **2024**, *16*, 333.
12. Lopes, S.A.; Roque-Borda, C.A.; Duarte, J.L.; Di Filippo, L.D.; Borges Cardoso, V.M.; Pavan, F.R.; Chorilli, M.; Meneguin, A.B. Delivery strategies of probiotics from nano-and Microparticles: Trends in the treatment of inflammatory bowel disease—An overview. *Pharmaceutics* **2023**, *15*, 2600.

References

1. Singh, S.; Sanwal, P.; Bhargava, S.; Behera, A.; Upadhyay, S.; Akhter, M.H.; Gupta, M.; Gupta, S.M. Smart advancements for targeting solid tumors via protein and peptide drug delivery (PPD). *Curr. Drug Deliv.* **2023**, *20*, 669–682. [CrossRef] [PubMed]
2. Chen, G.; Kang, W.; Li, W.; Chen, S.; Gao, Y. Oral delivery of protein and peptide drugs: From non-specific formulation approaches to intestinal cell targeting strategies. *Theranostics* **2022**, *12*, 1419. [CrossRef] [PubMed]
3. Nicze, M.; Borówka, M.; Dec, A.; Niemiec, A.; Bułdak, Ł.; Okopień, B. The current and promising oral delivery methods for protein-and peptide-based drugs. *Int. J. Mol. Sci.* **2024**, *25*, 815. [CrossRef] [PubMed]
4. Kashapov, R.; Ibragimova, A.; Pavlov, R.; Gabdrakhmanov, D.; Kashapova, N.; Burilova, E.; Zakharova, L.; Sinyashin, O. Nanocarriers for biomedicine: From lipid formulations to inorganic and hybrid nanoparticles. *Int. J. Mol. Sci.* **2021**, *22*, 7055. [CrossRef] [PubMed]
5. MWays, T.M.; Lau, W.M.; Khutoryanskiy, V.V. Chitosan and its derivatives for application in mucoadhesive drug delivery systems. *Polymers* **2018**, *10*, 267. [CrossRef] [PubMed]
6. Varum, F.; Freire, A.C.; Fadda, H.M.; Bravo, R.; Basit, A.W. A dual pH and microbiota-triggered coating (Phloral™) for fail-safe colonic drug release. *Int. J. Pharm.* **2020**, *583*, 119379. [CrossRef] [PubMed]
7. Al Tahan, M.A. Engineering a Novel Mesoporous Silica-Lipid Hybrid Carrier for Oral Peptide Delivery. Ph.D. Thesis, Aston University, Birmingham, UK, 2023.
8. Dan, N.; Samanta, K.; Almoazen, H. An update on pharmaceutical strategies for oral delivery of therapeutic peptides and proteins in adults and pediatrics. *Children* **2020**, *7*, 307. [CrossRef] [PubMed]
9. Yang, B.; Gomes Dos Santos, A.; Puri, S.; Bak, A.; Zhou, L. The industrial design, translation, and development strategies for long-acting peptide delivery. *Expert Opin. Drug Deliv.* **2022**, *19*, 1233–1245. [CrossRef] [PubMed]

pharmaceutics

Article

Study on the Scale-Up Possibility of a Combined Wet Grinding Technique Intended for Oral Administration of Meloxicam Nanosuspension

Csilla Bartos [1], Anett Motzwickler-Németh [1], Dávid Kovács [1], Katalin Burián [2] and Rita Ambrus [1,*]

[1] Institute of Pharmaceutical Technology and Regulatory Affairs, Faculty of Pharmacy, University of Szeged, 6720 Szeged, Hungary; bartos.csilla@szte.hu (C.B.); nemeth.anett@szte.hu (A.M.-N.); kovacsdav97@gmail.com (D.K.)

[2] Department of Medical Microbiology, Albert Szent-Györgyi Medical School, University of Szeged, 6720 Szeged, Hungary; burian.katalin@med.u-szeged.hu

* Correspondence: ambrus.rita@szte.hu

Abstract: Background/Objectives: This article reports on the scalability of a combined wet grinding technique applying planetary ball mill and ZrO_2 pearls as the grinding medium. After the determination of the parameters in a laboratory scale, the tenfold scale-up method was set. Meloxicam (MEL) was used as a nonsteroidal anti-inflammatory drug (NSAID) intended for per os delivery. During grinding, the PVA solution was used as a dispersion medium. **Methods:** The influence of the scaling-up on the particle size, morphology, crystallinity, and intra- and interparticulate phenomena has been studied. Formulation investigations of the milled suspensions were carried out. The dissolution test and the cytotoxicity analyses were accomplished. **Results:** Submicron MEL particle-containing samples were produced in both grinding scales. After the particle size determination was achieved from the suspensions, the wet milled, dried products were studied. The particle size of the dried products fell into the same range for both scales of milling (the maximum particle size was about 580 nm). There was no significant difference in drug crystallinity after the grindings; 70% of MEL remained crystalline in both cases. A remarkable interaction between the components did not develop as a result of milling. The polarity of the products increased, which resulted in a better dissolution, especially in the case of intestinal fluid (~100% in the first 5 min). The products were not found to be toxic. **Conclusions:** This research demonstrates that the scaling-up of combined wet grinding technique is feasible by adjusting the milling parameters and the adequate amount of excipient.

Keywords: combined wet grinding/milling; scale-up method; meloxicam; nanonization; dissolution; cytotoxicity

1. Introduction

Nearly 40–60% of approved active pharmaceutical ingredients—which are most often administered through the oral route—are poorly water soluble. Solving this problem is a perennial challenge for the pharmaceutical industry [1,2]. Particle engineering techniques are generally applied to modify the physico-chemical and biopharmaceutical properties of drugs [3]. The various size reduction techniques include top-down methods, where the raw material is subsequently broken down until micro- or nanosized particles are produced [4]. The reduction in particle size of these drugs may change their crystalline structure, increasing their dissolution rate and absorption, and therefore ensuring better bioavailability, decreased therapeutic dose, and more a favorable side effect profile [5]. There is an overview of dry and wet grinding techniques (ball milling, media milling, high pressure homogenization, etc.) in the literature which discusses the grinding-induced amorphization and as a result the enhanced dissolution in the case of many drugs (furosemide, indomethacin, phenytoin, ibuprofen, glibenclamide, etc.) [6]. In the wet grinding procedure, a concentrated dispersion of drug particles in an aqueous or organic solvent liquid medium is performed. For wet grinding, additives are needed, independently of the preparation of micro- or nanoparticles. The choice of stabilizer is specific for each drug candidate and each formulation procedure. Stabilizers help minimize the aggregation of suspended particles via electrostatic and steric mechanisms [7]. In addition, the applied additives are usually hydrophilic in nature (such as polyvinylpyrrolidone, cellulose ethers, polyethylene glycol, polyvinyl alcohol, poloxamers, and cyclodextrins) and ensure hydrophilicity to the hydrophobic drug particle surfaces, which therefore results in better wettability and dissolution properties [8–10]. Applying wet milling, the preparation of suspensions is possible, which can be feasible for the development pharmaceutical formulations by means of drying or by direct processing [11].

Grinding is the most commonly used surface machining process, which is carried out with the aim of obtaining a result with a specific shape in the chosen material both in a laboratory scale and in the industry, because of its reproducibility, and the process is relatively easy to implement [12–14]. During the development of pharmaceutical formulations, lab-scale milling is followed by the scale-up of the process, which poses a challenge for the industry due to its complexity [15]. There is some research on the investigation of the scale-up of grinding based on mathematical models. Mannheim determined the power consumption of the stirred ball mill for scale-up by a method based on dimensional analysis [16]. Lehocký et al. have studied transferring the stirred media wet milling process from a batch to a flow-through arrangement during process scale-up. The parametric dependence of the particle breakage kinetics on the main process parameters has been systematically investigated. They were ascertained that the same terminal particle size could be obtained by several different combinations of the ball fill level, stirring rate, and overall process time [17]. Lestary et al. investigated the scalability of wet ball milling. He investigated factors including milling time, milling speed, and the type of mill. They determined that during the change in the milling mode from batch mode to recirculation mode, either the milling speed or milling duration needed to be adjusted to ensure that enough energy was given to break the particles into a smaller size [18]. The guidelines or a published method for the scaling-up of planetary ball mill are not yet known [19]. Grinding effects depend on different milling conditions such as the pot diameter, ball diameter, ball-filling ratio, revolution radius, and rotational speed, etc. First, the critical parameters of the lab-scale grinding need to be determined. Mio et al. have studied a computational simulation based on the Discrete Element Method for the scale-up of a planetary ball mill [20]. They established that the impact energy is a key factor in controlling the milling achievement; this indicates the guideline for the designing relationships of the directions and the speed ratio between the rotation of the pot and the revolution of the disk in a planetary ball mill. During the investigation of the scale-up method by using the impact energy of balls, it was determined that the milling rate increased with an increasing rotation speed and the specific impact energy, and it also increased with decreasing the sample weight. Using computational simulation, the relationship between the impact energy and the total scale-up ratio was defined. The impact energy of the balls in the planetary mill is proportional to the diameter and depth of the pot and the revolution radius [21].

Meloxicam (MEL) is an enolic acid that belongs to the oxicam class of NSAIDs that selectively inhibits COX-2 (cyclo-oxygenase-2). It is usually used in the treatment of pain or inflammation [22]. MEL has a crystalline structure, low water-solubility (4.4 μg/mL at 25 °C), and a low dissolution rate. Different particle size reduction techniques were previously applied in the literature in order to change the dissolution features of MEL. Co-grinding of MEL with PVP-C30 in a planetary ball mill resulted in a significant increase in the dissolution properties [23]. Formulation of the MEL nanosuspension by an emulsion–diffusion method also resulted in a significantly faster dissolution compared to the untreated particles [24]. The preparation of MEL nanocrystals by wet-milling technology and high-pressure homogenization improved its solubility, dissolution, and oral bioavailability [25]. The formulation of smartcrystals, applying a bead mill method, followed by high-pressure homogenization resulted in the efficient dissolution of the drug as well [26].

For nanoparticles, intended for utilization in therapeutic tools to treat human diseases, cytotoxicity studies are required to investigate their effects on the contacted cells. The cytotoxicity of nanoparticles depends on the experimental conditions and their physico-chemical properties [27]. You et al. determined that in case of MEL nanocrystals, the cell viability decreased in time- and dose-dependent manners; furthermore, the cytotoxicity increased with the increasing particle size [25]. MEL micro- and nanoparticles, produced by nanosecond laser ablation, showed a concentration-dependent cytotoxicity when different laser wavelengths were used [28]. Extra-fine particles containing nanosized meloxicam, prepared by nano spray-drying, revealed no cytotoxic effect in the studied concentration range [29].

To eliminate the weakness of the conventional grinding techniques, our research group has developed and optimized a new combined method for particle size reduction in MEL, combining planetary ball and pearl milling [30]. Due to the high efficiency of smaller beads sizes [31] and the high mechanical energy of the planetary mill [32], the particle size reduction to the nano range was implemented. For the nanonization of MEL, poly(vinyl alcohol) (PVA), as a stabilizing additive, was required, which promotes the milling efficiency. The process parameters of combined milling (pearl amount, milling time, and rotation speed) were optimized in a laboratory scale and the influence on the particle size distribution, crystallinity, and dissolution rate of MEL was also studied. The changes in polymer viscosity and the drug–polymer interaction were also determined [33]. For these investigations, a small milling chamber was applied, which had a volume of 50 mL. However, the following question arose: could the process be scaled-up using a ten-times larger chamber?

This article reports on a comparison of a laboratory scale and a 10-fold scaled-up combined wet grinding process, as a novel organic solvent-free technology, where the planetary ball mill was combined with the pearl grinding procedure using a small (50 mL) and a larger (500 mL) milling chamber. Our aim was to scale-up the nanonization of MEL in an aqueous dispersant medium, intended for oral administration. The effects of both millings on the particle size, physical-chemical features, resuspendability, holding time, drug content, and uniformity were analyzed. The in vitro dissolution of MEL was studied and evaluated after filling the suspensions into capsules. The cytotoxicity study of products was also performed. In our opinion, this work presents useful information, filling a gap between the laboratory and industrial scale production of nanoparticle-based formulations.

2. Materials and Methods

2.1. Materials

MEL (4-hydroxy-2-methyl-N-(5-methyl-2-thiazolyl)-2H-benzothiazine-3-carboxamide-1,1-dioxide) was attained from EGIS Ltd. (Budapest, Hungary). PVA (polyvinyl alcohol), was procured from Sigma Aldrich (St. Louis, MO, USA). Purified water was used to prepare the 5% PVA solution. The phosphate buffer (pH 7.4 $\pm$ 0.1) was made from $Na_2HPO_4 \cdot 2H_2O$ (Spektrum 3D, Debrecen, Hungary), the pH was adjusted with 85% o-phosphoric acid (Molar Chemicals Kft, Halásztelek, Hungary). The artificial gastric fluid (pH 1.2 $\pm$ 0.1) was made from NaCl (Molar Chemicals Kft., Halásztelek, Hungary) and 37% HCl (Merck Kft., Budapest, Hungary) while the intestinal fluid (pH 6.8 $\pm$ 0.1) was made from KH_2PO_4 (Molar Chemicals Kft, Halásztelek, Hungary) and NaOH (Spektrum 3D, Debrecen, Hungary). All these chemical reagents were of analytical grade.

2.2. Preparation of Suspensions

For investigating the possibility of scale-up in the case of combined wet grinding (a combination of planetary ball and bead grinding) (Figure 1), the suspension intended for per os application was prepared using the large grinding chamber (500 mL) of the planetary ball mill (Retsch PM 100) (Retsch GmbH, Haan, Germany). As a grinding medium, 0.3 mm

ZrO_2 beads were applied. A total of 20 g of MEL was first suspended in the 5% PVA solution (180 g). Rpm—required for scale-up—was calculated from rpm, determined for lab-scale milling ($\Omega_1{}^2 d_{M1} = \Omega_2{}^2 d_{M2}$, where Ω represents the revolutions per minite, and d_M the diameter of the chamber (mm). (Ω_1 = 500 rpm, d_{M1} = 4.5 cm, d_{M2} = 10 cm)) [21,29]. The calculated prm was 335. During the grinding procedure, samples were taken at times of 10, 30, 50, 70, 90, 110, 130, and 150 min in order to monitor the particle size changes. Pearls were removed using a 150 µm mesh size sieve. The sample milled in the large milling chamber (MELscup) was compared with the sample prepared in a small volume chamber (500 rpm, 50 min, 50 mL chamber) (MELlab). As references, the initial drug (rawMEL) and the suspension of untreated MEL in the PVA solution (MELsusp) were applied. The abbreviations used in the article are summarized in Table 1.

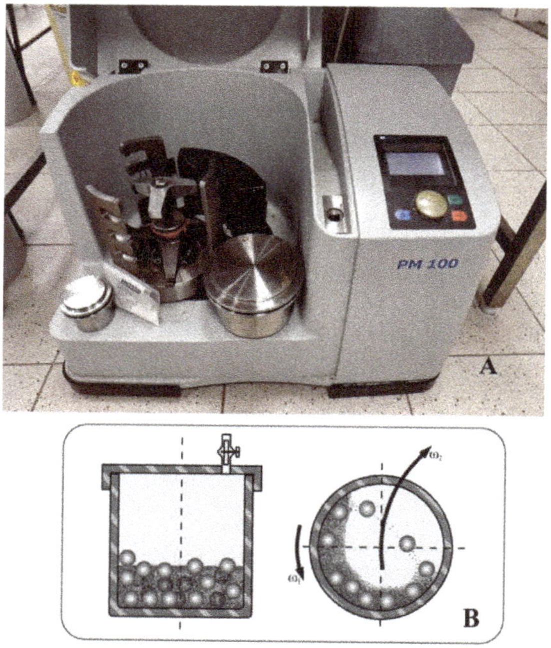

Figure 1. The picture of the planetary ball mill (**A**) and the schematic view of the ball mill (**B**).

Table 1. Abbreviations of samples in the text.

rawMEL	initial drug
MELsusp	untreated suspension of MEL
MELlab	sample milled in a laboratory scale for 50 min at 500 rpm
MELscup	scaled-up sample (335 rpm, 90 min)

2.3. Determination of Particle Size Distribution

After grinding, the particle size of MEL in the suspensions was established. The volume-based particle size distribution (PSD) was determined by laser diffraction (Mastersizer 2000, Malvern Instruments Ltd., Worcestershire, UK) with the following parameters: 300RF lens; small volume dispersion unit (2500 rpm); refractive index for dispersed particles 1.720; refractive index for dispersion medium 1.330. The Dynamic Laser Light Scattering method was applied to determine the PSD. The particle size of MEL was determined immediately from the ground suspension. The size analysis was repeated three times. Water was used as the dispersant medium, and the obscuration was in the range 11–16% for all measurements. The volume-based- particle size distributions, D10, D50, and D90 (where, for example, D90 is the maximum particle diameter below which 90% of the sample volume exists), were determined.

2.4. Preparation of Solid-Phase Products for Physical-Chemical Investigations of Products

The chosen suspensions were dried in a vacuum dryer (Binder GmbH, Tuttlingen, Germany) at 40 °C in order to gain solid products for the physico-chemical analysis.

2.5. Image Analysis (SEM)

The morphological features of the ground dried products were analyzed applying a scanning electron microscope (Hitachi S4700, Hitachi Scientific Ltd., Tokyo, Japan). The patterns were sputter-coated with gold–palladium under an argon atmosphere, using a gold sputter module in a high-vacuum evaporator, and the samples were investigated at 15 kV and 10 μA. The air pressure was 1.3–13 MPa. For the particle size determination of MEL, a public domain image analyzer software, ImageJ, was applied (https://imagej.nih.gov/ij/index.html, accessed on 17 November 2024) [34].

2.6. Structural Analysis

In order to investigate the physical state of the drug in the solid products, a Bruker D8 Advance diffractometer (Bruker AXS GmbH, Karlsruhe, Germany) system was applied with Cu K λI radiation (λ = 1.5406 Å). The samples were scanned at 40 kV and 40 mA from 3° to 40°·2θ, at a scanning speed of 0.05°/s and a step size of 0.010°. The crystallinity (xc) of MEL in the solid-state samples was ascertained semi-quantitatively in the case of both millings by the mean of the decrease in the total area beneath the curve of 3 characteristic peaks ($A_{crystalline}$) compared to the rawMEL ($A_{crystalline} + A_{amorphous}$) as follows (Equation (1)):

$$\text{xc} = \frac{A_{crystalline}}{A_{crystalline} + A_{amorphous}} * 100 \quad (1)$$

A Mettler Toledo DSC 821e thermal analysis system with the STARe thermal analysis program V9.0 (Mettler Inc., Schwerzenbach, Switzerland) was used for the thermoanalytical investigations of samples. About 2–5 mg of pure drug or ground dried product was studied in the temperature range between 25 °C and 300 °C. The heating rate was 5 °C·min^{-1}. Argon gas was used as the carrier gas at a flow rate of 10 L·h^{-1} during the DSC investigations.

2.7. Fourier-Transformed Infrared Spectroscopy (FT-IR)

An AVATAR330 FT-IR spectrometer (Thermo Nicolet, Unicam Hungary Ltd., Budapest, Hungary) was applied for the investigation of the formation of secondary interactions or changes in bonds in the samples. Examination was performed in the interval 400–4000 cm^{-1} at an optical resolution of 4 cm^{-1}. Samples were ground and compressed into pastilles at 10 t with 0.15 g of KBr.

2.8. Determination of the Interparticle Interactions

Approximately 0.10 g of the samples was pressed on a 1-ton hydraulic press (Perkin Elmer hydraulic press, Specac Inc., Waltham, MA, USA). The prepared pastilles were dribbled with polar liquid (4.8 μL of purified water) and with non-polar solvent (2.0 μL of diiodomethane). A Dataphysics OCA 20 apparatus (Dataphysics Instrument GmbH, Filderstadt, Germany) was applied for the detection of the contact angle in an interval of 1 to 25 s. The contact angles of the two fluids were achieved. The surface free energy (γ^s) of the products, consisting of the polar part ($\gamma_s{}^p$) and the disperse part ($\gamma_s{}^d$); ($\gamma^s = \gamma_s{}^p + \gamma_s{}^d$) was determined based on the Wu equation [35]. The surface tension of the used liquids can be found in the literature as follows: distilled water γ^p = 50.2 mN/m, γ^d = 22.6 mN/m and diiodomethane γ^p = 1.8 mN/m, γ^d = 49 mN/m. Below, the Wu equation is shown

(Equation (2)), where θ = contact angle, γ = surface free energy, s = solid phase, l = liquid phase, d = dispersion component, and p = polar component.

$$(1 + cos\theta)\gamma_l = \frac{4(\gamma_s{}^d\gamma_l{}^d)}{\gamma_s{}^{d+}\gamma_l{}^d} + \frac{4(\gamma_s{}^p\gamma_l{}^p)}{\gamma_s{}^{p+}\gamma_l{}^p} \quad (2)$$

The polarity (Pol) was calculated as the ratio of the surface free energy of the polar component and the surface free energy multiplied by 100 (Equation (3)).

$$Pol = \frac{\gamma^p}{\gamma^s} * 100 \quad (3)$$

2.9. *Characterizations of the Suspensions*

Suspensions were characterized before filling into capsules.

2.9.1. Resuspendability

The resuspendability of suspensions was evaluated qualitatively using a measuring cylinder of 25.0 mL. The test was performed by rotating the cylinder using a laboratory resuspending device. The number of rotations required for the complete elimination of sediment from the bottom was recorded. The suspensions were stored in a refrigerator at a temperature of 15 ± 1 °C.

2.9.2. Holding Time Determination

The holding time of the samples was determined after storage for one month. The PSD of MEL in the ground suspensions was detected using laser diffraction (Malvern Mastersizer S 2000) (Malvern Instruments Ltd., Worcestershire, UK). The suspensions were stored in a refrigerator at 15 ± 1 °C. In order to resuspend the samples, a magnetic stirrer was applied. Three parallel measurements were carried out and the average values were compared with the particle sizes of the initial suspensions.

2.9.3. Drug Content and Uniformity

The drug content of the suspensions was investigated by dissolving the samples containing 5.00 mg of MEL in a 25.0 mL phosphate buffer (pH 7.4 ± 0.1). The samples were stirred with a magnetic stirrer at room temperature (25 °C). After filtration (0.1 µm, FilterBio PES Syringe Filter) (Labex Ltd., Budapest, Hungary), the dissolved drug content was analyzed spectrophotometrically at 364 nm (ATI Unicam UV/VIS) (Cambridge, UK). Each suspension was sampled from 3 different locations, and the uniformity of the drug content was obtained by the calculation of the standard deviation of parallel measurements.

2.10. *In Vitro Dissolution Test*

The paddle method USP (Pharma Test, Heinburg, Germany) was applied for investigation the release of MEL from the suspensions. Dispersions containing 7.5 mg of MEL (therapeutic dose) were filled into "00" size capsules 5 sec after grinding and put quickly into the dissolution medium. The medium contained 900 mL of artificial gastric fluid, at pH 1.2 ± 0.1, and intestinal fluid (pH 6.8 ± 0.1). The rotation speed of the paddle was 100 rpm, and samples were taken at intervals up to 60 min. A spectrophotometer (ATI-UNICAM UV/VIS Spectrophotometer) was used to determine the drug content of samples at 362 nm for gastric juice and 364 nm for enteric fluid. The number of parallel runs was 3.

Dissolution efficiency (D.E.) (Equation (4)) is given by the area under a dissolution curve between defined time points and the mean dissolution time (M.D.T.) (Equation (5)) [36,37]. To facilitate the calculations, DDSolver program was applied [38].

$$\mathrm{DE} = \frac{\int_0^t \mathrm{y}*\mathrm{dt}}{\mathrm{y}100*\mathrm{t}}*100\% \quad (4)$$

$$MDT = \frac{\sum_{i=1}^{n} t_i * \Delta M_i}{\sum_{i=1}^{n} \Delta M_i} \quad (5)$$

In the formulas above, n is the number of sampling points; t_i is the ith sampling time point; y is the percentage of drug dissolved at time t; ΔM_i is the additional amount of drug dissolved between i and i − 1; and y100 is the maximum percentage of drug dissolved over the time period 0–t.

2.11. Cytotoxicity Studies

The cytotoxicity of the prepared suspensions was investigated on a Caco-2 cell line (immortalized cell line of human colorectal adenocarcinoma cells, the Caco-2 cell line was purchased from American Types Culture Collection ((ATCC) (Manassas, VA, USA)), in the range of concentration of 0.002 mg/mL–1.000 mg/mL). Cells were seeded in 96-well culture microplates (SPL Life Sciences Co., Pocheon-si, Republic of Korea) at a density of 4×10^4 cells/well in DMEM (Dulbecco's Modified Eagle's Medium) (Sigma-Aldrich Co., St. Louis, MO, USA), supplemented with 10% FBS ((Fetal Bovine Serum) (Sigma-Aldrich Co., St. Louis, MO, USA)). The samples were incubated with the cells for 24 h at 37 °C. MTT (Sigma-Aldrich Co., St. Louis, MO, USA), dissolved in PBS (Phosphate-Buffered Saline), at a 20 µL volume was added to the wells and incubated for 4 h. Later, 10% sodium dodecyl sulfate (Reanal Laborvegyszer Kft., Budapest, Hungary), dissolved in distilled water (100 µL), was added to the wells, and the optical density (OD) was measured after a 12 h incubation at 550 nm (ref. 630 nm) with EZ REAS 400 ELISA reader (Biochrom, Cambridge, UK). Untreated cells with 100% viability served as the control. Three parallel measurements were carried out for each sample.

3. Results

3.1. Particle Size Distribution of Milled Suspensions

After the optimization of the parameters in a laboratory scale [33,39], for scaling-up, a 10-fold amount of pearls of a ground composition was used. The rotation speed was calculated based on a formula previously applied in the literature [21]. Our main purpose was to determine and compare the milling times needed for the production of nanosized MEL particles at both milling scales. First, the effect of grinding time on the particle size distribution of MEL was determined for the scale-up conditions. Based on the laser diffraction results, grinding for 70 min resulted in micronized MEL particles (D90 = 1.013 µm) (Table 2). After 90 min of milling, the particle size of the drug decreased to the submicron range (D90 = 0.697 µm) due to the high mechanical forces of the planetary ball mill and the high efficiency of the small bead size [13]. Additionally, this was aided by the PVA, which inhibits particle aggregation. Further milling did not result in a significant decrease in particle size.

Table 2. PSD of MEL in suspensions prepared by scale-up method.

Samples	D10 (µm)	D50 (µm)	D90 (µm)
rawMEL	11.40	34.26	73.59
10 min	2.115	3.112	3.690
30 min	0.150	0.204	0.255
50 min	1.101	1.218	1.329
70 min	0.810	0.905	1.013
90 min	0.517	0.590	0.697
110 min	0.518	0.594	0.696
130 min	0.517	0.589	0.696
150 min	0.517	0.589	0.695

After that the effects of the lab-scale milling and the scaled-up milling on the particle size were compared (Table 3). Initial MEL, untreated suspended MEL, and MEL milled at different scales are shown in Figure 2. It can be established that the particle size of the suspended untreated MEL was lower compared with the raw drug due to the surface dissolution in the presence of PVA [40]. In these cases, the particle size was in the micrometer range. Grinding resulted in nanosized particles (D50 < 600 nm) in both cases; however, while 50 min of grinding was sufficient for nanonization in a laboratory scale, 90 min were required at the scaled-up conditions. In the case of the scaled-up milling, a 2.5-fold larger particle size was measured compared to the laboratory scale (D90 = 0.270 μm). Due to the measurement methodology of laser diffraction, particles moving together may be detected as aggreagates during size distribution determination. As a check, further investigaiotns were carried out using ImageJ software.

Table 3. PSD of initial MEL, of untreated suspended MEL, and of MEL milled at different scales.

Samples	D10 (μm)	D50 (μm)	D90 (μm)
rawMEL	11.40	34.26	73.59
MELsusp	11.01	20.407	35.28
MELlab	0.093	0.177	0.270
MELscup	0.517	0.590	0.697

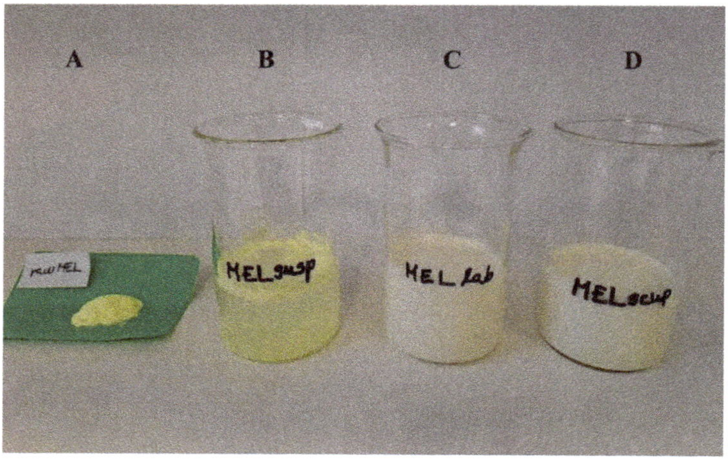

Figure 2. The photo of initial MEL (**A**), untreated suspended MEL (**B**), and MEL milled at different scales (**C**,**D**).

3.2. Morphology of MEL

The morphology of the ground particles is presented in the SEM images. After taking samples from the suspensions milled for 50 min (MELlab) and for 90 min (MELscup), samples were dried and characterized. The surfaces and shape changes were investigated.

RawMEL and the suspension of rawMEL contained mostly rough, lamellar crystals with a broad size distribution (Figure 3). However, ground products consisted of particles with a smooth surface and a rounded shape, as a result of the surface abrasion effect of milling beads [41]. Nanoparticles were embedded in the PVA film. Due to the presence of PVA, no aggregation was noticed in the case of the milled products. PVA coated the particles and worked to keep them away from each other [42,43].

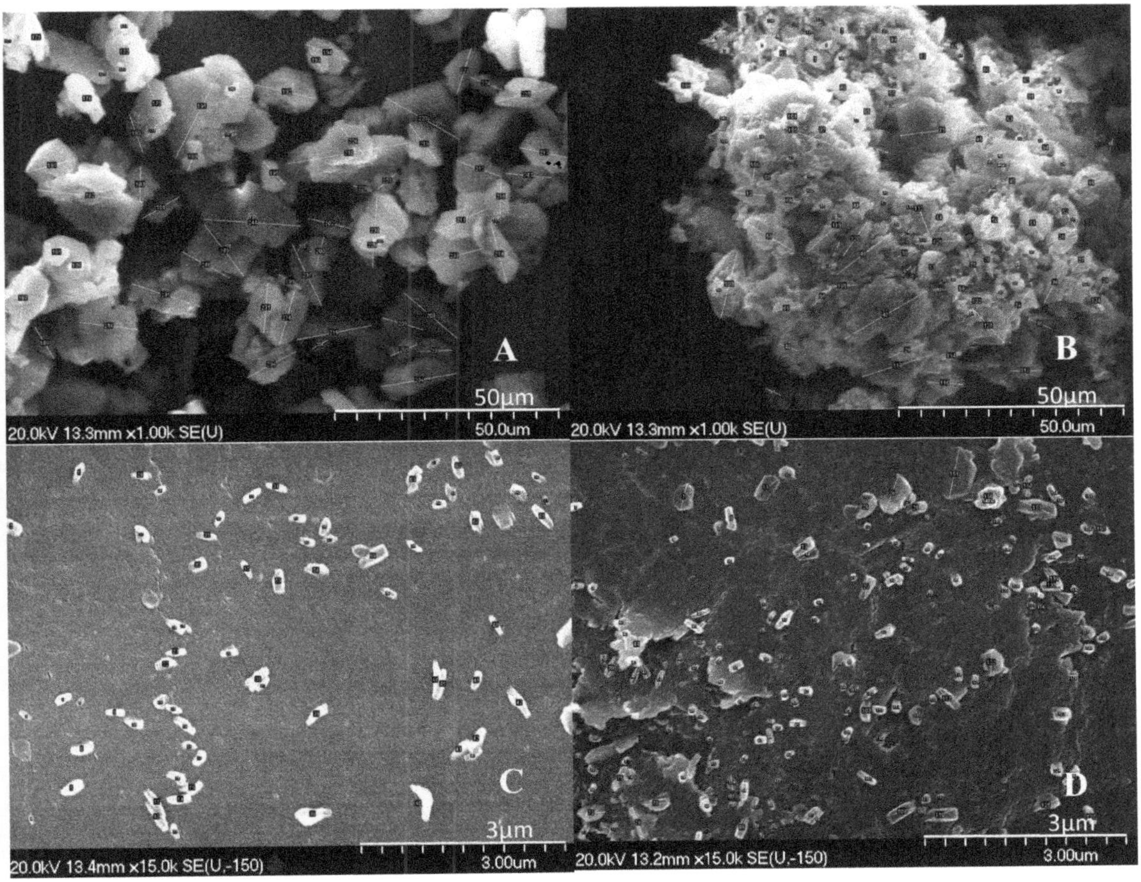

Figure 3. SEM pictures of rawMEL (**A**), of dried untreated suspension of MEL (**B**), of MEL milled in laboratory scale (**C**), and of MEL milled at scaled-up conditions (**D**).

Based on the values determined by the image analysis program ImageJ, it was established that in the dried suspension form, the particles of rawMEL (MELsusp) were separated from each other, resulting in a lower particle size in comparison with tge powder form of rawMEL, in which case the particles were stuck together (Table 4). However, in the case of dried suspensions produced by grinding (MELlab; MELscup), these values were significantly lower and more reliable (smaller standard deviation (SD)), and the average particle size of these samples was in the submicron range (<600 nm). In the SEM images, the individual particles could be analyzed separately.

Table 4. PS data of rawMEL, of dried untreated suspension of MEL, and of MEL milled at different scales determined by ImageJ.

Samples	Minimum (µm)	Maximum (µm)	Average (µm)
rawMEL	3.19 ± 1.32	27.05 ± 8.15	12.01 ± 6.07
MELsusp	0.60 ± 0.09	16.06 ± 6.36	4.62 ± 3.05
MELlab	0.14 ± 0.01	0.57 ± 0.02	0.33 ± 0.01
MELscup	0.09 ± 0.02	0.58 ± 0.05	0.24 ± 0.03

3.3. Structural Analyses (XRPD and DSC)

For the characterization of the crystalline state of MEL after the grinding processes, X-ray powder diffraction was applied. RawMEL, the dried untreated suspension of MEL, and MEL milled at different scales were characterized. The XRPD diffractograms of rawMEL showed its crystalline structure. The characteristic 2θ data of MEL were 13.22, 15.06, 26.46, and 26.67. In the case of the dried untreated MEL suspension, the intensities of the characteristic peaks decreased due to the semicrystalline structure of the PVA, which covered the MEL particles [44] (Figure 4). Further grinding resulted in the same decrease in the crystallinity of the drug. After the suspendation of MEL in the PVA solution, its crystallinity decrease from 100 to 72%. This value did not change in either the laboratory scale or during scaled-up milling; the drug retained 70% of its crystalline structure (Table 5) [45].

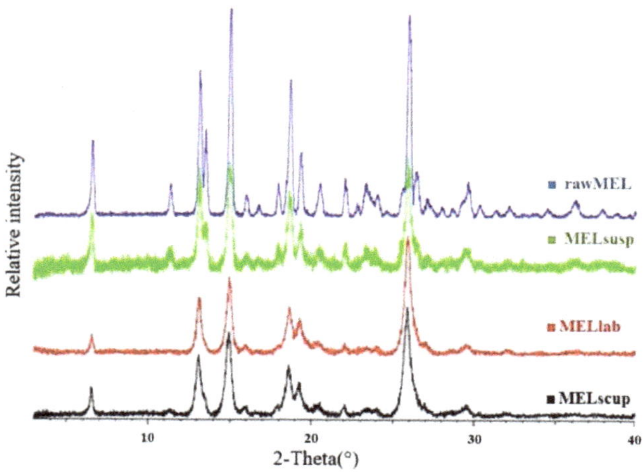

Figure 4. XRPD patterns of rawMEL, of dried untreated suspension of MEL, and of MEL milled at different scales.

Table 5. The degree of MEL crystallinity (%) before and after milling procedures.

Sample	Crystallinity (%)
rawMEL	100
MELsusp	71.8
MELlab	70.2
MELscup	71.2

DSC was employed to investigate the melting of MEL in the raw form, in the dried untreated suspension, and in the dried ground products (Figure 5). The DSC curve of rawMEL showed a sharp endothermic peak at 263.55 °C, representing its melting point and verifying its crystalline structure. The DSC curve revealed a broad endothermic peak for MEL in the case of the initial suspension (MELsusp: 252.23 °C) and for the milled products (MELlab: 244.94 °C and MELscup: 242.60 °C), indicating that the crystallinity of the drug was decreased. In these cases, MEL crystals melted at a lower temperature than the crystals of rawMEL. This phenomenon is due to the PVA, which covered the MEL particles during grindings and softened at 85 °C, as the glass transition temperature (Tg) value induces the melting of the drug at a lower temperature [46].

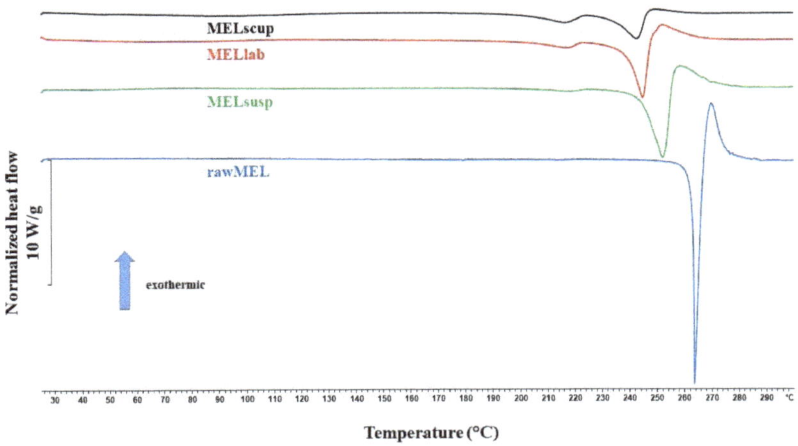

Figure 5. DSC thermograms of rawMEL, of dried untreated suspension of MEL, and of MEL milled at different scales.

3.4. FT-IR Investigations

Using FT-IR spectroscopy, we investigated whether the grinding process has any effect on the formation of secondary interactions or changes in the bonds in the samples. Figure 6 presents the FT-IR spectra of the following four samples: the rawMEL, MELsusp after drying, the ground sample (MELlab), and the scaled-up ground sample (MELscup). The most characteristic vibrations of MEL [47,48] were observed at 3288.8 cm^{-1} (N-H stretching), 1620.7 cm^{-1} (C=O stretching), 1549.8 cm^{-1} (C=N stretching), 1455.8 cm^{-1} (C=C stretching of the aromatic ring), 1344.6 cm^{-1}, and 1161.6 cm^{-1} (S=O stretching vibrations of the sulfonyl groups). These characteristic peaks appeared in MELsusp as well as in the ground samples (MELlab and MELscup). There were no shifts, fusions, losses, or broadenings that would suggest the formation of new interactions, nor were there any new peaks recorded. A decrease in the intensity of the peaks was observed in samples MELlab and MELscup, which occurred due to the decrease in crystallinity and particle size [45,49]. The results of the FT-IR measurements indicated that the MEL remained in the milled preparations in an unchanged form without decomposition. The FTIR measurements proved that the milling process did not affect the molecular structure of the MEL, furthermore confirming the stability of the formulations during the milling process.

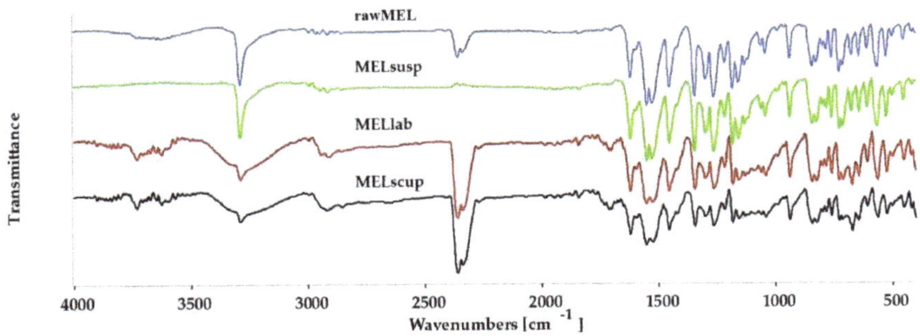

Figure 6. FTIR spectra of rawMEL, of dried untreated suspension of MEL, and of MEL milled at different scales.

3.5. Interparticular Interactions

The polarity and the cohesive work (Wc) characteristics of the materials were determined on the basis of the contact angle measurements. The wettability study showed that the milled dried samples (MELlab and MELscup) had decreased values of the contact angle with water (θwater), indicating a more hydrophilic character as compared with hydrophobic rawMEL and MELsusp. Milling created a new hydrophobic drug surface that was hydrophilized with PVA, which is a hydrophilic polymer, and therefore, wettability could be increased [50]. The polarity of the milled products, calculated as the ratio of surface free energy of the polar component and the surface free energy, also increased, forecasting the better dissolution results (Table 6).

Table 6. The polarity, the surface free energy (γ), and the contact angle values of the rawMEL, dried untreated, and dried milled suspensions.

Samples	θ Water (°)	θ Diiodomethane (°)	γ (mN/m)	Polarity (%)
rawMEL	68.99	13.33	57.10	20.96
MELsusp	67.47	9.46	58.29	21.56
MELlab	61.97	27.02	58.76	26.67
MELscup	54.40	21.03	62.40	31.07

3.6. Investigations of Milled Suspnesions

3.6.1. Resuspendability Test and Holding Time Determination

Resuspendability and the uniformity in particle size are essential in suspension formulation. During the resuspendability test of the investigated suspensions, it was found that both samples produced at laboratory (MELlab) and at scaled-up (MELscup) conditions proved to be stable even after 1 month of storage, as the sediment from the bottom disappeared after only two revolutions, and homogeneous suspensions were obtained. In contrast, the suspension containing untreated MEL (MELsusp) needed 45 revolutions to achieve homogeneity (Table 7). PVA increased the viscosity of the dispersion medium, thereby ensured a slow sedimentation of the nanosized particles [51].

Table 7. Resuspendability of the untreated and milled suspensions.

Sample	Number of Revolutions
MELsusp	45
MELlab	2
MELscup	2

During the holding time determination, it was obtained that no aggregation occurred after 1 month of storage (Table 8). This can be explained by the presence of PVA, which—forming the coating layer as a steric barrier around particles—could prevent aggregation and stabilize the suspension [30,52].

Table 8. Average particle size of milled suspensions after 1 month of storage.

Sample	Average Particle Size (nm)	
	Day 0	Day 30
MELlab	296.1 ± 20.3	299.3 ± 17.1
MELscup	424.7 ± 25.6	428.6 ± 45.2

3.6.2. Drug Content and Uniformity Determination

During the drug content investigations, a loss of more than 10% was experienced in both millings (Table 9), which can be explained by the fact that the drug may stick to the surface of the milling beads during milling, and we could not completely remove the samples from the milling chamber. The uniformity of the drug content was improved in the case of the milled samples compared to the untreated suspension.

Table 9. Drug content and uniformity of the untreated and milled suspensions.

Sample	Drug Content and Uniformity (mg)	Drug Content (%)
MELsusp	5.00 ± 0.35	100 ± 7.07
MELlab	4.41 ± 0.06	88.12 ± 1.36
MELscup	4.44 ± 0.03	88.80 ± 0.63

3.7. Results of In Vitro Dissolution Test

First, the in vitro dissolution test was carried out in an artificial gastric fluid at pH 1.2 ± 0.1 (Figure 7A). Suspnesions of MEL were filled into the capsules and promptly put into the medium. MELsusp was compared with the ground products. The investigation exhibited the slow and gentle dissolution of the drug from the untreated MELsusp, and after 60 min, approximately 7% of the drug was liberated. MEL has a weak acidic character (pKa 4.08), which results in a very low solubility in gastric fluid (1.6 ± 0.2 mg/L, at 37 °C) [53]. Grinding in both laboratory and scaled-up cases resulted in a 10-fold increase in the dissolution rate of the drug. In the case of the MELlab sample, 20% of the drug was dissolved in the first 10 min. In case of MELscup, this value was 10%; however, after 30 min, 20% of MEL was dissolved in this case too. This increase in the dissolved amount resulted in the small particle size and the wetting effect of PVA, which improves the wettability of poorly soluble drugs, enhancing their dispersion in aqueous environments [51].

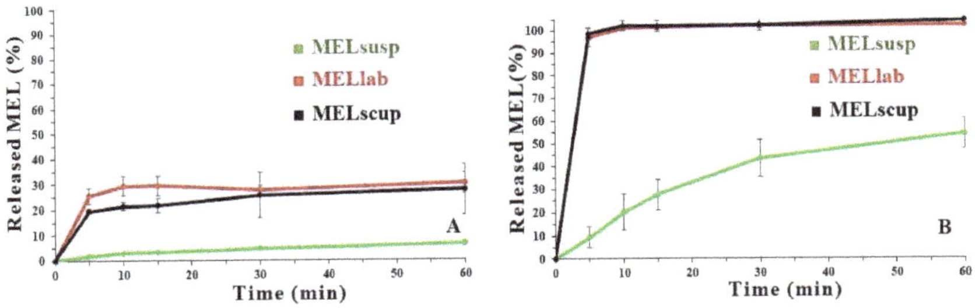

Figure 7. In vitro dissolution profile of initial and milled suspensions filled into capsules in artificial gastric fluid (**A**) and in artificial intestinal fluid (**B**).

After the dissolution test in the artificial gastric fluid, dissolution investigations were carried out in an artificial intestinal fluid (pH 6.8 ± 0.1) (Figure 7B). In this case, the liberated amount of the drug was higher because of the higher solubility of MEL (0.272 ± 0.001 mg/mL, at 37 °C). It was established that in case of MELsusp, the rate of dissolution of raw MEL, with particles in the micrometer size range, was lower compared with ground products; only 10% of the drug was dissolved in the first 5 min and approximately 50% after 60 min. Milled products had a significantly better drug release than the reference sample. Furthermore, it can be observed that there was no significant difference between the liberated drug amount from the samples prepared in laboratory scale and at scaled-up conditions. About 100% of the drug released from both ground samples in the first 5 min due to the small particle size and the enhanced wettability increased with the use of PVA [54].

During the determination of dissolution kinetics, the dissolution efficiency (DE) and the mean dissolution time (MDT) were determined. The calculated values in the table clearly show that the dissolution of MEL and the average dissolution time in the case of ground samples are coincident for intestinal fluid and significantly better than those of the reference for both digestive media. More than 50% lower values were calculated for MDT in the case of the intestinal fluid compared with gastric fluid (Table 10).

Table 10. Dissolution kinetics of the untreated and milled suspensions.

	Gastric Fluid		Intestinal Fluid	
Samples	**DE (%)**	**MDT (min)**	**DE (%)**	**MDT (min)**
MELsusp	4.37	20.05	37.03	19.17
MELlab	27.48	6.96	97.37	3.14
MELscup	23.57	8.70	98.48	3.63

3.8. Cytotoxicity Studies

The therapeutic dose of MEL in marketed medicines is 7.5 or 15.0 mg per os [55]; hence, in this study, suspensions containing 7.5 mg of MEL were chosen for further investigations. In order to recognize the effect of nanoparticles on cells, cytotoxicity analyses were performed. The cytotoxicity of the prepared suspensions (MELsusp, MELlab and MELscup) was determined on a Caco-2 cell line (Figure 8). It was observed that the degree of cell death appreciably increased above 0.5 mg/mL MEL concentration, especially in case of samples prepared by grinding. However, below concentration values of 0.5 mg/mL, it can already be stated that the suspensions can be used safely; there is no need to expect a significant toxic effect. Our capsules contained the drug in a concentration of 0.1 mg/mL; therefore, no cytotoxic effect was expected in the case of the investigated samples.

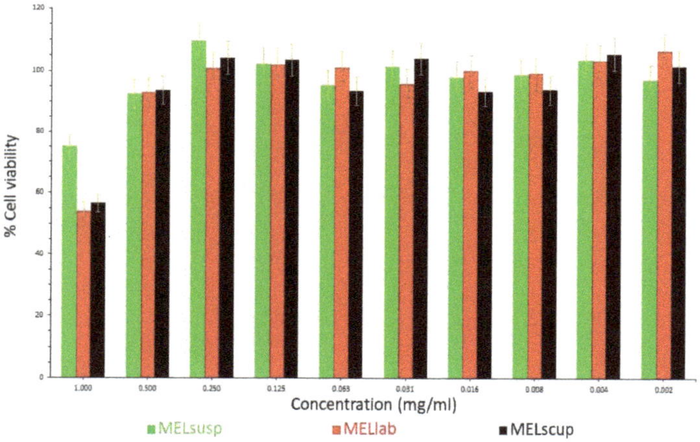

Figure 8. Cytotoxicity of the untreated and milled suspensions as a function of concentration on a Caco-2 cell line.

4. Conclusions

In our work, the possibility of a scaling-up of a combined wet grinding technique—previously optimized by our research group—was investigated. MEL was used as a NSAID. MEL-containing samples were prepared at laboratory and at tenfold scaled-up conditions. Water was used as a grinding medium; therefore, the procedure was considered green technology, while the product was organic solvent-free. The effect of millings on the physico-chemical properties of the products were determined. The resuspendability, holding time, drug content, and uniformity of suspensions were established. The results of the dissolution tests were compared. For both lab-scale milling and scaled-up milling, the particle size of the suspensions was in the submicron range. For nanonization, 50 min of milling at laboratory conditions, and 90 min of milling at scaled-up conditions were needed. Both grindings resulted in rounded particles with a smooth surface. The maximum particle size determined by ImageJ analyses program was almost the same (MELlab = 0.57 µm; MELscup = 0.58 µm) in both cases. A 30% decrease in the drug crystallinity was confirmed by DSC and XRPD during the grinding procedures. No secondary interaction could be detected between the compounds in the investigated products for any milling. The polarity of the milled products increased compared with the untreated drug. Formulation investigations proved the physical stability of ground suspensions. In the intestinal fluid, the dissolved amount of MEL was the same for any sampling points under laboratory conditions and under scaled-up conditions too. The liberated drug amount was significantly higher compared with the results of the gastric fluid. The samples investigated were not found to be cytotoxic.

We can declare based on our results that, although there is no suggested protocol for scaling-up the grinding process and a lot of experiments are needed even under laboratory conditions, the settings of the grinding speed and the grinding time are essential during the scale-up procedure. Furthermore, the application of hydrophilic additives is usually required to ensure the desired particle size reduction. Despite the size limitation of our planetary ball mill compared to industrial-scale grinding equipment, this report provides useful information and can be a starting point for the industry, where the scale-up of different processes—including grinding—is essential to attain cost-effective production.

Author Contributions: Methodology, C.B. and R.A.; Investigation, C.B., A.M.-N., D.K., K.B. and R.A.; Writing—original draft, C.B. and D.K.; Writing—review and editing, R.A.; Supervision, R.A. All authors have read and agreed to the published version of the manuscript.

Funding: This research was supported by National Research, Development and Innovation Office, NKFIH_OTKA K_146148.

Institutional Review Board Statement: Not applicable.

Informed Consent Statement: Not applicable.

Data Availability Statement: Data are contained within the article.

Acknowledgments: Csilla Bartos was supported by the Hungarian Academy of Science's grant for the support of researchers raising children.

Conflicts of Interest: The authors declare no conflicts of interest. The funding sponsors had no role in the design of the study; in the collection, analyses, or interpretation of data; in the writing of the manuscript; and in the decision to publish the results.

References

1. Liu, X.; Zhao, L.; Wu, B.; Chen, F. Improving Solubility of Poorly Water-Soluble Drugs by Protein-Based Strategy: A Review. *Int. J. Pharm.* **2023**, *634*, 122704. [CrossRef] [PubMed]
2. Tran, T.T.-D.; Tran, K.A.; Tran, P.H.-L. Modulation of Particle Size and Molecular Interactions by Sonoprecipitation Method for Enhancing Dissolution Rate of Poorly Water-Soluble Drug. *Ultrason. Sonochem* **2015**, *24*, 256–263. [CrossRef]
3. Marushka, J.; Brokešová, J.; Ugo Ogadah, C.; Kazemi, A.; Duintjer Tebbens, J.; Šklubalová, Z. Milling of Pharmaceutical Powder Carrier Excipients: Application of Central Composite Design. *Adv. Powder Technol.* **2022**, *33*, 103881. [CrossRef]
4. Méndez Cañellas, F.; Al-Rifai, N.; Padrela, L.; Tajber, L.; Khamiakova, T.; Otava, M.; Geertman, R. A Comparative Study of Dry and Wet Top-down Milling Approaches for the Preparation of Microparticle Suspensions. *Powder Technol.* **2023**, *428*, 118829. [CrossRef]
5. Kumar, R.; Thakur, A.K.; Chaudhari, P.; Banerjee, N. Particle Size Reduction Techniques of Pharmaceutical Compounds for the Enhancement of Their Dissolution Rate and Bioavailability. *J. Pharm. Innov.* **2022**, *17*, 333–352. [CrossRef]
6. Loh, Z.H.; Samanta, A.K.; Sia Heng, P.W. Overview of Milling Techniques for Improving the Solubility of Poorly Water-Soluble Drugs. *AJPS* **2015**, *10*, 255–274. [CrossRef]
7. Zulbeari, N.; Holm, R. Is Roller Milling—The Low Energy Wet Bead Media Milling—A Reproducible and Robust Milling Method for Formulation Investigation of Aqueous Suspensions? *Int. J. Pharm.* **2024**, *651*, 123733. [CrossRef]
8. Varghese, S.; Ghoroi, C. Improving the Wetting and Dissolution of Ibuprofen Using Solventless Co-Milling. *Int. J. Pharm.* **2017**, *533*, 145–155. [CrossRef]
9. Karde, V.; Ghoroi, C. Influence of Surface Modification on Wettability and Surface Energy Characteristics of Pharmaceutical Excipient Powders. *Int. J. Pharm.* **2014**, *475*, 351–363. [CrossRef]
10. Penkina, A.; Semjonov, K.; Hakola, M.; Vuorinen, S.; Repo, T.; Yliruusi, J.; Aruväli, J.; Kogermann, K.; Veski, P.; Heinämäki, J. Towards Improved Solubility of Poorly Water-Soluble Drugs: Cryogenic Co-Grinding of Piroxicam with Carrier Polymers. *Drug Dev. Ind. Pharm.* **2016**, *42*, 378–388. [CrossRef]

11. Cerdeira, A.M.; Mazzotti, M.; Gander, B. Formulation and Drying of Miconazole and Itraconazole Nanosuspensions. *Int. J. Pharm.* **2013**, *443*, 209–220. [CrossRef] [PubMed]
12. Mithu, M.D.S.H.; Ross, S.A.; Hurt, A.P.; Douroumis, D. Effect of mechanochemical grinding conditions on the formation of pharmaceutical cocrystals and co-amorphous solid forms of ketoconazole—Dicarboxylic acid. *J. Drug Deliv. Sci. Technol.* **2021**, *63*, 102508. [CrossRef]
13. Shin, H.; Lee, S.; Jung, H.S.; Kim, J.-B. Effect of Ball Size and Powder Loading on the Milling Efficiency of a Laboratory-Scale Wet Ball Mill. *Ceram. Int.* **2013**, *39*, 8963–8968. [CrossRef]
14. Seibert, K.D.; Collins, P.C.; Luciani, C.V.; Fisher, E.S. *Chemical Engineering in the Pharmaceutical Industry: Active Pharmaceutical Ingredients*, 2nd ed.; John Wiley & Sons, Inc.: Hoboken, NJ, USA, 2019; pp. 861–879.
15. Altun, O.; Sert, T.; Altun, D.; Toprak, A.; Kwade, A. Scale-up of Vertical Wet Stirred Media Mill (HIGmill) via Signature Plots, Stress Analyses and Energy Equations. *Miner. Eng.* **2024**, *205*, 108460. [CrossRef]
16. Mannheim, V. Empirical and scale-up modeling in stirred ball mills. *Chem. Eng. Res. Des.* **2011**, *89*, 405–409. [CrossRef]
17. Lehocký, R.; Pěček, D.; Štěpánek, F. Scale-up from Batch to Flow-through Wet Milling Process for Injectable Depot Formulation. *Eur. J. Pharm. Sci.* **2016**, *95*, 122–129. [CrossRef]
18. Lestari, M.L.A.D.; Müller, R.H.; Möschwitzer, J.P. The Scalability of Wet Ball Milling for The Production of Nanosuspensions. *PNT* **2019**, *7*, 147–161. [CrossRef]
19. Srivalli, K.M.R.; Mishra, B. Drug Nanocrystals: A Way toward Scale-Up. *SPJ* **2016**, *24*, 386–404.
20. Mio, H.; Kano, J.; Saito, F.; Kaneko, K. Effects of Rotational Direction and Rotation-to-Revolution Speed Ratio in Planetary Ball Milling. *Mater. Sci. Eng. A* **2002**, *332*, 75–80. [CrossRef]
21. Mio, H.; Kano, J.; Saito, F. Scale-up Method of Planetary Ball Mill. *Chem. Eng. Sci.* **2004**, *59*, 5909–5916. [CrossRef]
22. Bolourchian, N.; Nili, M.; Foroutan, S.M.; Mahboubi, A.; Nokhodchi, A. The Use of Cooling and Anti-Solvent Precipitation Technique to Tailor Dissolution and Physicochemical Properties of Meloxicam for Better Performance. *J. Drug Deliv. Sci. Technol.* **2020**, *55*, 101485. [CrossRef]
23. Kürti, L.; Kukovecz, Á.; Kozma, G.; Ambrus, R.; Deli, M.A.; Szabó-Révész, P. Study of the Parameters Influencing the Co-Grinding Process for the Production of Meloxicam Nanoparticles. *Powder Technol.* **2011**, *212*, 210–217. [CrossRef]
24. Ambrus, R.; Kocbek, P.; Kristl, J.; Šibanc, R.; Rajkó, R.; Szabó-Révész, P. Investigation of Preparation Parameters to Improve the Dissolution of Poorly Water-Soluble Meloxicam. *Int. J. Pharm.* **2009**, *381*, 153–159. [CrossRef] [PubMed]
25. Yu, Y.; Tian, Y.; Zhang, H.; Jia, Q.; Chen, X.; Kang, D.; Du, Y.; Song, S.; Zheng, A. The Evaluation of Meloxicam Nanocrystals by Oral Administration with Different Particle Sizes. *Molecules* **2022**, *27*, 421. [CrossRef]
26. Ambrus, R.; Alshweiat, A.; Szabó-Révész, P.; Bartos, C.; Csóka, I. Smartcrystals for Efficient Dissolution of Poorly Water-Soluble Meloxicam. *Pharmaceutics* **2022**, *14*, 245. [CrossRef]
27. Lewinski, N.; Colvin, V.; Drezek, R. Cytotoxicity of Nanoparticles. *Small* **2008**, *4*, 26–49. [CrossRef]
28. Nagy, E.; Homik, Z.; Smausz, T.; Kopniczky, J.; Náfrádi, M.; Alapi, T.; Kokai, D.; Burián, K.; Szabó-Révész, P.; Ambrus, R.; et al. A Comprehensive Analysis of Meloxicam Particles Produced by Nanosecond Laser Ablation as a Wet Milling Technique. *Sci. Rep.* **2022**, *12*, 12551. [CrossRef]
29. Party, P.; Bartos, C.; Farkas, Á.; Szabó-Révész, P.; Ambrus, R. Formulation and In Vitro and In Silico Characterization of "Nano-in-Micro" Dry Powder Inhalers Containing Meloxicam. *Pharmaceutics* **2021**, *13*, 211. [CrossRef]
30. Bartos, C.; Ambrus, R.; Sipos, P.; Budai-Szűcs, M.; Csányi, E.; Gáspár, R.; Márki, Á.; Seres, A.B.; Sztojkov-Ivanov, A.; Horváth, T.; et al. Study of Sodium Hyaluronate-Based Intranasal Formulations Containing Micro- or Nanosized Meloxicam Particles. *Int. J. Pharm.* **2015**, *491*, 198–207. [CrossRef]
31. Zulbeari, N.; Holm, R. Wet bead milling by dual centrifugation—An approach to obtain reproducible and differentiable suspensions. *Int. J. Pharm.* **2023**, *646*, 123455. [CrossRef]
32. Alshora, D.; Ibrahim, M.; Elzayat, E.; Almeanazel, O.T.; Alanazi, F. Defining the process parameters affecting the fabrication of rosuvastatin calcium nanoparticles by planetary ball mill. *Int. J. Nanomed.* **2019**, *14*, 4625–4636. [CrossRef] [PubMed]
33. Bartos, C.; Jójárt-Laczkovich, O.; Katona, G.; Budai-Szűcs, M.; Ambrus, R.; Bocsik, A.; Gróf, I.; Deli, M.; Szabó-Révész, P. Optimization of a Combined Wet Milling Process in Order to Produce Poly(Vinyl Alcohol) Stabilized Nanosuspension. *DDDT* **2018**, *12*, 1567–1580. [CrossRef] [PubMed]
34. Beidokhti, H.R.N.; Ghaffarzadegan, R.; Mirzakhanlouei, S.; Ghazizadeh, L.; Dorkoosh, F.A. Preparation, Characterization, and Optimization of Folic Acid-Chitosan-Methotrexate Core-Shell Nanoparticles by Box-Behnken Design for Tumor-Targeted Drug Delivery. *AAPS Pharm. Sci. Tech.* **2017**, *18*, 115–129. [CrossRef] [PubMed]
35. Fröhlich, E.; Mercuri, A.; Wu, S.; Salar-Behzadi, S. Measurements of Deposition, Lung Surface Area and Lung Fluid for Simulation of Inhaled Compounds. *Front. Pharmacol.* **2016**, *7*, 181. [CrossRef]
36. Anderson, N.H.; Bauer, M.; Boussac, N.; Khan-Malek, R.; Munden, P.; Sardaro, M. An Evaluation of Fit Factors and Dissolution Efficiency for the Comparison of in Vitro Dissolution Profiles. *JPBA* **1998**, *17*, 811–822. [CrossRef]
37. Costa, P.; Sousa Lobo, J.M. Modeling and Comparison of Dissolution Profiles. *Eur. J. Pharm. Sci.* **2001**, *13*, 123–133. [CrossRef]
38. Zhang, Y.; Huo, M.; Zhou, J.; Zou, A.; Li, W.; Yao, C.; Xie, S. DDSolver: An Add-In Program for Modeling and Comparison of Drug Dissolution Profiles. *AAPS J.* **2010**, *12*, 263–271. [CrossRef]

39. Bartos, C.; Szabó-Révész, P.; Bartos, C.; Katona, G.; Jójárt-Laczkovich, O.; Ambrus, R. The Effect of an Optimized Wet Milling Technology on the Crystallinity, Morphology and Dissolution Properties of Micro- and Nanonized Meloxicam. *Molecules* **2016**, *21*, 507. [CrossRef]
40. Pandey, K.U.; Poornachary, S.K.; Dalvi, S.V. Insights to the Action of Additives for Stabilization of Ultrafine Particles of Fenofibrate in Aqueous Suspensions Produced by Sonoprecipitation. *Powder Technol.* **2020**, *363*, 310–325. [CrossRef]
41. Li, C.; Gao, Z. Effect of Grinding Media on the Surface Property and Flotation Behavior of Scheelite Particles. *Powder Technol.* **2017**, *322*, 386–392. [CrossRef]
42. Isaac, J.; Ganguly, S.; Ghosh, A. Co-Milling of Telmisartan with Poly(Vinyl Alcohol)—An Alkalinizer Free Green Approach to Ensure Its Bioavailability. *Eur. J. Pharm. Biopharm.* **2016**, *101*, 43–52. [CrossRef] [PubMed]
43. Peltonen, L.; Hirvonen, J. Pharmaceutical Nanocrystals by Nanomilling: Critical Process Parameters, Particle Fracturing and Stabilization Methods. *J. Pharm. Pharmacol.* **2010**, *62*, 1569–1579. [CrossRef] [PubMed]
44. Nagarkar, R.; Patel, J. Polyvinyl Alcohol: A Comprehensive Study. *ASPS* **2019**, *3*, 34–44.
45. Mártha, C.; Kürti, L.; Farkas, G.; Jójárt-Laczkovich, O.; Szalontai, B.; Glässer, E.; Deli, M.A.; Szabó-Révész, P. Effects of Polymers on the Crystallinity of Nanonized Meloxicam during a Co-Grinding Process. *Eur. Polym. J.* **2013**, *49*, 2426–2432. [CrossRef]
46. Thomas, D.; Zhuravlev, E.; Wurm, A.; Schick, C.; Cebe, P. Fundamental Thermal Properties of Polyvinyl Alcohol by Fast Scanning Calorimetry. *Polymer* **2018**, *137*, 145–155. [CrossRef]
47. Todoran, N.; Antonoaea, P.; Rusu, A.; Ciurba, A.; Birsan, M.; Redai, E. DSC and FT-IR Analysis for the Formulation of Dermal Films with Meloxicam in Bioadhesive Polymeric Matrices. *Rev. Chim.* **2019**, *69*, 3692–3697. [CrossRef]
48. Rus, L.M. Development of meloxicam oral lyophilisates: Role of thermal analysis and complementary techniques. *Farmacia* **2019**, *67*, 56–67. [CrossRef]
49. Etman, M.; Shekedef, M.; Nada, A.; Ismail, A. In Vitro and In Vivo Evaluation of Tablets Containing Meloxicam- PEG 6000 Ball-Milled Co-Ground Mixture. *J Appl Pharm Sci* **2017**, *7*, 031–039.
50. Rasenack, N.; Müller, B.W. Micron-Size Drug Particles: Common and Novel Micronization Techniques. *Pharm. Dev. Technol.* **2004**, *9*, 1–13. [CrossRef]
51. Abdollahi, S.; Raissi, H.; Farzad, F. Examine Stability Polyvinyl Alcohol-Stabilized Nanosuspensions to Overcome the Challenge of Poor Drug Solubility Utilizing Molecular Dynamic Simulation. *Sci. Rep.* **2024**, *14*, 17386. [CrossRef]
52. Buttini, F.; Soltani, A.; Colombo, P.; Marriott, C.; Jones, S.A. Multilayer PVA Adsorption onto Hydrophobic Drug Substrates to Engineer Drug-Rich Microparticles. *Eur. JPharm Sci.* **2008**, *33*, 20–28. [CrossRef] [PubMed]
53. Friuli, V.; Urru, C.; Ferrara, C.; Conti, D.M.; Bruni, G.; Maggi, L.; Capsoni, D. Design of Etched- and Functionalized-Halloysite/Meloxicam Hybrids: A Tool for Enhancing Drug Solubility and Dissolution Rate. *Pharmaceutics* **2024**, *16*, 338. [CrossRef] [PubMed]
54. Rahmani, F.; Ziyadi, H.; Baghali, M.; Luo, H.; Ramakrishna, S. Electrospun PVP/PVA Nanofiber Mat as a Novel Potential Transdermal Drug-Delivery System for Buprenorphine: A Solution Needed for Pain Management. *Appl. Sci.* **2021**, *11*, 2779. [CrossRef]
55. Yocum, D. Safety and Efficacy of Meloxicam in the Treatment of Osteoarthritis: A 12-Week, Double-Blind, Multiple-Dose, Placebo-Controlled Trial. *Arch. Intern. Med.* **2000**, *160*, 2947. [CrossRef]

pharmaceutics

MDPI

Article

Pharmacometrics to Evaluate Dosing of the Patient-Friendly Ivermectin CHILD-IVITAB in Children ≥ 15 kg and <15 kg

Klervi Golhen [1,*], Michael Buettcher [1,2,3], Jörg Huwyler [4], John van den Anker [1,5], Verena Gotta [1], Kim Dao [6], Laura E. Rothuizen [6], Kevin Kobylinski [7] and Marc Pfister [1]

1 Pediatric Pharmacology and Pharmacometrics, University Children's Hospital Basel (UKBB), University of Basel, 4056 Basel, Switzerland; michael.buettcher@luks.ch (M.B.); jvandena@childrensnational.org (J.v.d.A.); verena.gotta@ukbb.ch (V.G.); marc.pfister@ukbb.ch (M.P.)
2 Pediatric Infectious Diseases, Children's Hospital of Central Switzerland (KidZ), Lucerne Cantonal Hospital, 6000 Luzern, Switzerland
3 Faculty of Health Sciences and Medicine, University of Lucerne, 6000 Luzern, Switzerland
4 Department of Pharmaceutical Sciences, Division of Pharmaceutical Technology, University of Basel, 4056 Basel, Switzerland; joerg.huwyler@unibas.ch
5 Division of Clinical Pharmacology, Children's National Hospital, Washington, DC 20001, USA
6 Clinical Pharmacology Service, Lausanne University Hospital, University of Lausanne, 1011 Lausanne, Switzerland; kim.dao@chuv.ch (K.D.); laura.rothuizen@chuv.ch (L.E.R.)
7 Mahidol Oxford Tropical Medicine Research Unit (MORU), Bangkok 10400, Thailand; kevin@tropmedres.ac
* Correspondence: klervi.golhen@ukbb.ch

Abstract: The antiparasitic drug ivermectin is approved for persons > 15 kg in the US and EU. A pharmacometric (PMX) population model with clinical PK data was developed (i) to characterize the effect of the patient-friendly ivermectin formulation CHILD-IVITAB on the absorption process and (ii) to evaluate dosing for studies in children < 15 kg. Simulations were performed to identify dosing with CHILD-IVITAB associated with similar exposure coverage in children ≥ 15 kg and < 15 kg as observed in adults receiving the reference formulation STROMECTOL®. A total of 448 ivermectin concentrations were available from 16 healthy adults. The absorption rate constant was 2.41 h^{-1} (CV 19%) for CHILD-IVITAB vs. 1.56 h^{-1} (CV 43%) for STROMECTOL®. Simulations indicated that 250 μg/kg of CHILD-IVITAB is associated with exposure coverage in children < 15 kg consistent with that observed in children ≥ 15 kg and adults receiving 200 μg/kg of STROMECTOL®. Performed analysis confirmed that CHILD-IVITAB is associated with faster and more controlled absorption than STROMECTOL®. Simulations indicate that 250 μg/kg of CHILD-IVITAB achieves equivalent ivermectin exposure coverage in children < 15 kg as seen in children ≥ 15 kg and adults.

Keywords: ivermectin; STROMECTOL®; dosing; pharmacometrics; absorption; variability; orodispersible tablet (ODT); TIP-based technology; oral drug delivery; novel delivery systems

1. Introduction

Ivermectin has been a cornerstone in the treatment and control of parasitic infections since its introduction in the 1980s, providing broad-spectrum efficacy against a wide range of conditions including lymphatic filariasis, onchocerciasis, head lice, intestinal helminths, strongyloidiasis, and scabies [1]. Ivermectin is on the World Health Organization's List of Essential Medicines, underscoring its significance in global health [2]. Approximately 400 million ivermectin treatments are distributed annually by mass drug administration (MDA) to control and eliminate onchocerciasis and lymphatic filariasis [3]. In addition, since 2023, a conventional ivermectin tablet formulation (Subvectin) has been registered in Switzerland for the treatment of scabies in adults, and high priority has been given to research on child-friendly treatment modalities [4,5]. Despite its extensive use in adults, there is a significant gap in knowledge regarding its pharmacokinetic profile in young children, particularly those with a weight of less than 15 kg. Children weighing less than

15 kg are excluded from official MDA treatment programs; thus, they do not receive the benefits of ivermectin to control numerous neglected tropical diseases (NTDs) that afflict young children [6–8]. Further, this contraindication leads to off-label use of ivermectin without a robust evidence base for appropriate dosing in children weighing less than 15 kg.

Traditional ivermectin tablet formulations are not suitable for children weighing less than 15 kg, necessitating innovative approaches to ensure acceptability, safety and efficacy. There is a need for new, child-friendly formulations of ivermectin that can ensure accurate dosing, improved acceptability, palatability, safety during administration, and stability suitable for diverse environmental conditions where these NTDs occur. Young children are an extremely important population suffering a disproportionate health burden from helminth and scabies infection [6]. Previous studies have highlighted significant inter-individual variability in drug exposure with STROMECTOL® [9,10], prompting a detailed comparison to ensure that new formulations can provide consistent and reliable therapeutic outcomes. Indeed, children weighing less than 15 kg that were treated with ivermectin doses less than 200 μg/kg were less likely to achieve therapeutic success for scabies compared to children treated with doses 200 μg/kg and above [11]. To address these needs, a novel orodispersible tablet (ODT) formulation of ivermectin, called CHILD-IVITAB, has been developed utilizing multifunctional template inverted particle (TIP) technology, designed to provide rapid disintegration, controlled absorption, and enhanced taste masking [12–15]. The rapid disintegration time (less than 10 s) of CHILD-IVITAB greatly improves ease of administration, virtually eliminates any choking risk, and removes need for potable water, which would facilitate use of ivermectin in children under 15 kg in MDA programs. To inform the pediatric program of CHILD-IVITAB, 16 healthy adults were enrolled in a phase I, single-center, open-label, randomized, two-period, cross-over, single-dose trial which aimed to compare the palatability, tolerability, and bioavailability and pharmacokinetics (PK) of CHILD-IVITAB compared against the marketed ivermectin tablets (STROMECTOL®) at a single dose of 12 mg in a fasting state. Non-compartmental analysis (NCA) demonstrated that CHILD-IVITAB yielded controlled absorption associated with reduced variability in drug exposure as compared to STROMECTOL® [16]. The objective of the present study is to develop a population PK model to characterize the absorption profile and variability of the ivermectin CHILD-IVITAB formulation compared to the reference formulation STROMECTOL®. In addition, the developed model will be applied to simulate and evaluate dosing for a planned pediatric study in children $\geq$ 15 kg and those < 15 kg. By addressing these aspects, the goal is to contribute to optimizing ivermectin dosing strategies for children, ensuring consistent exposure and effective treatment outcomes across different age groups [7].

2. Materials and Methods

2.1. Study Design

The data originate from a previously published phase I, single-center, open-label, randomized, two-period, cross-over, single-dose trial (NCT05477810) [16], which aimed to compare the palatability, tolerability, bioavailability and pharmacokinetics of ivermectin ODT (CHILD-IVITAB) against the marketed ivermectin tablets (STROMECTOL®) at a single dose of 12 mg in a fasting state [10]. Subjects were instructed to place four ODTs of CHILD-IVITAB (3 mg) between the gum and the cheek for 30 s, then rinse and swallow with 150 mL of water. Subjects were instructed to immediately swallow four tablets of STROMECTOL® (3 mg) with 150 mL of water. Both periods were separated by a washout period of at least 7 days. Palatability, tolerability, safety, pharmacokinetics and their variability were assessed in 16 healthy adult subjects. Power estimation can be found in the study by Dao et al. [16]. During each period, venous blood samples were collected in EDTA tubes pre-dose, and at 0.5, 1, 2, 3, 4, 5, 6, 8, 10, 24, 48, 72 and 96 h post-dose. Blood was centrifuged at 10 °C and 3220 g for 30 min and plasma was separated and stored at −20 °C until bioanalytical analysis. Plasma ivermectin samples were quantified by liquid chromatography tandem mass spectrometry (LC-MS/MS) [17]. The lower limit of quantification (LLOQ) and upper limit of quantification (ULOQ) of ivermectin plasma samples were 0.5 ng/mL and 250 ng/mL, respectively.

2.2. Pharmacometric Population PK Modeling

All participants who received the study drug during the study were included in the pharmacometric PK analysis of ivermectin, which used nonlinear mixed-effects modeling within the pharmacometric PK software Monolix (version 2023, Lixoft SAS, a Simulations Plus company, Antony, France). Model simulations were performed with the pharmacometric PK software Simulx (version 2023, Lixoft SAS, a Simulations Plus company). R version 4.3.1 was used within RStudio (version 2023.06.1, Vienna, Austria) for data handling, graphical visualization, and numerical calculations. Ivermectin plasma concentrations below the LLOQ and above the ULOQ were censored, except for pre-dose samples which were set to 0. Here, the CENSORING column in Monolix was used, corresponding to the M3 method in NONMEM [18].

2.3. Base Pharmacokinetic (PK) Model

For model building purposes, the population PK model developed by Brussee et al., using PK data obtained from 200 children 2–12 years of age and 11 adults, was used as the baseline structural model [7]. Brussee et al.'s model is a two-compartment PK model including two transit compartments to account for a delay in absorption, which was initially assumed for both formulations [19]. To align with the previously reported model from Brussee et al., body weight was included as a covariate for clearance CL, intercompartmental clearance Q, and volume of distribution in the central Vc and peripheral Vp compartment, and allometric scaling centered to 18 kg was applied, with the coefficients fixed to 0.75 for clearance and 1 for volume (Figure 1). Ivermectin typical oral clearance (CL) was described as a nonlinear function of weight ($CL = 5.8 \times (\text{weight}/18)^{0.75}$). The model included two transit compartments with $k_{tr} = k_a$, leading to a computed mean transit time $MTT = 3/k_{tr}$. The choice of two transit compartments as the baseline model structure has been made because of a previously published model-based analysis in pediatric patients. However, another study in healthy volunteers has found an increased number of transit compartments to describe ivermectin absorption data best (N = 6) [9,10]. A sensitivity analysis for the number of transit compartments for each formulation, with up to 6 transit compartments tested, was conducted. Population parameters were estimated, using estimates from Brussee et al. as initial values. Again, as per Brussee et al., inter-individual variability (IIV) was included for the absorption rate constant, clearance, and both volume parameters (central and peripheral compartment), with individual parameters assumed to be log-normally distributed. Initially, a mixed residual error model was assumed. The covariance matrix of random effects was initially set to a diagonal matrix (no correlation between random effects assumed).

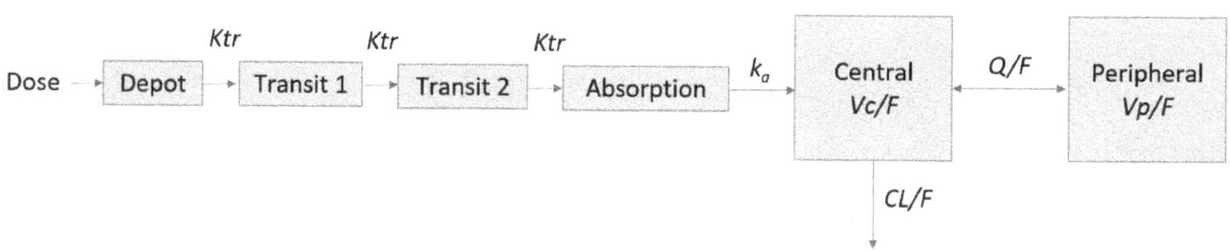

Figure 1. Graphical representation of the two-compartment PK model best describing the ivermectin data for both CHILD-IVITAB and STROMECTOL® formulations. The model included weight-dependent clearance and distribution (allometric scaling centered to 18 kg) and two transit compartments. CL/F: apparent clearance, F: bioavailability, k_a: absorption rate constant, k_{tr}: transfer rate constant ($k_{tr} = k_a$), MTT: mean transit time ($MTT = 3/k_{tr}$), Q/F: apparent intercompartmental clearance, Vc/F: apparent volume of the central compartment, Vp/F: apparent volume of the peripheral compartment.

2.4. Alternative Investigated Model Structures

As structural models, one- and three-compartment models with first-order elimination were also evaluated. Additive, proportional and combined (i.e., additive and proportional) residual error models were investigated to describe the residual variability.

2.5. Correlation between Parameters

After selecting the structural model, the covariance matrix of random effects was built, starting from a diagonal matrix and then progressively assessing the significance of correlation terms by assessing scatterplots of the random effects and Pearson correlation coefficients. Screening for correlations was performed using "conditional distribution mode" in Monolix.

2.6. Investigation of a Formulation Effect and Potential Other Covariates

A potential formulation effect (CHILD-IVITAB or STROMECTOL®) on absorption rate k_a (and resulting *MTT*) and/or relative bioavailability *Frel* (with *Frel* set to 1 for the reference formulation STROMECTOL® and estimated *Frel* for CHILD-IVITAB) was evaluated with formulation-specific IIV. As the age range in Dao et al.'s trial was narrow (i.e., healthy young adults), this covariate was not investigated. Additionally, a gender covariate was investigated on the model parameter *CL*.

2.7. Evaluation of Population PK Model

A sensitivity analysis was conducted to evaluate the impact of specific individuals on model fit. Goodness of fit was graphically evaluated using standard plots (prediction vs. observations, randomness of residual scatter plots versus time/predictions and of random effects versus covariates) and a simulation-based visual predictive check of key models. Model development considered reductions in the objective function between candidate models (ΔOFV = $-2 \times$ log-likelihood), reductions in the inter-subject variability and residual error, and parameter precision and the clinical relevance of estimated effects. A visual predictive check (VPC) was performed, with n = 1000 simulations to evaluate whether the model can accurately predict the observed concentrations and capture the observed variability. A convergence assessment was conducted to assess the reproducibility of the results.

2.8. Model-Based Simulations to Evaluate Dosing of CHILD-IVITAB in Persons $\geq$ 15 kg and Children < 15 kg

Simulations were conducted to compare simulated ivermectin exposure $AUC_{0\text{–}96h}$ (i.e., up to the last measured PK timepoint) and $AUC_{0\text{–}168h}$ (i.e., extrapolated *AUC* up to 7 days after first dosing) following a single administration of 200 µg/kg of the reference formulation STROMECTOL® in adults, and simulated ivermectin exposure ($AUC_{0\text{–}96h}$ and $AUC_{0\text{–}168h}$) in persons $\geq$ 15 kg and children < 15 kg following a single administration of various doses of CHILD-IVITAB. Different dosing scenarios were simulated with a dose of (i) 200 µg/kg; (ii) 250 µg/kg and (iii) 300 µg/kg. Monte Carlo simulations were performed using the developed PK model and population parameters to generate 1000 concentration–time profiles of ivermectin for each scenario, after which $AUC_{0\text{–}96h}$ and $AUC_{0\text{–}168h}$ were calculated by integration of simulated observed concentrations. Simulations of reference exposure (adults, STROMECTOL® formulation, 200 µg/kg) were conducted for a population with a weight distribution (normal distribution) of N (mean, μ = 85.1 kg, standard deviation, σ = 11.7 kg), to yield a weight range of approximately 50.1 to 120.0 kg (comprising $\pm$ three standard deviations). Simulations of expected CHILD-IVITAB exposure in children under varying doses were similarly conducted in each weight group as follows: (i) for 5.0–7.5 kg, weight ~ N (μ = 6.3 kg, σ = 0.4 kg); (ii) 7.6-10.0 kg: weight ~ N (μ = 8.8 kg, σ = 0.4 kg); (iii) 10.1–14.9 kg: weight ~ N (μ = 12.5 kg, σ = 0.8 kg); (iv) 15.0-30.0 kg: weight ~ N (μ = 22.5 kg, σ = 2.5 kg); and (v) 30.1–50.0 kg: weight ~ N (μ = 40.1 kg, σ = 3.3 kg). As

CHILD-IVITAB is dosed in 1 mg and 3 mg tablets, we established matching between fixed CHILD-IVITAB dosing and weight-based dosing, stratified by weight group.

3. Results

All sixteen healthy volunteers were included in the data analysis. Baseline demographics are shown in Table 1.

Table 1. Demographic characteristics of study participants included in population PK analysis. Represented as median [IQR, inter-quartile range] or n (%). BMI, body mass index.

Demographic Characteristics of Study Participants (N = 16)	
Age (years)	24.0 [20.8, 28.0]
Weight (kg)	63.7 [58.0, 71.5]
Height (cm)	171 [168, 178]
BMI (kg/m^2)	22.3 [19.7, 23.1]
Gender	
Female	7 (43.8%)
Male	9 (56.3%)
Ethnicity	
African	2 (12.5%)
Caucasian	10 (62.5%)
Hispanic/Latin American	1 (6.3%)
Multiracial	3 (18.8%)

A total of 448 ivermectin venous plasma concentrations were available and included in the population PK analysis, of which 40 (8.9%) concentrations were below the limit of quantification (BLQ), all during the absorption phase, and 16 were pre-dose samples. The remaining plasma concentrations of ivermectin following CHILD-IVITAB and STROMECTOL® dosing were in the range of 0.53–92.45 ng/mL and 0.51–82.79 ng/mL, respectfully (Figure 2).

3.1. Pharmacometric Population PK Modeling

Similar to Brussee et al. [7], a two-compartment PK model including two transit compartments to account for a delay in absorption, first-order elimination kinetics, weight-dependent clearance and distribution (allometric scaling centered to 18 kg), and a combined error model described the ivermectin data well for both CHILD-IVITAB and STROMECTOL® formulations (Figure 1, Supplementary Materials Figures S2–S4). Estimated PK parameters of the fitted two-compartment model are shown in Table 2. There are notable differences in the study design and patient demographics between the data included in this study and the data used to develop the referenced model. Brussee et al.'s analysis included extensive PK data from 200 children aged 2–12 years and 11 adults. Despite these differences in the demographics, the estimation of ivermectin clearance, the peripheral volume of distribution, and the absorption rate constant and transit rate constant were similar. De novo parameter estimation of central volume of distribution was ~52% lower, associated with ~67% higher intercompartmental clearance than in the model from Brussee et al. [7].

Decreasing variability in absorption parameters by approximately 50% was observed with CHILD-IVITAB (19%, RSE = 22%) compared to STROMECTOL® (43%, RSE = 19%). Inter-individual variability in *CL, Vc, Vp,* and *Frel* of CHILD-IVITAB were estimated at 67%, 84%, 57%, and 61%, respectively (Table 2). Correlations between parameters with variability were suggested (p-value < 0.05) and set between *CL, Vc, Vp* and *Frel* in the correlation matrix, with estimated correlation values of 0.95 between *Vc* and *CL*, 0.89 between *Vp* and *CL*, 0.8 between *Frel* and *CL*, 0.92 between *Vc* and *Vp*, 0.84 between *Frel* and Vc, and 0.92 between *Frel* and *Vp*. Incorporating correlations between random effects improved the VPC (Figure 3).

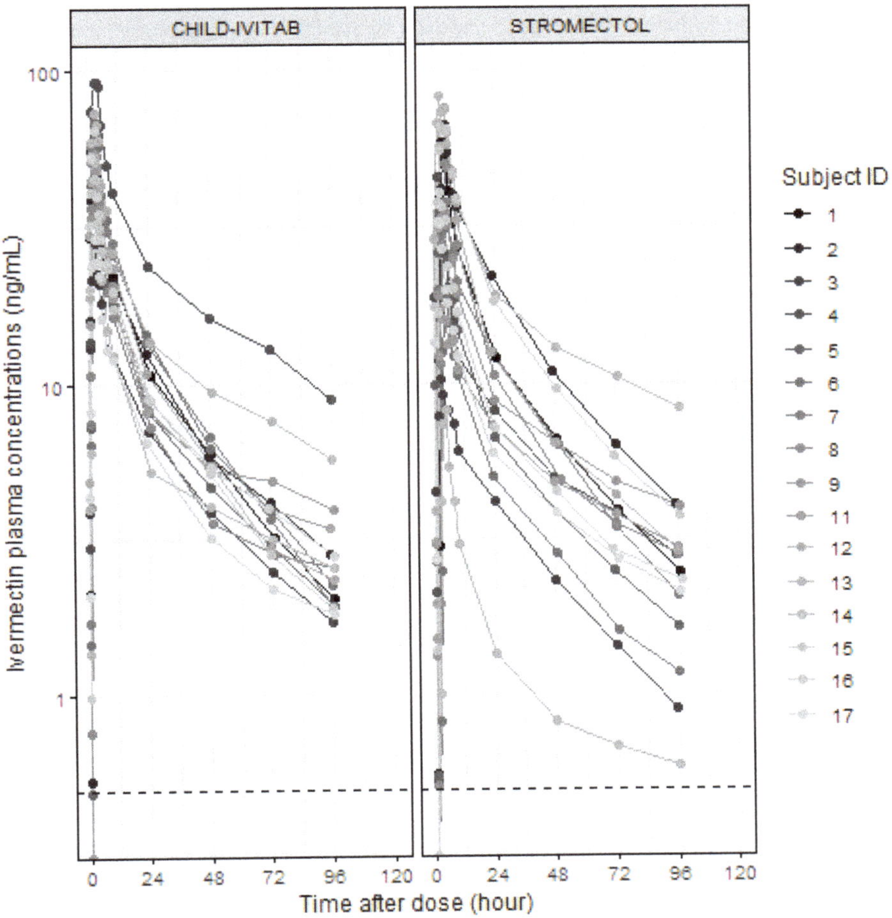

Figure 2. Individual observed plasma concentrations versus time after single oral dose of 12 mg ivermectin. Dotted horizontal line corresponds to LLOQ = 0.5 ng/mL. Note: one screening failure occurred (individual #10) because of positive cannabis drug screen.

Table 2. Population PK parameter estimates for ivermectin. Proportional and additive errors are reported as variance estimates (σ^2). *CL*, clearance; *Frel*, relative bioavailability (*Frel* set to 1 for the reference formulation STROMECTOL® and estimated *Frel* for CHILD-IVITAB); IIV, inter-individual variability, reported as coefficient of variation (CV%); *Q*, intercompartmental clearance; k_a, absorption rate constant; k_{tr}, transfer rate constant; RSE, relative standard error; *Vc*, volume of distribution in the central compartment; *Vp*, volume of distribution in the peripheral compartment. Additive error (mg/L): 0.69 (15%); proportional error: 0.16 (7%).

Parameter (Unit)		Value (RSE %) (Shrinkage)
CHILD-IVITAB absorption rate constant and transit rate constant (h^{-1})	$k_a = k_{tr}$	2.41 (6%)
STROMECTOL® absorption rate constant and transit rate constant (h^{-1})		1.56 (12%)

Table 2. *Cont.*

Parameter (Unit)		Value (RSE %) (Shrinkage)
Clearance (L/h)	*CL*	5.8 (17%) × (WT/18)$^{0.75}$
Volume of distribution (L)	V_c	60.29 (24%) × (WT/18)
	V_p	103.56 (16%) × (WT/18)
Intercompartmental clearance (L/h)	*Q*	9.73 (18%) × (WT/18)$^{0.75}$
CHILD-IVITAB relative bioavailability	*Frel*	1.30 (16%)
IIV $k_{a\ CHILD\text{-}IVITAB}$ (CV%)		0.19 (22%) (14%)
IIV $k_{a\ STROMECTOL}$ (CV%)		0.43 (19%) (0.70%)
IIV CL (CV%)		0.67 (27%) (1.6%)
IIV V_c (CV%)		0.84 (28%) (1.1%)
IIV V_p (CV%)		0.57 (41%) (5.9%)
IIV *Frel* (CV%)		0.61 (24%) (2.3%)

3.2. Alternative Investigated Model Structures

A one-compartment model did not appropriately capture the elimination phase of ivermectin for both formulations. A three-compartment model did not yield an analytical solution for most PK parameters. A reduced model without transit compartments did not appropriately capture the maximal concentration C_{max} for both ivermectin formulations. As expected, estimating distinct k_{tr} and k_a yielded model instability (RSE > 100%) due to over-parametrization. No IIV on *Frel* resulted in large RSE on random effects of *CL*, k_a and *Vp* (>100%).

3.3. Investigation of a Formulation Effect and Potential Other Covariates

Ivermectin absorption was faster with CHILD-IVITAB than with STROMECTOL® with typical k_a values of 2.4 (95% CI: 2.17–2.68) and 1.6 (95% CI: 1.27–1.92) per hour, respectively, leading to a mean transit time (*MTT*) of 1.2 (95% CI: 1.12–1.38) hours with CHILD-IVITAB and 1.9 (95% CI: 1.56–2.36) hours with STROMECTOL® (Table 2). The absence of allometric scaling in the model worsened the model fit (*p*-value of likelihood ratio test, LRT > 0.05 and residual standard errors (RSEs) of the random effects on *CL*, *Vc*, *Vp* and *Frel* > 100%). There was no formulation effect on apparent clearance (*CL*), with estimated *CL* of 5.2 (95% CI: 4.00–6.83) L/h and 5.9 (95% CI: 3.94–8.94) L/h for CHILD-IVITAB and STROMECTOL®, respectively, and therefore, this was not retained in the final population PK model. The effect of formulation on relative ivermectin bioavailability was not significant, with *Frel* of CHILD-IVITAB (1.30%, 95% CI: 0.97–1.74) not significantly differing from STROMECTOL® (F fixed to 1, for no information from intravenous administration) (Table 2). Gender effect on *CL* was not a significant covariate to be included in the model (RSE > 100%).

3.4. Evaluation of Population PK Model

No subject was excluded from the main analysis. Individual clearance values ranged from IQR: 10.60 to 20.85 L/h. Individual #14 was excluded from the model sensitivity analysis, as particularly high oral clearance (65.83 L/h) and high (approximately 4-fold increased) relative bioavailability were estimated. Exclusion did not impact population parameter estimates significantly (overlapping 95% CI, Supplementary Materials Table S4), but resulted in reduced observed IIV and a slightly better description of concentrations measured. The goodness-of-fit plots (individual and population predicted vs. observed concentrations, individual fits, individual parameter distribution plots and conditionally weighted residuals vs. population predications and time after dose) showed that the model in the sensitivity analysis described the data well (Supplementary Materials Figure S1). A sensitivity analysis for the number of transit compartments, with up to six transit compartments tested, showed that four transit compartments yielded the best model fit (lowest OFV). However, there was no change in estimated clearance compared to the base PK model with two transit compartments, and hence no effect on simulated *AUCs*. Adding a distinct number of transit compartments per formulation did not improve the model fit (Supplementary Materials Table S3).

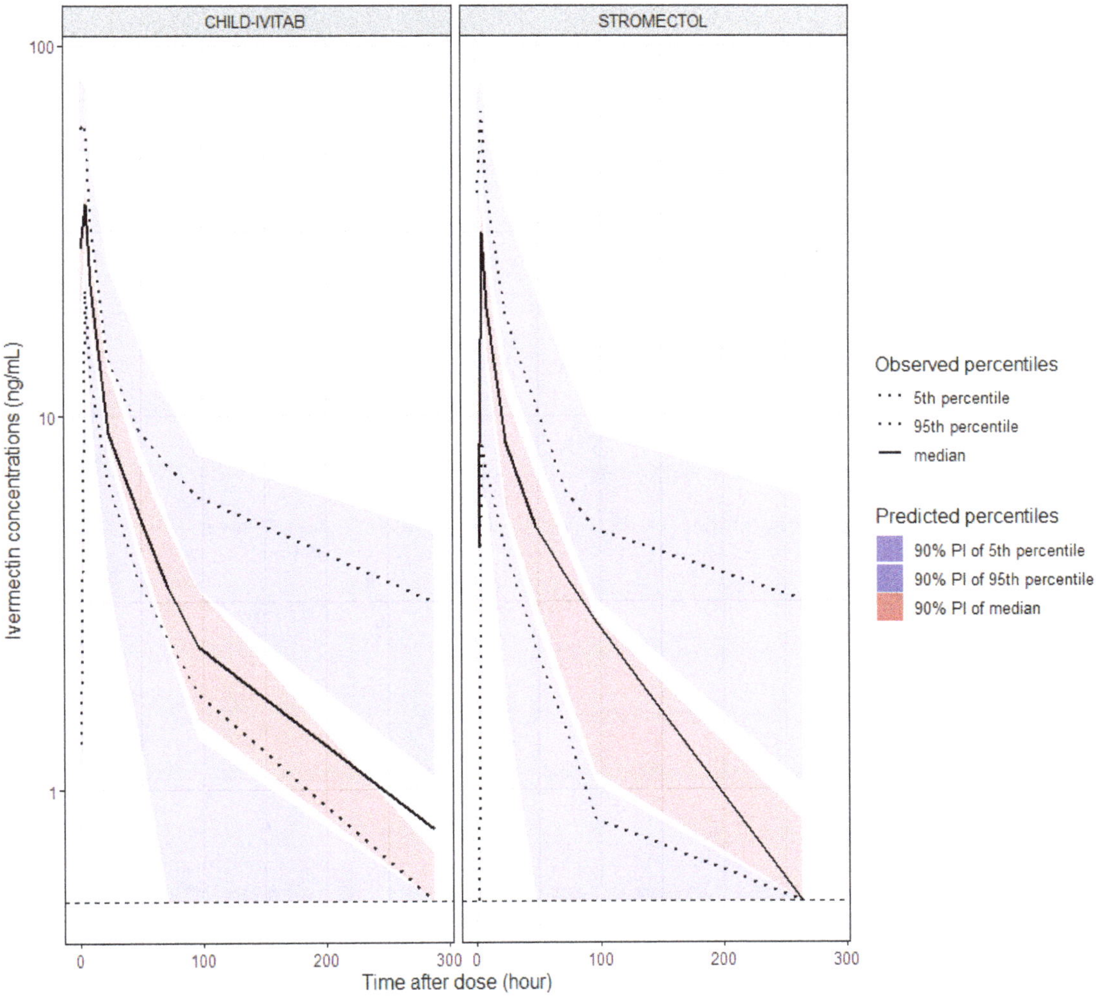

Figure 3. Visual predictive checks for PK model presented in Table 2 for ivermectin concentrations (ng/mL) on *y*-axis (log scale) and time after dose (h) on *x*-axis. Dotted horizontal line corresponds to LLOQ = 0.5 ng/mL. Pre-dose samples of next dosing from cross-over trial were included in the VPC.

3.5. Model-Based Simulations to Evaluate Dosing of CHILD-IVITAB in Persons ≥ 15 kg and Children < 15 kg

From model-based simulations a reference exposure $AUC_{0\text{–}96h}$ and $AUC_{0\text{–}168h}$ following a single administration of 200 μg/kg of the reference formulation STROMECTOL® in adults was calculated to a median of 800 (inter-quartile range, IQR: 516–1230) μg·h/L and 884 (IQR: 572–1380) μg·h/L, respectively (Table 3).

Table 3. Simulated ivermectin exposures (area under the concentration–time curve, AUC_{0-96h} and AUC_{0-168h}) according to weight-based ivermectin dosing regimen. Simulated ivermectin exposures in 1000 adults following a single administration of 200 µg/kg of the reference STROMECTOL® formulation and according to defined dose recommendations of 250 µg/kg in children < 15 kg and 200 µg/kg in children ≥ 15 kg following a single CHILD-IVITAB administration. IQR, inter-quartile range.

	Weight-Based Ivermectin Dosing Regimen			
Ivermectin Formulation	**Body Weight (kg)**	**Recommended Dosing Regimen (µg/kg)**	**Simulated Median AUC_{0-96h} [IQR] (µg·h/L)**	**Simulated Median AUC_{0-168h} [IQR] (µg·h/L)**
STROMECTOL® (reference in adults)	50.1–120	200	800 [516, 1230]	884 [572, 1380]
CHILD-IVITAB	5.0–7.5	250	752 [574, 1010]	770 [589, 1040]
	7.6–10.0	250	822 [635, 1070]	853 [651, 1120]
	10.1–14.9	250	879 [661, 1150]	919 [682, 1220]
	15.0–30.0	200	780 [612, 1010]	832 [639, 1080]
	30.1–50.0	200	899 [698, 1140]	971 [740, 1260]

A single dose of 200 µg/kg ivermectin CHILD–IVITAB was predicted to lead to 24.8%, 17.8% and 12.1% lower exposure (AUC_{0-96h}) in children weighing 5.0–7.5 kg, 7.6–10.0 kg and 10.1–14.9 kg compared with adults receiving STROMECTOL®, respectively (Supplementary Materials Figure S5). Therefore, a dose adjustment in children < 15 kg was deemed necessary to achieve equivalent exposure coverage as in children ≥ 15 kg and adults. Model-based simulations indicated that a single dose administration of 250 µg/kg of CHILD-IVITAB is associated with equivalent exposure coverage in children < 15 kg compared with children ≥ 15 kg and adults receiving 200 µg/kg STROMECTOL® (Supplementary Materials Figure S5). Evaluating the 300 µg/kg dosing regimen with CHILD-IVITAB yielded 12.9%, 23.4% and 31.3% over-exposure in children weighing 5.0–7.5 kg, 7.6–10.0 kg and 10.1–14.9 kg compared with adults receiving the reference 200 µg/kg of STROMECTOL®, respectively (Supplementary Materials Figure S5). Therefore, Table 3 and Figure 4 show ivermectin target exposure values obtained with the recommended dosing regimen using CHILD-IVITAB.

From Table 4, matching was established between the CHILD-IVITAB fixed-dosing regimen (given as 1 mg and 3 mg tablets) and weight-based dosing, stratified by weight group.

Table 4. CHILD-IVITAB dose sliding scale stratified by weight group.

Body Weight (kg)	**CHILD-IVITAB 1 mg Tablets**	**CHILD-IVITAB 3 mg Tablets**	**Effective Dose Range (µg/kg/dose)**
5.0–7.5	1 to 2	-	133–400
7.6–10.0	2	-	200–263
10.1–14.9	-	1	201–297
15.0–30.0	-	2	200–400
30.1–50.0	-	3	180–300
50.1–120	-	4	100–240

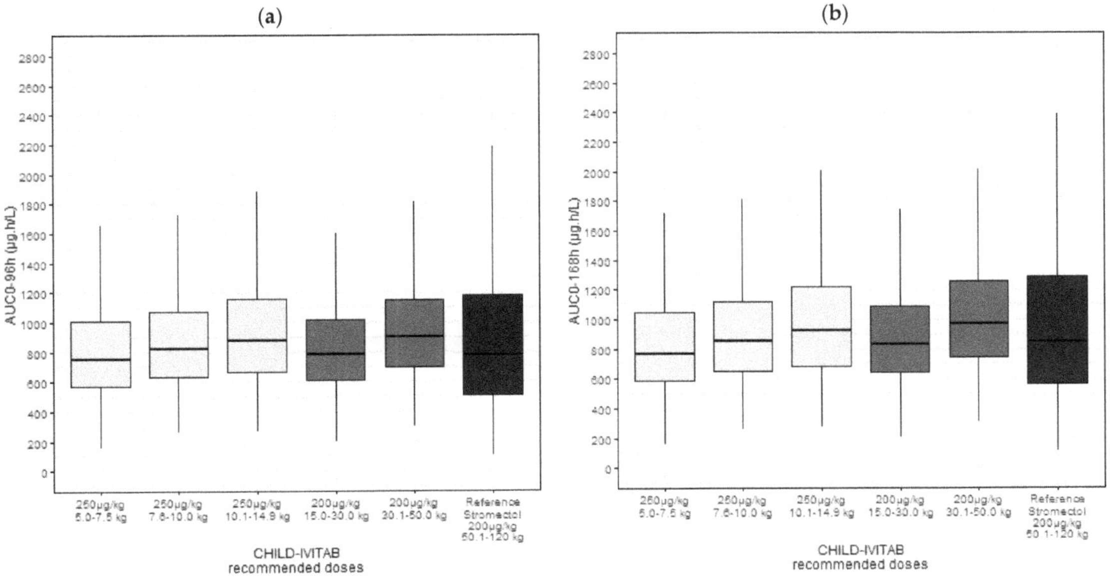

Figure 4. Simulated ivermectin exposure (N = 1000) according to weight-based ivermectin dosing regimen in adults following a single administration of 200 µg/kg of the reference STROMECTOL® formulation and according to defined dose recommendations of 250 µg/kg in children < 15 kg and 200 µg/kg in children ≥ 15 kg following a single CHILD-IVITAB administration. (**a**) Simulated ivermectin exposure 96h after dosing (area under the concentration–time curve, $AUC_{0\text{–}96h}$). (**b**) Simulated ivermectin exposure 168h after dosing ($AUC_{0\text{–}168h}$). IQR, inter-quartile range.

4. Discussion

Currently, there is a lack of a child-friendly, age-appropriate ivermectin formulation for young children, and ivermectin is currently not approved for children and infants < 15 kg [6,20,21]. Current oral administrations of ivermectin (crushed tablets in water or locally produced suspensions) for young children are prone to imprecise dosing due to loss of product after crushing and sedimentation of product after suspension. Furthermore, these methods are cumbersome and thus not appropriate for administration at scale during MDAs [22,23]. These factors may result in reduced drug adherence and effectiveness of ivermectin-based treatments in pediatric patient populations. As such, a child-friendly oral ivermectin formulation is needed. In a recent study in healthy adults [16], it was shown that palatability with CHILD-IVITAB was enhanced as compared to STROMECTOL® which would improve acceptability during MDA. CHILD-IVITAB was well tolerated, and there were no adverse events reported in the study. Further, CHILD-IVITAB was associated with considerably reduced inter-individual variability in overall exposure ($AUC_{0\text{–}96h}$ and $AUC_{0\text{-}inf}$) with close to equivalent exposure coverage as compared to STROMECTOL®.

In this study, a previously published population PK model of oral ivermectin was used to characterize the absorption profile of the two formulations CHILD-IVITAB and STROMECTOL® in healthy adults [7]. All PK parameter estimates were comparable with previously published results in children aged 2–12 years old [7]. Absorption with CHILD-IVITAB was faster than with STROMECTOL® with typical k_a (set equal to k_{tr}) values of 2.4 (95%CI: 2.17–2.68) vs. 1.6 (95% CI: 1.27–1.92) per hour, respectively, and corresponding shorter calculated mean transit time (MTT) with values of 1.2 (95% CI: 1.12–1.38) vs. 1.9 (95% CI: 1.56–2.36) hours, respectively. Some differences in model parameter estimates were observed when compared to values previously reported in children [7]. In particular, a 52% lower central volume of distribution and ~67% higher intercompartmental clearance were estimated, resulting in faster (×5) initial decline (alpha: 0.56 h^{-1} in the present study and 0.11 h^{-1} in Brussee et al. [7]), but a similar terminal elimination phase (beta: 0.028 h^{-1} in the present study and 0.023 h^{-1} in Brussee et al. [7]) (Supplementary Materials Table S1). We hypothesize that these differences in the initial exposure profile could mainly be the result of different study designs, including different formulations used (ELEA ivermectin 3 mg or mini-tablets 0.5 mg produced at the Hospital Pharmacy of Basel University), administration in a fed versus fasted state in the present study, a different blood sampling approach (capillary versus venous blood sampling in the present study) and timing (more dense early sampling in the present study, and an additional late measurement at 96 h) [8]. A decreasing variability of absorption parameters (k_a) by ~50% was seen with CHILD-IVITAB compared to STROMECTOL® with the population PK model, in line with previous findings from non-compartmental PK analysis [16]. Age-dependent variation in the PK of ivermectin has been reported in previous studies. Decreased intestinal motility in children is thought to cause limited transit time (3–7.5 h in children vs. 3–4 h in adults), which in turn might explain the increased relative bioavailability [8]. In the near future, we plan to collect PK data in children to further characterize absorption in pediatric patients. From the planned pediatric PK study, we may be able to investigate potential age-dependent effects of ivermectin absorption. The marginally ~20% increased relative bioavailability estimated, as well as faster absorption process, could represent a small fraction of ivermectin absorbed buccally. However, we did not consider model-based analysis of such a possible parallel buccal absorption process, which may be defined in terms of the fraction of dose absorbed buccally with the corresponding buccal absorption rate constant. In fact, on an individual level, lower relative bioavailability was also estimated for CHILD-IVITAB for 7/16 subjects (Supplementary Materials Table S2), which would imply an unphysiological negative fraction absorbed buccally. The faster absorption observed for CHILD-IVITAB (in the fasted state) could also be related to faster dissolution and gastric emptying, especially since absorption for ivermectin is assumed to be limited by solubility rather than permeability (classified as BCS class II). In the fed state, increased bile micelle-mediated solubility appears to explain faster and more complete absorption [24]. Further preclinical and clinical studies are being designed to focus on characterizing trans-buccal absorption process of the ODT. There was no formulation effect on apparent clearance (p-value > 0.05). A trend towards higher (~30%) ivermectin relative bioavailability with CHILD-IVITAB compared to STROMECTOL® was observed, also confirming results from the trial [16]. One subject (#14) showed potentially low absolute bioavailability resulting in high oral clearance. Sensitivity analysis excluding subject #14 showed a significant decrease in relative bioavailability. Unknown and potentially variable absolute oral bioavailability may also explain the high correlation between estimated individual PK parameters. Inspection of individual profile plots (Figure 1) suggested that IIV is necessary to be included in models due to mostly higher CHILD-IVITAB profiles, but in a few instances, also lower profiles compared to STROMECTOL®. As such, variability in ivermectin exposure between these two formulations does not seem to originate from differences in drug clearance but is driven by a more controlled absorption process with CHILD-IVITAB. This would result in more homogeneous response to ivermectin, limiting under- and over-exposed patients, and may consequently be beneficial in a clinic or in MDA settings.

4.1. Modeling and Simulation to Facilitate Dose Selection for a Pediatric Study in Children with Scabies

Clinical trials are being set up in LMICs (EPIC-15 trial in Brazil, NCT06404333) and Europe to assess palatability, tolerability, safety, efficacy, and exposure coverage of CHILD-IVITAB in pediatric patients with a parasitic disease, including children weighing more than 5 and less than 15 kg. The objectives of this clinical study were to determine drug exposure coverage after oral administration of CHILD-IVITAB applying weight-adjusted dosing in children > 5 kg and <15 kg compared to children $\geq$ 15 kg treated for scabies. The popPK model developed by Brussee et al. for standard ivermectin in children 2–12 years of age indicated that an increased dose of 250 and 300 μg/kg would be needed in school-aged children (6–12 years) and pre-school-aged children (2–5 years), respectively, to achieve equivalent exposure coverage in children compared to adults [7]. The current developed popPK model was used to perform simulations to support the design of such a clinical trial, with the objective to determine ivermectin concentration profiles and drug exposure coverage for 200 μg/kg, 250 μg/kg and 300 μg/kg, in children ≥ 15 kg and <15 kg following a single administration of CHILD-IVITAB. Outputs from simulations in children < 15 kg revealed that a dose of 250 μg/kg CHILD-IVITAB is associated with consistent exposure coverage as compared to a dose of 200 μg/kg in children ≥ 15 kg and adults, up to 7 days post administration. CHILD-IVITAB will be developed at 1 mg and 3 mg strengths, allowing for fine-tuned dosing depending on body weight in children < 15 kg by combining both fixed-dose regimens of 1 mg and 3 mg [25]. Altogether, these results suggest that CHILD-IVITAB is a suitable formulation for clinical or MDA settings to prevent and/or treat NTDs (e.g., scabies, helminth, onchocerciasis), not just in adults, but also in adolescents and children ≥ 15 kg and children and infants < 15 kg.

4.2. Limitations

One of the limitations of this study is the relatively small sample size. Nevertheless, the rich sampling design enabled parameter estimation with good precision. Further pediatric studies will be conducted to collect safety data in children. In this study, we considered weight (allometric scaling) to predict exposure in pediatric patients up to the age of 6 months (i.e., approximately 5 kg), while age might generally play a role in the metabolization pathway due to maturation processes in the smallest age group. However, cytochrome P450 3A4 (CYP3A4) is the predominant isoform responsible for the metabolism of ivermectin by human liver microsomes, and after 2 years of age, CYP3A4 exhibits 100% of its activity [26]. In addition, no particular effect of age on P-glycoprotein (P-gp) is expected [27]. Therefore, while age might be an important covariate to consider below 2 years, age will likely have a limited impact on ivermectin elimination in the considered target population (from 2 years of age, i.e., approximately 10 kg), as found previously [7]. Further clinical studies are warranted to expand knowledge on ivermectin exposure in pediatric patients < 10 kg. While VPC showed overall adequate model fit, some trend for underprediction of late concentrations measured at 96h may need to be acknowledged (residual plots, Supplementary Materials Figure S1B–D). The presented model should therefore be used with caution for extrapolation to later timepoints (e.g., 7 days after administration). The trend of underprediction of late concentrations may be reduced by fitting a three-compartmental model; however, we could not estimate corresponding parameters reliably (RSE > 100%, OFV = 2704 vs. 2341 for base population PK model, CV > 100% on parameter estimates). Further clinical studies may help to identify such a model structure, with planned concentration measurements after 96 h. Elimination of the need for water administration is one of the main advantages of CHILD-IVITAB. However, in the settings of the presented trial in healthy adults, CHILD-IVITAB was administered for 30 s in the buccal cavity, then rinsed and swallowed with water. In the case of CHILD-IVITAB, the drug may partly be absorbed trans-buccally within the first 30 s after uptake, before water intake. Further preclinical and clinical studies are being designed to focus on characterizing the sublingual, trans-buccal and gastro-intestinal absorption process of the ODT. Nevertheless, the faster absorption process, as seen with the novel template inverted particle (TIP) technology loaded with ivermectin CHILD-IVITAB, shows significant potential for other APIs that require a fast onset of action.

5. Conclusions

This pharmacometric analysis confirmed that CHILD-IVITAB shows faster and more controlled absorption than STROMECTOL® in the fasting state, explaining previously reported reduced variability in ivermectin exposure with CHILD-IVITAB. Model-based simulations indicated that a CHILD-IVITAB dose of 250 μg/kg in children < 15 kg is expected to achieve equivalent ivermectin exposure coverage in these children as compared to children ≥ 15 kg and adults treated with a dose of 200 μg/kg.

Supplementary Materials: The following supporting information can be downloaded at https://www.mdpi.com/article/10.3390/pharmaceutics16091186/s1: Table S1: Comparison between de novo parameter estimates and parameters from referenced model by Brussee et al. CI, confidence interval; Vc, central volume of distribution; Vp, peripheral volume of distribution. Table S2: Individual parameter estimates (empirical bayes estimates): CL, clearance; Frel, relative bioavailability; IQR, inter-quartile range. Table S3: Objective function value (OFV) according to number of transit compartments per formulation. Table S4: Population PK parameter estimates for ivermectin, for base population PK model and sensitivity analysis (excluding subject #14). Proportional and additive errors are reported as variance estimates (σ^2). CL, clearance; Frel, relative bioavailability (Frel set to 1 for the reference formulation STROMECTOL® and estimated Frel for CHILD-IVITAB); IIV, inter-individual variability, reported as coefficient of variation (CV%); Q, intercompartmental clearance; k_a, absorption rate constant; k_{tr}, transfer rate constant; RSE, relative standard error; Vc, volume of distribution in the central compartment; Vp, volume of distribution in the peripheral compartment. Figure S1: Goodness-of-fit plots for PK model presented in Table 2 for ivermectin concentrations by formulation. A. Observed ivermectin concentrations (mg/L) versus population predicted ivermectin concentrations (μg/L). B. Population-weighted residuals (PWRESs) versus time after dose. C. Individual weighted residuals (IWRESs) versus time after dose. D. Normalized prediction distribution errors (NPDEs) versus time after dose. Pre-dose samples of next dosing (after wash-out period of 7 days) from cross-over trial were included in the GOFs. Light grey circles correspond to censored data (BLQ, with LLOQ = 0.05 mg/L). Figure S2: Individual fits (grey lines) of ivermectin concentrations (ng/mL) on y-axis and time after dose (hour) on x-axis. Black dots correspond to observed data. Note: one screening failure occurred (individual #10) because of positive cannabis drug screen. Figure S3: Zoom on absorption phase. Individual fits (grey lines) of ivermectin concentrations (ng/mL) on y-axis and time after dose (hour) on x-axis. Black dots correspond to observed data. Note: one screening failure occurred (individual #10) because of positive cannabis drug screen. Figure S4: Individual parameter (conditional mode, i.e., empirical Bayesian estimates, EBEs) distribution, represented as histograms for the probability density function. Theoretical individual parameter distribution is represented as continuous black line. Shrinkage value of each individual parameter is displayed on top of the histograms. ka_0, absorption rate constant of CHILD-IVITAB; ka_1, absorption rate constant of STROMECTOL®; CL, clearance; V1, volume of distribution in the central compartment; V2, volume of distribution in the peripheral compartment; relF1, relative bioavailability. Figure S5: Simulated ivermectin exposures (N = 1000) 96 h (AUC_{0-96h}) and 168 h (AUC_{0-168h}) after dosing according to weight-based ivermectin dosing regimen in adults following a single administration of 200 μg/kg of the reference STROMECTOL® formulation and 200, 250 or 300 μg/kg in children < 15 kg and ≥ 15 kg following a single CHILD-IVITAB administration. Supplementary Materials S10: Model code.

Author Contributions: M.B., M.P., J.H., L.E.R. and K.D. designed the study, while K.D. and L.E.R. performed the study and interpreted data. K.G., V.G. and M.P. performed the pharmacometric PK analysis. K.G., J.v.d.A., K.K. and M.P. drafted the manuscript. All authors have read and agreed to the published version of the manuscript.

Funding: This study was funded by the Pediatric Pharmacology and Pharmacometrics Research Center at the University Children's Hospital Basel (UKBB) and the Division of Pharmaceutical Technology, University of Basel.

Institutional Review Board Statement: The study was conducted in accordance with the Declaration of Helsinki and the ICH-GCP, and the protocol was approved by Swissmedic and Swissethics (Trial Registration Number: NCT05477810).

Informed Consent Statement: Informed consent was obtained from all subjects involved in the study.

Data Availability Statement: The data that support the findings of this study are available from the corresponding author upon reasonable request.

Acknowledgments: We thank Galvita AG for the right to use their proprietary TIP technology, which was needed to produce the study medication CHILD-IVITAB. We thank Stefanie Deuster and Uli Loesch (Hospital Pharmacy Basel) for support with respect to the preparation of the CHILD-IVITAB study medication under GMP. We thank Gilbert Koch and Andrew Atkinson from the Department of Pediatric Pharmacology, UKBB, for reviewing the manuscript.

Conflicts of Interest: J.H. is a board member of Galvita AG. The authors declare no conflicts of interest.

References

1. Molyneux, D.; Taylor, H.R. The Discovery of Ivermectin. *Trends Parasitol.* **2015**, *31*, 1. [CrossRef] [PubMed]
2. World Health Organization. *Model List of Essential Medicines for Children*; WHO: Geneva, Switzerland, 2019.
3. Sodahlon, Y. 2022 Annual Highlights. Available online: https://mectizan.org/wp-content/uploads/2023/05/2022-Annual-Highlights-of-Mectizan-Donation-Program.pdf (accessed on 1 July 2024).
4. Buettcher, M.; Stebler, A.K.; Theiler, M.; Kobylinski, K.; Pfister, M. National Survey in Switzerland Calls for Improved Diagnosis and Treatment in Children with Scabies. *Swiss. Med. Wkly.* **2023**, *153*, 40129. [CrossRef] [PubMed]
5. Compendium. Subvectin. Available online: https://compendium.ch (accessed on 23 July 2024).
6. Jittamala, P.; Monteiro, W.; Smit, M.R.; Pedrique, B.; Specht, S.; Chaccour, C.J.; Dard, C.; Del Giudice, P.; Khieu, V.; Maruani, A.; et al. A Systematic Review and an Individual Patient Data Meta-Analysis of Ivermectin Use in Children Weighing Less than Fifteen Kilograms: Is It Time to Reconsider the Current Contraindication? *PLoS Negl. Trop. Dis.* **2021**, *15*, e0009144. [CrossRef]
7. Brussee, J.M.; Schulz, J.D.; Coulibaly, J.T.; Keiser, J.; Pfister, M. Ivermectin Dosing Strategy to Achieve Equivalent Exposure Coverage in Children and Adults. *Clin. Pharmacol. Ther.* **2019**, *106*, 661–667. [CrossRef]
8. Schulz, J.D.; Coulibaly, J.T.; Schindler, C.; Wimmersberger, D.; Keiser, J. Pharmacokinetics of Ascending Doses of Ivermectin in Trichuris Trichiura-Infected Children Aged 2–12 Years. *J. Antimicrob. Chemother.* **2019**, *74*, 1642–1647. [CrossRef] [PubMed]
9. Duthaler, U.; Suenderhauf, C.; Karlsson, M.O.; Hussner, J.; Meyer zu Schwabedissen, H.; Krähenbühl, S.; Hammann, F. Population Pharmacokinetics of Oral Ivermectin in Venous Plasma and Dried Blood Spots in Healthy Volunteers. *Br. J. Clin. Pharmacol.* **2019**, *85*, 626–633. [CrossRef] [PubMed]
10. Duthaler, U.; Leisegang, R.; Karlsson, M.O.; Krähenbühl, S.; Hammann, F. The Effect of Food on the Pharmacokinetics of Oral Ivermectin. *J. Antimicrob. Chemother.* **2020**, *75*, 438–440. [CrossRef]
11. Levy, M.; Martin, L.; Bursztejn, A.; Chiaverini, C.; Miquel, J.; Mahé, E.; Maruani, A.; Boralevi, F.; Groupe de Recherche de la Société Française de Dermatologie Pédiatrique. Ivermectin Safety in Infants and Children under 15 Kg Treated for Scabies: A Multicentric Observational Study. *Br. J. Dermatol.* **2020**, *182*, 1003–1006. [CrossRef]
12. Kost, J.; Huwyler, J.; Puchkov, M. Calcium Phosphate Microcapsules as Multifunctional Drug Delivery Devices. *Adv. Funct. Mater.* **2023**, *33*, 2303333. [CrossRef]
13. Wagner-Hattler, L.; Kiene, K.; Bielicki, J.; Pfister, M.; Puchkov, M.; Huwyler, J. High Acceptability of an Orally Dispersible Tablet Formulation by Children. *Children* **2021**, *8*, 194. [CrossRef]
14. Wagner-Hattler, L.; Wyss, K.; Schoelkopf, J.; Huwyler, J.; Puchkov, M. In Vitro Characterization and Mouthfeel Study of Functionalized Calcium Carbonate in Orally Disintegrating Tablets. *Int. J. Pharm.* **2017**, *534*, 50–59. [CrossRef]
15. Wagner-Hattler, L.; Schoelkopf, J.; Huwyler, J.; Puchkov, M. Stability Investigation of FCC-Based Tablets for Oral Suspension with Caffeine and Oxantel Pamoate as Model Drugs. *Drug Dev. Ind. Pharm.* **2019**, *45*, 222–230. [CrossRef] [PubMed]
16. Dao, K.; Buettcher, M.; Golhen, K.; Kost, J.; Schittny, A.; Duthaler, U.; Atkinson, A.; Haefliger, D.; Guidi, M.; Bardinet, C.; et al. Novel Patient-Friendly Orodispersible Formulation of Ivermectin Is Associated with Enhanced Palatability, Controlled Absorption, and Less Variability: High Potential for Pediatric Use. *J. Clin. Pharmacol.* **2024**. [CrossRef] [PubMed]
17. Duthaler, U.; Suenderhauf, C.; Gaugler, S.; Vetter, B.; Krähenbühl, S.; Hammann, F. Development and Validation of an LC-MS/MS Method for the Analysis of Ivermectin in Plasma, Whole Blood, and Dried Blood Spots Using a Fully Automatic Extraction System. *J. Pharm. Biomed. Anal.* **2019**, *172*, 18–25. [CrossRef] [PubMed]
18. Bergstrand, M.; Karlsson, M.O. Handling Data below the Limit of Quantification in Mixed Effect Models. *AAPS J.* **2009**, *11*, 371–380. [CrossRef] [PubMed]
19. Koch, G.; Krzyzanski, W.; Pérez-Ruixo, J.J.; Schropp, J. Modeling of Delays in PKPD: Classical Approaches and a Tutorial for Delay Differential Equations. *J. Pharmacokinet. Pharmacodyn.* **2014**, *41*, 291–318. [CrossRef]
20. Nicolas, P.; Maia, M.F.; Bassat, Q.; Kobylinski, K.C.; Monteiro, W.; Rabinovich, N.R.; Menéndez, C.; Bardají, A.; Chaccour, C. Safety of Oral Ivermectin during Pregnancy: A Systematic Review and Meta-Analysis. *Lancet Glob. Health* **2020**, *8*, e92–e100. [CrossRef]
21. Kimland, E.; Odlind, V. Off-Label Drug Use in Pediatric Patients. *Clin. Pharmacol. Ther.* **2012**, *91*, 796–801. [CrossRef]
22. Vallet, T.; Elhamdaoui, O.; Berraho, A.; Cherkaoui, L.O.; Kriouile, Y.; Mahraoui, C.; Mouane, N.; Pense-Lheritier, A.-M.; Ruiz, F.; Bensouda, Y. Medicines Acceptability in Hospitalized Children: An Ongoing Need for Age-Appropriate Formulations. *Pharmaceutics* **2020**, *12*, 766. [CrossRef]
23. Wohlrab, J.; Stadie, L.; Neubert, R.H.H.; Bosse, K. Development of an Ivermectin-Containing Syrup as an Extemporaneous Preparation for Treatment of Scabies in Children. *Hautarzt* **2021**, *72*, 720–728. [CrossRef]

24. Rowland Yeo, K.; Wesche, D. PBPK Modeling of Ivermectin—Considerations for the Purpose of Developing Alternative Routes to Optimize Its Safety Profile. *CPT Pharmacomet. Syst. Pharmacol.* **2023**, *12*, 598–609. [CrossRef] [PubMed]
25. Gwee, A.; Duffull, S.; Zhu, X.; Tong, S.Y.C.; Cranswick, N.; McWhinney, B.; Ungerer, J.; Francis, J.; Steer, A.C. Population Pharmacokinetics of Ivermectin for the Treatment of Scabies in Indigenous Australian Children. *PLoS Negl. Trop. Dis.* **2020**, *14*, e0008886. [CrossRef] [PubMed]
26. Johnson, T.N.; Rostami-Hodjegan, A.; Tucker, G.T. Prediction of the Clearance of Eleven Drugs and Associated Variability in Neonates, Infants and Children. *Clin. Pharmacokinet.* **2006**, *45*, 931–956. [CrossRef] [PubMed]
27. Brouwer, K.; Aleksunes, L.; Brandys, B.; Giacoia, G.; Knipp, G.; Lukacova, V.; Meibohm, B.; Nigam, S.; Rieder, M.; de Wildt, S. Human Ontogeny of Drug Transporters: Review and Recommendations of the Pediatric Transporter Working Group. *Clin. Pharmacol. Ther.* **2015**, *98*, 266–287. [CrossRef]

pharmaceutics

MDPI

Article

Archaeosomes for Oral Drug Delivery: From Continuous Microfluidics Production to Powdered Formulations

Ivan Vidakovic [1,†], Karin Kornmueller [1,†], Daniela Fiedler [2], Johannes Khinast [3], Eleonore Fröhlich [4], Gerd Leitinger [5], Christina Horn [6], Julian Quehenberger [6,7], Oliver Spadiut [7] and Ruth Prassl [1,*]

1 Division of Medical Physics and Biophysics, Gottfried Schatz Research Center for Cell Signaling, Metabolism and Aging, Medical University of Graz, 8010 Graz, Austria; ivan.vidakovic@medunigraz.at (I.V.); karin.kornmueller@medunigraz.at (K.K.)
2 Institute of Process and Particle Engineering, Graz University of Technology, 8010 Graz, Austria; daniela.fiedler@miex.cc
3 Research Center Pharmaceutical Engineering, 8010 Graz, Austria; khinast@tugraz.at
4 Center for Medical Research, Medical University of Graz, 8010 Graz, Austria; eleonore.froehlich@medunigraz.at
5 Division of Cell Biology, Histology and Embryology, Gottfried Schatz Research Center for Cell Signaling, Metabolism and Aging, Medical University of Graz, 8010 Graz, Austria; gerd.leitinger@medunigraz.at
6 NovoArc GmbH, 1120 Vienna, Austria; christina.horn@novoarc.at (C.H.); julian.quehenberger@tuwien.ac.at (J.Q.)
7 Institute of Chemical, Environmental and Bioscience Engineering, TU Wien, 1060 Vienna, Austria; oliver.spadiut@tuwien.ac.at
* Correspondence: ruth.prassl@medunigraz.at; Tel.: +43-316-385-71695
† These authors contributed equally to this work.

Abstract: Archaeosomes were manufactured from natural archaeal lipids by a microfluidics-assisted single-step production method utilizing a mixture of di- and tetraether lipids extracted from *Sulfolobus acidocaldarius*. The primary aim of this study was to investigate the exceptional stability of archaeosomes as potential carriers for oral drug delivery, with a focus on powdered formulations. The archaeosomes were negatively charged with a size of approximately 100 nm and a low polydispersity index. To assess their suitability for oral delivery, the archaeosomes were loaded with two model drugs: calcein, a fluorescent compound, and insulin, a peptide hormone. The archaeosomes demonstrated high stability in simulated intestinal fluids, with only 5% of the encapsulated compounds being released after 24 h, regardless of the presence of degrading enzymes or extremely acidic pH values such as those found in the stomach. In a co-culture cell model system mimicking the intestinal barrier, the archaeosomes showed strong adhesion to the cell membranes, facilitating a slow release of contents. The archaeosomes were loaded with insulin in a single-step procedure achieving an encapsulation efficiency of approximately 35%. These particles have been exposed to extreme manufacturing temperatures during freeze-drying and spray-drying processes, demonstrating remarkable resilience under these harsh conditions. The fabrication of stable dry powder formulations of archaeosomes represents a promising advancement toward the development of solid dosage forms for oral delivery of biological drugs.

Keywords: archaeosomes; archaeal lipids; oral drug delivery; insulin; dry powder formulation; solid dosage form

1. Introduction

Archaea are a group of single-celled prokaryotic microorganisms. In the phylogenetic tree, they represent—besides bacteria and eukaryotes—the third domain of life. Concerning their ancient evolutionary history, archaea can typically withstand extreme conditions such as high temperatures, acidic pH values, elevated pressure, or high salinity [1]. For example, *Sulfolobus acidocaldarius*, one representative of the thermophilic subgroup of archaea commonly occurring near hydrothermal sources, can endure temperatures as high as 80 °C and acidic pH values as low as 2 [2]. Figure 1a,b show representative transmission electron microscopic (TEM) and scanning electron microscopic (SEM) micrographs of *Sulfolobus acidocaldarius* cells, which were used for the isolation of archaeal lipids applied in this study. The exceptional resistance of archaea against high temperatures and acidic conditions stems from their unique plasma membrane composition, characterized by two main components: diether lipids (DELs) and tetraether lipids (TELs) [3,4]. As their names imply, these lipids contain ether bonds connecting prevalent isoprenoid sidechains to glycerol. This is in contrast to ester bonds in phospholipids and amide bonds found in sphingolipids connecting non-branched fatty acid chains to glycerol in bacterial and eukaryotic membranes. The structures of the most prominent ether lipids extracted from cultivated *Sulfolobus acidocaldarius* are shown in Figure 1c,d.

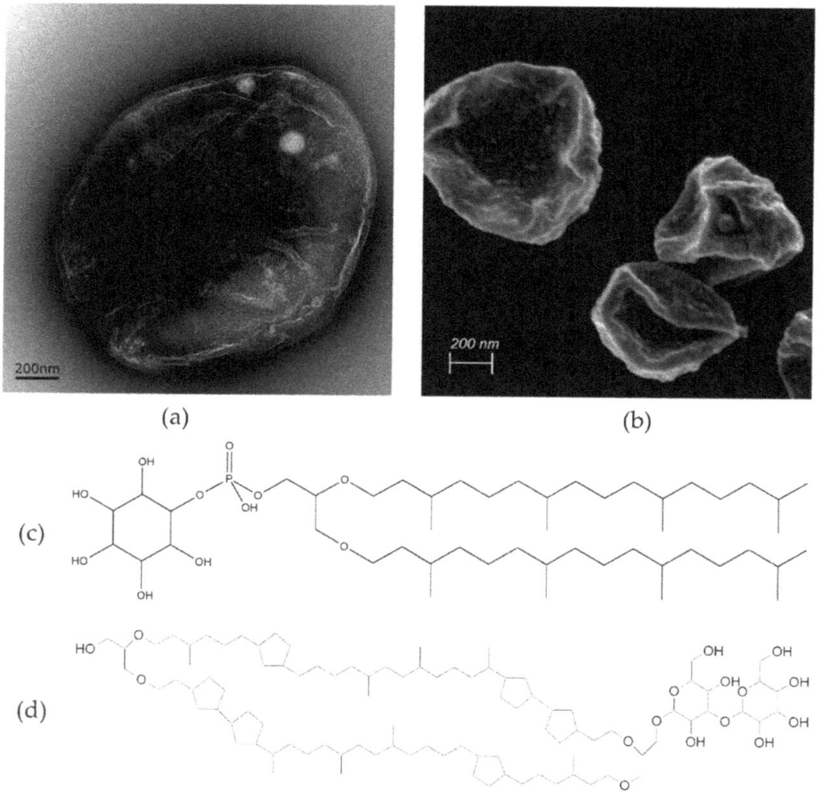

Figure 1. Visualization of *Sulfolobus acidocaldarius* cells using (**a**) TEM and (**b**) SEM. The scale bar represents 200 nm. The sample preparation for SEM includes water displacement through a series of ethanol treatments that can cause cell shrinkage as evident in (**b**). The molecular structures of two ether lipid species isolated from the archaeal membrane are presented in (**c**,**d**), highlighting structural differences. (**c**) Features archaeol—the principal representative of DEL containing two isoprenoid chains and (**d**) caldarchaeol—a prominent representative of TEL, which is almost double in length having two polar groups connected with two isoprene-like chains containing 6 cyclic structures.

Similar to conventional phospholipid molecules isolated from eukaryotes, ether lipids extracted from archaea form vesicular structures in aqueous solution [5]. Diether-based archaeal lipids are known to build less permeable and more condensed lipid bilayer membranes compared to those found for conventional diester-based eukaryotic lipids.

Tetraether lipids are membrane-spanning lipids that form a monolayer structure that is densely packed due to the presence of the isoprenoid methyl groups and rigid saturated hydrocarbon chains [6–8]. Owing to their unique chemical structures and physical characteristics, archaeal lipids can self-assemble into highly stable and stress-resistant liposome-like particles, known as archaeosomes. Concerning structural features, the monolayer-forming tetraether lipids are believed to enhance the membrane packing density, making archaeosomes more stable and less permeable for ions and compounds compared to conventional liposomes [9–11]. Thus, archaeosomes are extensively investigated as drug delivery systems for proteins, peptides, gene delivery, or delivery of natural antioxidant compounds [12,13]. In this context, archaeosomes are considered particularly promising for oral drug delivery. When ingested, the compounds encounter a similar hostile environment present in the gastric system of the human body as the archaea face in their natural habitat, not in terms of high temperatures but regarding the acidic pH value and degrading enzymes present in the gastrointestinal (GI) tract. Likewise, archaeosomes are also stable in the presence of bile salts and lipases [12]. While some studies report on the use of archaeosomes as oral delivery systems for various drug molecules [12–14], limited information exists on how archaeosomes behave under different physiological conditions, interact with cells mimicking the GI tract, and whether archaeosomes, due to their pronounced stability, can be transformed into a solid dosage form. Dry powders can, for example, be produced by lyophilization [15,16] or spray-drying processes as already shown for liposomes or solid lipid nanoparticles [17,18]. However, heat and shear stress during manufacturing may lead to instability, enhanced particle aggregation, and rapid drug release, which limits pharmaceutical production on a large scale.

This study aimed to establish a continuous manufacturing process of archaeosomes using isolated archaeal lipids from *Sulfolobus acidocaldarius*. The developed preparation process involves a microfluidics-controlled system enabling the concurrent production of archaeosomes and drug loading within a single-step procedure. Two model compounds were chosen for drug encapsulation. One was calcein, a small inorganic molecule serving as a fluorescent marker to estimate the release behavior of encapsulated compounds from archaeosomes. The second one was human insulin, a pharmaceutically relevant example of a peptide drug molecule. The drug-loaded archaeosomes underwent thorough characterization in terms of particle size, zeta potential, membrane structure, and morphology. The stability of archaeosomes was evaluated in both simulated gastric and intestinal fluid. Loading efficiency and release behavior were determined. The interaction and adhesion behavior with the intestinal barrier were evaluated in a trans-well system using a Caco-2 and HT29-MTX co-culture system as a model for the intestinal epithelium. Finally, freeze-drying and spray-drying procedures were implemented to create a solid dosage form.

2. Materials and Methods

2.1. Materials

1,2-Dioleoyl-sn-glycero-3-phosphoethanolamine-*N*-(lissamine rhodamine B sulfonyl) ammonium salt (DOPE-rhodamine), (*p-tert*-Octylphenoxy)polyethoxyethanol (Triton X-100), cholesterol, fluorescein-bis-(methyliminodiacetic acid) (calcein), paraformaldehyde, glutaraldehyde, pancreatin, pepsin, and human insulin were obtained from Sigma® Aldrich Handels GmbH, Vienna, Austria. Sodium cacodylate was purchased from Science Services GmbH (München, Germany). Caco-2 cells (ACC169, HTB-37 clone from the German Collection of Microorganisms and Cell Cultures) were provided by E. Fröhlich (Medical University of Graz, Austria) and HT29-MTX-E12 cells were kindly provided by T. Lesuffleur (INSERM UMR S 938, Paris, France). All components used for the in vitro experiments were purchased from ThermoFisher Scientific (Waltham, MA, USA): high-glucose Dulbecco's modified Eagle medium (DMEM), fetal bovine serum (FBS), a mixture of penicillin and streptomycin (Pen-Strep), non-essential amino acids, TrypLe as the synthetic substitution for trypsin, as well as the fluorescent stains Phalloidin Alexa Fluor 488, Phalloidin Rhodamine 565, and Hoechst 33258. Fluorescence mounting medium DAKO was purchased from Agilent (Santa Clara, CA, USA). Phosphate buffered saline (PBS; pH 7.4, ionic strength of 162.7 mM) was purchased from Gibco, Life Technologies Corporation (Painsley, UK). Translucent membranes with pores of 3 μm in 12-well plates were obtained from Greiner Bio-One (Kremsmünster, Austria). The following filters and membranes were used in the production process: 20 nm Whatman Anotop 25 syringe filters and polycarbonate membranes of various pore sizes purchased from Cytiva Europe GmbH (Vienna, Austria) and Membra-cel dialysis membranes (Viskase, Lombard, IL, USA). All other chemicals such as dimethylsulfoxide (DMSO), 2-propanol (iPA), trichloromethane (chloroform), methanol, absolute ethanol, and HEPES buffer were obtained from Carl Roth GmbH (Karlsruhe, Germany).

Archaeosomes were produced using mixtures of diether and tetraether lipids that were directly isolated from *S. acidocaldarius* [19] and kindly provided in the form of a crude lipid extract by NovoArc GmbH (Vienna, Austria).

2.2. Methods

2.2.1. Particle Preparation Using Microfluidics with Simultaneous Loading of Calcein or Insulin

The crude extract containing a DEL:TEL mixture isolated from the archaea was dissolved either in DMSO: iPA (2:1 vol/vol) or absolute ethanol at a total lipid concentration of 20–21 mg/mL depending on the individual batches. Before microfluidic mixing, the suspension was filtered through a 200 nm syringe filter to remove any solid residues that could obstruct the channels of the microfluidics cartridge. As aqueous phase, 10 mM HEPES buffer pH 7.4 (filtered through a 20 nm syringe filter) was used. A single step production of archaeosomes was performed with a NanoAssemblr® microfluidics mixing device (Precision Nanosystems, Vancouver, BC, Canada) using a staggered herringbone mixer [20–23]. Process parameters were optimized and set as follows: flow rate ratio 2:1 (aqueous to organic phase) and a total flow rate of 1.7 mL/min. This setup resulted in a final lipid concentration of 7 mg/mL.

For drug encapsulation, calcein, which is a green fluorescent marker with the ability to self-quench at higher concentrations, was used [24,25]. To achieve the quenching effect in our preparations the concentration of calcein was set to 60 mM, corresponding to 37.35 mg/mL calcein dissolved in 10 mM HEPES buffer (pH 7.4). The calcein solution was used as an aqueous phase in the microfluidics system. The process parameters were kept constant as described before. Removal of non-encapsulated calcein along with the organic solvent was performed by dialysis with a 14 kDa membrane tube in two steps against 10 mM PBS (0.15 M NaCl, pH 7.4) buffer. An exchange with a buffer of higher salt concentration was necessary to counteract sample dilution due to the high hypertonic effect of dissolved calcein during dialysis.

The second model drug was the human peptide insulin. In this case, the aqueous phase contained an insulin solution in 10 mM HEPES adjusted to a pH of 2.0 using 1 M hydrochloric acid [26]. Due to the incompatibility between insulin and DMSO the lipids were dissolved in absolute ethanol. Retaining all the process parameters as described before, the final insulin concentration in the prepared formulations was approximately 3 mg/mL. Non-encapsulated insulin was rinsed twice with prefiltered 10 mM HEPES buffer (pH 7.4) within a Satorius Vivaspin 20 (Satorius Lab Instruments GmbH, Göttingen, Germany) centrifuge tube with a 100 kDa cut-off membrane. The encapsulation efficiency (EE%) of insulin was determined using the bicinchoninic acid (BCA) protein assay (BCA™Protein Assay, Thermo Scientifc, Rockford, IL, USA) according to the manufacturer's instructions. Briefly, sample dilutions were pipetted in triplicates together with an albumin solution of known concentration as standard in a 96-well plate format. After the addition of the reagent mixture and incubation at 37 °C, absorbance measurement at 562 nm of the created colored product was performed using the CLARIOstar plate reader (BMG LABTECH GmbH, Ortenberg, Germany). To verify insulin loading into archaeosomes a native gel electrophoresis using a native acrylamide gradient gel (4–12%) was performed in a Mini-

ProteanTetra vertical electrophoresis cell (Bio-Rad Laboratories, Feldkirchen, Germany). The gel was stained with Coomassie blue staining solution for 40 min and destained overnight. Imaging of the stained gels was performed using the Gel Doc EZ Imager (Bio-Rad Laboratories, Feldkirchen, Germany).

2.2.2. Particle Size Analysis

To determine the particle size, photon correlation spectroscopy (PCS) was performed using a Zetasizer HS3000 (Malvern Panalytical, Malvern, Worcestershire, UK) which operates with a 10 mW helium–neon laser at a wavelength of 633 nm. The scattered light was measured at an angle of 90°. All samples were previously diluted with buffer to a concentration of approximately 0.3 mg/mL lipids and measured in a quartz cuvette (Hellma GmbH, Müllheim, Germany) at room temperature. The distribution width and the homogeneity of the particle preparation are given by a polydispersity index (PDI) ranging from 0 (for totally homogeneous samples) to 1 (for highly heterogeneous mixtures).

2.2.3. Zeta Potential

To estimate the surface charge of the archaeosomes, the zeta potential was measured using a Zetasizer NANO ZS (Malvern Panalytical, Malvern, Worcestershire, UK). The samples were diluted 1:10 with distilled water (previously filtered through a 20 nm syringe filter) and measured at room temperature in a special cuvette with a folded capillary cell fitted with the electrodes.

2.2.4. Small-Angle X-ray Scattering (SAXS)

To obtain information on the lipid layer organization in terms of layer thickness and lamellarity, SAXS experiments were performed with a SAXSpace system (Anton Paar, Graz, Austria), equipped with a 30 W-Genix 3D microfocus X-ray generator (Xenocs, Sassenage, France) with a Cu anode and an Eiger R 1 M detector system (Dectris, Baden-Daettwil, Switzerland). SAXS patterns were recorded in a q-range from 0.2 to 6.0 nm^{-1}, where $q = (4\pi \sin \theta)/\lambda$ is the scattering vector, 2θ the scattering angle, and $\lambda = 0.154$ nm the wavelength of the X-ray beam. The data were buffer background corrected, normalized, and corrected for slit collimation geometry. The electron density profile was calculated with the global analysis program (GAP) [27,28], in which ρ represents the local electron density at the distance z from the center plane in the middle of the lipid layer. From the position of the Gaussian modeling of the electron dense lipid headgroup regions, a direct measure for the membrane thickness can be derived defining the head-to-headgroup distance. SAXS measurements were performed at 25 °C with an exposure time of 1.800 s at an archaeosome concentration of 30 mg/mL.

2.2.5. Transmission Electron Microscopy (TEM)

For negative staining TEM, either archaea or solutions of archaeosomes at a concentration of 0.07 mg/mL were dropped onto a glow-discharged (PELCO easiGlow, Plano GmbH, Wetzlar, Germany) carbon-coated copper grid (EMResolutions, C400Cu100, mesh 400), blotted, and stained for 1 min with 1% (*w*/*w*) uranyl acetate solution. Imaging was performed using a Fei Tecnai G^2 20 transmission electron microscope (Eindhoven, The Netherlands), operating at an acceleration voltage of 120 kV. Digital images were captured with a Gatan US1000 CCD camera at 2 K × 2 K resolution using the Digital Micrograph software (Version 1.93.1362, Gatan Inc., Pleasanton, CA, USA) [29].

2.2.6. Scanning Electron Microscopy (SEM)

Archaeosomes or archaea samples were pipetted onto a poly-L-lysine-coated glass slide. After incubation, the samples were gently rinsed with water and immediately fixed using a mixture of 2% paraformaldehyde, 2.5% glutaraldehyde, and 0.1 M cacodylate buffer (pH 7.4). After an incubation period of 30 min, the fixative solution was exchanged with cacodylate buffer for another 30 min, followed by a dehydration step using a series of ethanol to remove water from the sample. The ethanol concentration was increased stepwise with short incubation periods in between. At the very end, the 100% ethanol solution was exchanged with pure acetone and the samples underwent a critical point drying step. In another set of samples, the spray-dried and lyophilized powders containing archaeosomes were deposited onto an SEM holder (Plano G301) covered with adhesive carbon tape (Plano G3347). Liquid conductive silver was applied on the rim of each sample holder and dried for several minutes. Both sets of samples were then sputter coated using a BalTec SCD 500 sputter coater (Balzers, Liechtenstein). Imaging was performed using a Zeiss Sigma 500 VP scanning electron microscope (Zeiss, Oberkochen, Germany) operated at 2 kV, using an Everhart–Thornley secondary and backscattered electron detector. Images were acquired with the Zeiss SmartSEM V05.06 imaging software.

2.2.7. Stability in Simulated Gastric and Intestinal Fluid

To estimate the stability of the archaeosomes in the microenvironment of the stomach and intestine, the following simulated fluids were used. Gastric simulated fluid (GSF) was prepared using sodium chloride, pepsin, and hydrochloric acid with a pH adjusted to 1.2. For the simulated intestinal fluid (SIF) with a pH of 6.8, monobasic potassium phosphate, pancreatin, and sodium hydroxide were used [25]. The solutions were prepared according to the U.S. Pharmacopeia. Then, 1 mL of archaeosome solution (7 mg/mL) loaded with calcein dye was mixed with simulated body fluids in a volume ratio of 2:1 and inserted in a dialysis tube with a 100 kDa molecular cut-off membrane. The filled tube was immersed in 15 mL PBS buffer and continuously stirred using a magnetic stirrer. The experiments were performed at room temperature. Every hour for the first 6 h and after 24 h a 100 µL sample was taken from the surrounding PBS buffer. The displaced volume was refilled using the same amount of PBS buffer. After 24 h, a disruption of the archaeosomes was induced by adding 10 µL of 10% Triton X-100 to release calcein quantitatively. The fluorescence intensities were measured in a 96-well plate with a CLARIOstar plate reader (BMG LABTECH GmbH, Ortenberg, Germany) at excitation and emission wavelengths of 475 nm and 530 nm, respectively.

2.2.8. In Vitro Uptake Studies

To simulate the intestinal barrier a Caco-2 and HT29-MTX co-culture model was used. Caco-2 cells are epithelial-like cells isolated from a patient with colorectal carcinoma, while the HT29-MTX are differentiated into mature goblet cells with primary mucus-secreting function. Cell lines were combined at a ratio of 7 to 3 of Caco-2 to HT29-MTX and seeded in a total amount of 500,000 cells/well onto the translucent membrane of a Thincert cell culture insert of a 12 trans-well plate system (Greiner Bio-One, Kremsmünster, Austria). Further cultivation was necessary until reaching the full confluency of the monolayer. To determine the integrity of the cellular barrier the transepithelial electrical resistance (TEER of $427 \pm 18\ \Omega/cm^2$; n = 12) was measured using the Millicell ERS-2 system (Millipore Corp., Burlington, MA, USA) [30]. Following this, samples were loaded on top of the cell layer within the apical compartment and incubated at 37 °C for 4 h, resembling the typical environment and duration of digestion. The basal compartment was filled with 1 mL high-glucose DMEM solution without phenol red. Three different archaeosome formulations were used. The first formulation was loaded with calcein, the second was labeled with 0.003 mol% fluorescent DOPE-rhodamine lipid, and the third formulation contained both calcein and the fluorescent DOPE-rhodamine lipid within the lipid layer. All formulations were diluted to a final concentration of 500 µg/mL lipid. As a positive control a 0.05 mg/mL calcein solution was used, while the negative control consisted of only PBS buffer [31]. After a 4 h incubation period the contents of both compartments were collected and calcein-labeled (green) and rhodamine-labeled (red) archaeosomes were quantified by fluorescence assays at wavelength pairs of excitation/emission of 475/530 nm and 560/597 nm, respectively. This approach enabled a detailed examination of the efficacy of archaeosome formulations to cross the cellular barrier or to adhere to and penetrate the cell layer, allowing for the separate analysis of lipid components and entrapped drugs (calcein).

Within the same set of experiments, the cell monolayer was fixed onto the trans-well membrane using 10% formaldehyde. Subsequently, the cells were stained with Hoechst 33,258 (blue) and two sets of phalloidin dyes: Phalloidin Rhodamine 565 (red) and Phalloidin Alexa Fluor 488 (green) depending on the specific formulation used. After 30 min of incubation the cells were washed twice with buffer. Visualization of the prepared and stained specimen was performed using a Zeiss LSM 510 confocal laser scanning microscope (Carl Zeiss AG, Oberkochen, Germany). For every randomly chosen area a stack of approximately 20 images was captured, changing the focal height systematically and thus recording variations in the color intensities along the *z*-axis, covering a distance of about 10 µm. From these data, a 3D depth profile was created [32].

2.2.9. Lyophilization

Archaeosomes loaded with insulin were transformed into a solid dosage form. The lipid concentration was maintained at 7 mg/mL and the insulin concentration was about 3 mg/mL. The formulation was enriched with lactose at a final amount of 5% (*w*/*w*). Lactose served as a cryoprotectant during the drying process forming a matrix in which the archaeosomes are incorporated. Aliquots of 5 mL of archaeosomes were transferred into 50 mL lyophilization glass vials, which were then frozen overnight at −80 °C. The lyophilization step was carried out using the Benchtop 3L Sentry device (VirTis, Gardiner, NY, USA). The device operates under reduced pressure causing the sublimation of frozen water, leaving behind a dry powder containing the archaeosomes. The powder particles were then characterized using SEM. After the reconstitution of the dried particles in purified water SEM, PCS, native gel electrophoresis, and a BCA protein assay were performed.

2.2.10. Spray Drying

The same formulations as those for the lyophilization process along with 5% (*w*/*w*) lactose were employed for spray drying. The Büchi B-90 Nano Spray Dryer (BÜCHI Labortechnik AG, Flawil, Switzerland) was used. The drying parameters were kept constant at an inlet temperature of 120 °C and an air flow of 120 L/min, resulting in a pressure of 45 mbar(g). To enable a stationary state, the whole system was conditioned by spraying the pure solvent (i.e., water) before each sample run for a minimum of 20 min. This ensured a constant temperature of the spraying head of approximately 84 °C. The spray rate was set at 30%, generating a fine constant cone of spraying mist. Being dispersed in hot air, the droplets evaporated, leaving behind fine powdered particles that adhered to the cylindrical collecting electrode situated at the bottom of the device. The analysis of the powdered particles and rehydrated archaeosomes was performed in the same way as after the lyophilization process.

2.2.11. Statistical Analysis

Results presented are expressed as mean values ± standard deviation (SD). If not stated otherwise, n = 3. For statistical analysis of the data, a Student's *t*-test was performed, and differences were considered significant at levels of $p \leq 0.05$.

3. Results

3.1. Manufacturing and Physicochemical Characterization of Archaeosomes

Efficient production of archaeosomes, derived from diether and tetraether lipids isolated from *Sulfolobus acidocaldarius*, was achieved using microfluidic mixing methods after carefully adjusting the process parameters, including the total flow rate (TFR) and the flow rate ratio (FRR) between the aqueous and the organic phase. Constrained by the solubility of the archaeal lipids, the highest achievable lipid concentration was 20–21 mg/mL in both DMSO-iPA and absolute ethanol, which were used as organic phase. To establish the microfluidics mixing protocol we first varied the FRR of aqueous to organic phase from 2:1 to 5:1 and 10:1. For any of these conditions, TFR was varied from 1, 2, 5, 10, to 12 mL/min. Increasing the FRR in favor of water resulted in a decrease in particle size to 10–20 nm for a ratio of 10:1 aqueous to organic phase. These archaeosomes showed a low encapsulation efficiency and were unstable in solution regardless of the TFR. Thus, an FRR of 2:1 was used for the following experiments, again varying the TFR from 1 to 12 mL/min as described above. It was found that with increasing TFR the particle size decreases while the PDI value tends to increase. Using a TFR of 1 and 2 mL/min, the particle sizes were below 200 nm. Thus, to attain a particle size of about 100 nm the TFR was adjusted to 1.7 mL/min. The FRR was set and kept constant at 2:1 in favor of the aqueous phase, but still resulted in high amounts (about 30%) of organic solvents within the formulation. Immediate dialysis against HEPES buffer effectively reduced this solvent content. The size of the empty archaeosomes determined after dialysis by PCS was 85.4 ± 0.6 nm with a PDI value of 0.34 ± 0.02. The archaeosomes showed a highly negative zeta potential ($\zeta = -31.8 \pm 0.2$ mV), indicative of a pronounced physical particle stability. This premise was also supported by the long-term stability experiments, which were conducted over a period of 6 months. During storage at 4 °C the average size of the archaeosomes changed only slightly to 93.22 ± 2.7 nm, with a PDI of 0.42 ± 0.24, consistent with an unchanged transparency of the sample. A summary of all size data is provided in Table 1. It is important to note that for the stability assays, cellular uptake studies, and powder production, different batches of natural lipid extracts have been used, nevertheless, the process parameters remained the same. The data suggest that archaeosomes can be efficiently produced through microfluidics when employing optimized operational parameters [33]. Accordingly, using a continuous flow pump system in conjunction with an array of mixing channels would enable the continuous large-scale manufacturing of archaeosomes relevant for clinical applications [34,35]. The size data were affirmed by TEM measurements of negatively stained air-dried archaeosomes. The TEM images showed single particles in a proper size range around 100 nm (Figure 2a). By SAXS measurements, information on the internal structure, lamellarity, and lipid layer thickness of archaeosomes could be derived. The SAXS scattering profile (Figure 2b) showed the characteristics of an uncorrelated layer structure typical for unilamellar vesicles. Thus, the data were fitted to a unilamellar vesicle model by using a single bilayer electron density model. The thickness of the archaeal lipid bilayer was derived from the positions of the maxima in the electron density profile (Figure 2b, inset). Defined as lipid headgroup-to-headgroup distance an average value of ~4.5 nm was obtained for the membrane thickness of the archaeosomes. This value is in good agreement with published data, which revealed a thickness of the central hydrophobic part of 3.0 nm plus an outer hydrophilic shell thickness of ~1.5 nm for archaeal lipid layers [36]. Compared to liposomes composed of conventional phosphatidylcholines whose bilayer thickness is in the range of 3.0–4.1 nm depending on lipid composition, temperature, and salt content [37], archaeosomal membranes are substantially thicker.

Table 1. Overview of key experiments (stability assays, cellular uptake studies, powder production) with the respective archaeosome formulations used. All formulations were produced with the same process parameters, however, different batches of natural lipid extracts have been used. This might explain small deviations in size and polydispersity index (PDI) for identical formulations.

Organic Solvent	Loading	Mean Particle Size [nm]	PDI
Stability assays			
EtOH	-	85.4 ± 1.1	0.336 ± 0.017
DMSO-iPA (2:1 *v*/*v*)	-	86.3 ± 0.7	0.423 ± 0.140
DMSO-iPA (2:1 *v*/*v*)	calcein	111.6 ± 1.3	0.070 ± 0.002

Table 1. *Cont.*

Organic Solvent	Loading	Mean Particle Size [nm]	PDI
Cellular uptake studies			
DMSO-iPA (2:1 v/v)	calcein	129.6 ± 0.7	0.119 ± 0.013
DMSO-iPA (2:1 v/v)	calcein + DOPE-rhodamine	127.0 ± 0.2	0.107 ± 0.006
DMSO-iPA (2:1 v/v)	DOPE-rhodamine	137.7 ± 0.5	0.220 ± 0.050
Powder production			
EtOH	insulin	97.5 ± 1.7	0.285 ± 0.031
EtOH	insulin *	103.1 ± 1.2	0.348 ± 0.079
EtOH	insulin **	105.9 ± 2.1	0.324 ± 0.064

* Spray-dried insulin formulation, re-dissolved in water.** Freeze-dried insulin formulation, re-dissolved in water.

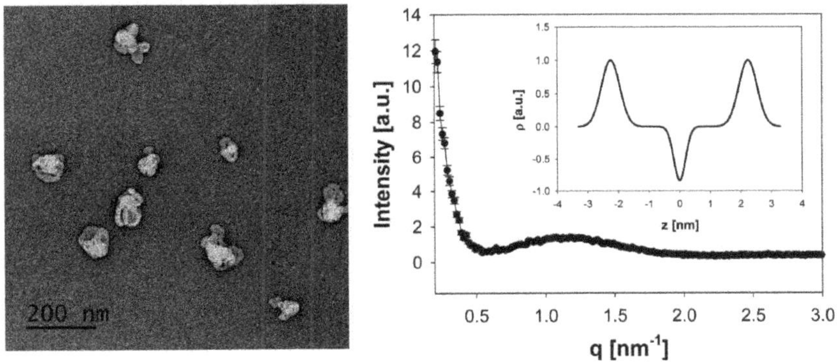

(a) (b)

Figure 2. (**a**) TEM image of negatively stained archaeosomes using 1% uranyl acetate. The image of the air-dried archaeosomes shows single particles with fairly uniform size distribution. The scale bar represents 200 nm. (**b**) Global fit of the SAXS pattern of archaeosomes indicating unilamellar structures. The inset gives the corresponding electron density profile, in which the distance between the two maxima of the Gaussian modeling of the electron dense headgroup regions gives a measure for the lipid layer thickness.

3.2. Archaeosome Stability in Simulated Intestinal Fluids and Drug Release Behavior

Stability, leakage, and in vitro release kinetics were probed using calcein as a model drug. The calcein molecules were incorporated into the archaeosomes directly during the manufacturing process. Calcein loading induced a noticeable modification of the particle size distribution, resulting in larger but highly uniformly sized particles with a very low PDI value (Table 1). One possible explanation for this effect could be the high calcein concentration, which increases the ionic strength of the solution, potentially enhancing the electrostatic repulsion between the single particles or even changing the curvature of the lipid bilayer. Notably, the particle size and homogeneity remained unchanged after dialysis and removal of the organic solvent and non-encapsulated calcein. To study the permeability of the lipid membrane and particle stability in different media, we monitored the fluorescence signal intensity of calcein. At the initial relatively high concentration of calcein encapsulated within the archaeosomes, the intrinsic fluorescent signal of calcein is self-quenched and the fluorescence intensity is low. Upon leakage and release of calcein from the archaeosomes to the surrounding aqueous environment, the fluorophore becomes diluted and the fluorescence intensity increases in a concentration-dependent manner. This behavior allowed us to follow the release profile of calcein under different environmental conditions. In particular, we investigated the release properties of archaeosomes in PBS buffer (pH 7.4), simulated intestinal fluid (SIF) (pH 6.8), and simulated gastric fluid (SGF) (pH 1.2), with and without the addition of the characteristic digestive enzymes pancreatin and pepsin, respectively. A modified protocol for the in vitro digestion of food in the gastric and intestinal phase, which recommends an incubation for 2 h at 37 °C, was applied [38]. As we did not see any release after 2 h, we repeated the whole experiment for 24 h but this time at 20 °C to follow particle stability over time rather than digestion. This approach allowed us to better understand the behavior of archaeosomes under different conditions and time scales. Across all samples, a minor release was observed within the first few hours, which was minimal for samples incubated at pH 7.4 in buffer and at pH 6.8 in SIF, regardless of the presence of pancreatin. At pH 1.2 the overall release rate was slightly higher but still remained below 3%, irrespective of the presence of pepsin. After a certain time, the release curves flattened out, indicating no further release of calcein from the particles (Figure 3). The very low release rate observed over 24 h demonstrated the high stability of the archaeosomes, even when exposed to extreme pH conditions. Just after chemical destruction of the lipid membrane with solubilizing detergents (addition of 10 µL, 10% Triton X-100) an immediate and rapid release of the payload could be induced, considered as 100% release. For oral drug delivery the elevated stability implies that the particles readily survive the harsh conditions of the stomach (simulated by SGF), however, the particles are equally stable in the intestinal environment (simulated by SIF). Additionally, degrading enzymes had no marked impact on the membrane stability of the archaeosomes as observed in vitro using a commercially available porcine pancreatin extract. This extract is commonly used and contains a mixture of proteases, amylases, and lipases with well-characterized enzyme activities. However, the phospholipase activity in the porcine pancreatin extract is four times lower than that found in human pancreatic juices, where degradation is more likely to occur [39]. Nevertheless, our data support the general consensus that archaeosomes are less susceptible to enzymatic digestion by lipases when compared to conventional liposomes composed of ester lipids [12,40].

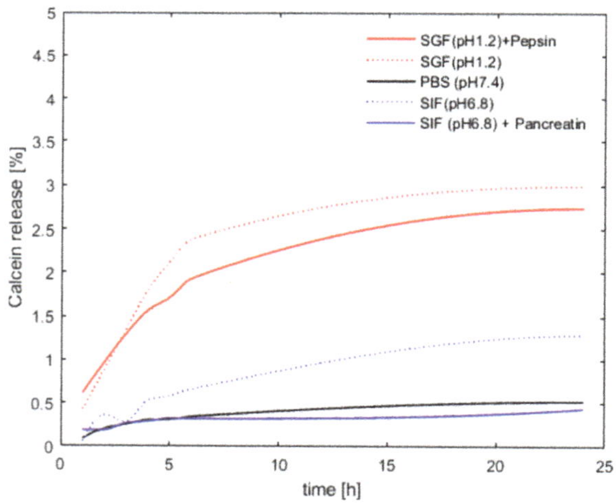

Figure 3. Archaeosome stability in different media. The presented values are given as percentages of released calcein compared to the maximum fluorescence signal obtained after detergent-induced membrane disruption (defined as 100% release).

3.3. In Vitro Release and Cellular Uptake Behavior

For the in vitro release and uptake studies a co-culture cell system mimicking the intestinal epithelium in combination with fluorescence spectroscopy and confocal laser scanning microscopy (CLSM) was used. For the fluorescent uptake assay, freshly prepared formulations were pipetted on an already confluent co-culture (Caco-2 and HT29MTX) cell layer within the trans-well system. After 4 h of incubation, resembling the duration of digestion, fluids were collected from both the apical and the basal compartment. Quantification of archaeosomes was made possible by the use of rhodamine-labeled lipids. The fluorescence intensities were measured at the beginning for all formulations which had been pipetted on the cells (insert) and after incubation from the apical and basal compartments. The intensity measured for the formulation initially placed in the trans-well system was defined as 100% of particles available for the interaction with the cell layer. The percentage from the apical compartment corresponded to the portion of recovered particles not interacting with the cells, while the percentage of particles in the basal compartment represented the amount that went through the cell layer and the polycarbonate membrane, corresponding to the archaeosomes that passed through the model membrane of the intestinal barrier. The portion of archaeosomes that were either attached to or taken up by the cells was calculated by subtracting the percentages in both apical and basal compartments from the initial total amount determined in the insert. The results (Table 2) revealed that approximately 27–29% of both calcein-loaded (TR_C) and empty (TR) archaeosomes were associated with the cells. The percentage of the archaeosomes found in the basal compartment was negligible. Taken together these findings suggest that intact archaeosomes cannot pass through the cell layer, but a substantial proportion (about 30%) of the archaeosomes is associated with the cells.

Table 2. Quantification of archaeosomes labeled with DOPE-Rhodamine after the in vitro uptake assay using fluorescence spectroscopy (Ex 560 nm/Em 597.5 nm; n = 3). TR (archaeosomes labeled with DOPE-Rhodamine); TR_C (archaeosomes labeled with DOPE-Rhodamine and loaded with calcein).

	Inserted	Apical	Basal	Cell Attached
TR [%]	100	72.982 ± 1.672	0.063 ± 0.007	~27
TR_C [%]	100	70.994 ± 13.036	0.065 ± 0.009	~29

To determine the in vitro release kinetics of encapsulated calcein, the same experimental setup was used as described above. After an incubation time of 4 h the fluids were collected in the apical and basal compartments and the concentration of calcein was determined before and after addition of Triton X-100 (10 µL of 10% (*v*/*v*) solution). The addition of detergent was required to quantitatively release calcein, thereby preventing signal quenching of calcein molecules entrapped within archaeosomes. Similar to the assay described above, the fluorescence intensity of the initially loaded calcein in the insert was defined as 100%. The percentages of calcein present in the apical and basal compartments were determined after collection by relating the measured fluorescence intensities to the initial fluorescence intensity. The results are presented in Table 3.

Table 3. Quantification of encapsulated and released calcein after the in vitro uptake assay using fluorescence spectroscopy (Ex 475 nm/Em 530 nm; n = 3). T_C (archaeosome loaded with calcein); TR_C (archaeosomes labeled with DOPE-Rhodamine and loaded with calcein).

		Inserted	Apical	Basal	Cell Attached
T_C	Calcein [%]	100	96.510 ± 0.382	0.418 ± 0.002	~3
TR_C	Calcein [%]	100	80.417 ± 0.385	0.443 ± 0.002	~19

The amount of calcein released from archaeosomes was relatively low, ranging from 1–3%. This finding is roughly consistent with the release behavior of calcein from archaeosomes incubated with simulated body fluids. However, when the formulations were additionally enriched with the fluorescently labeled lipid DOPE-Rhodamine, the release rate of encapsulated calcein increased to approximately 16–19%. These data suggest that the addition of conventional lipids, even at low concentrations, has an impact on the drug release properties of archaeosomes. Given that the DOPE phospholipid (0.003 mol%) was incorporated in the lipid membrane, it is tempting to speculate that the DOPE molecules, which contain two unsaturated fatty acid chains with cis double bonds that cause a kink in the hydrocarbon chain, introduce some disorder in the archaeal membrane. Defects in the lipid membrane could make it more permeable, thereby facilitating calcein release.

To study the localization of archaeosomes with respect to the cells more closely we employed confocal laser scanning microscopy (CLSM). Three different kinds of formulations containing differently colored fluorescent labels were prepared for double labeling of archaeosomes, alongside with blanks (PBS) and calcein solution serving as controls. The double labeling approach allowed the simultaneous visualization of calcein along with archaeosomes whose lipid membrane was labeled with a fluorescent DOPE lipid component. Focusing at varying depths along the z-axis allowed the visualization of distinct layers within the cell monolayer, as shown in Figure 4a–f. The cytoskeleton was stained with two phalloidin stains, either in red or in green, and served as control to provide information about the cell layer thickness. As seen (Figure 4a,b), the cells formed a continuous monolayer as described previously [30]. The differently colored cytoskeleton (green or red) enabled the distinction between the positions of archaeosomes (red) and calcein (green) in relation to the cytoskeleton. The blue color originated from the Hoechst stain bound to DNA, staining the nuclei of the cells. A free calcein solution was applied as control (Figure 4c). When calcein was loaded into archaeosomes, the green color was detected on top of the red stained layer of the cytoskeleton (Figure 4d) with very low penetration of calcein into the cell layer. Combining this information with the data from fluorescence spectroscopy (Table 3), it can be stated that the majority of the loaded calcein remained entrapped inside the archaeosomes. This finding is further confirmed by the co-localization (yellow) of archaeosomes (red) and calcein (green) as seen in Figure 4f. Here the cell membrane was not stained, but the nuclei seen in blue allowed an estimation of the spatial position of archaeosomes and calcein with respect to the cell membrane. When empty archaeosomes labeled with the fluorescent lipid DOPE-Rhodamine were used (Figure 4e), a co-localization (yellow) with the cytoskeleton is observed, indicating that the archaeosomes reach the upper part of the cells. These results align with the analytical data presented in Table 2, where almost 30% of the archaeosomes adhered to the cell membrane. The co-localization of red and green indicated that most calcein was still entrapped inside the archaeosomes, while empty archaeosomes after calcein release are visualized in red (Figure 4f). The results of the uptake images correlate nicely with data from fluorescence spectroscopy presented within Tables 2 and 3.

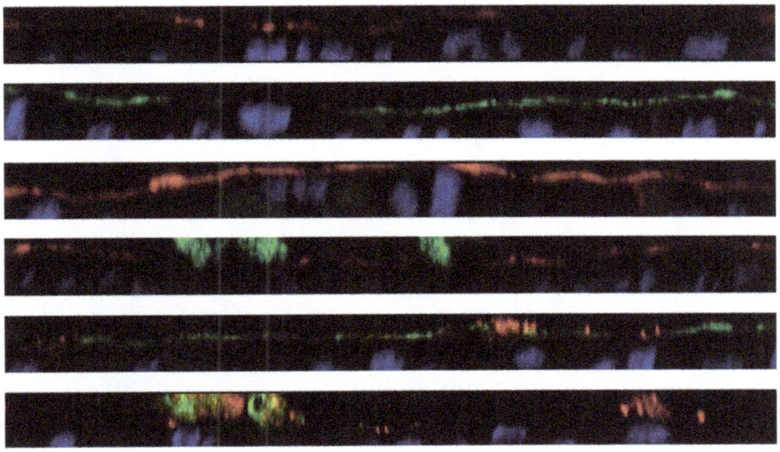

Figure 4. CLSM z-scans of co-culture (Caco-2/HT_29MTX of 7/3) cell layers incubated with different archaeosome formulations. (**a**,**b**) Blank samples incubated with pure buffer only. The cytoskeleton was labeled with phalloidin (either red or green), the nuclei were stained with Hoechst Blue. (**c**) Free calcein. (**d**) Calcein-loaded archaeosomes. The green stain detected on top of the red cytoskeleton layer implies that the calcein is found outside on top of the cell membrane with low penetration of calcein into the cell layer. (**e**) Co-localization (yellow) of red-labeled empty archaeosomes and the cell layer (in this case colored with a green phalloidin dye) indicates good adhesion of archaeosomes to the cell membrane. (**f**) shows the co-localization in yellow of calcein (green) still encapsulated within archaeosomes (red). In this case the cytoskeleton was not stained.

3.4. Dry Powder Formulations of Archaeosomes

To investigate the applicability of archaeosomes as dry powder formulations, both empty or insulin-loaded particles were either spray-dried or lyophilized in the presence of 5% lactose as cryoprotectant. The corresponding SEM images of the powdered formulations embedded in the sugar matrix are presented in Figure 5. The SEM images of the spray-dried archaeosomes showed differently sized single spherical particles (Figure 5a). Notably, when insulin was encapsulated in the spray-dried archaeosomes, the images revealed the presence of larger spherical particles exhibiting a distinctive crinkled pattern (Figure 5b). This unique appearance was not observed in the case of empty archaeosomes or those filled with calcein. Despite the observation of various spray-dried nanoparticles using lactose as sugar matrix, the underlying causes of the different morphologies observed for the spray-dried material remain unclear. One possible explanation for wrinkled surfaces may be attributed to temperature effects like rapid shrinkage of the powder during cooling [41]. Additionally, the interaction with the wall material has been suggested as another potential reason for diverse surface structures [42]. In contrast, the lyophilized powder showed a spongy bone-like structure that looked very fragile. The fragility was even more pronounced in the presence of insulin (Figure 5c,d). The dried powder formulations were not further processed except for rehydration with water. Figure 6 shows the SEM images of the rehydrated insulin-loaded archaeosomes, where individual particles of appropriate size are distinctly recognizable.

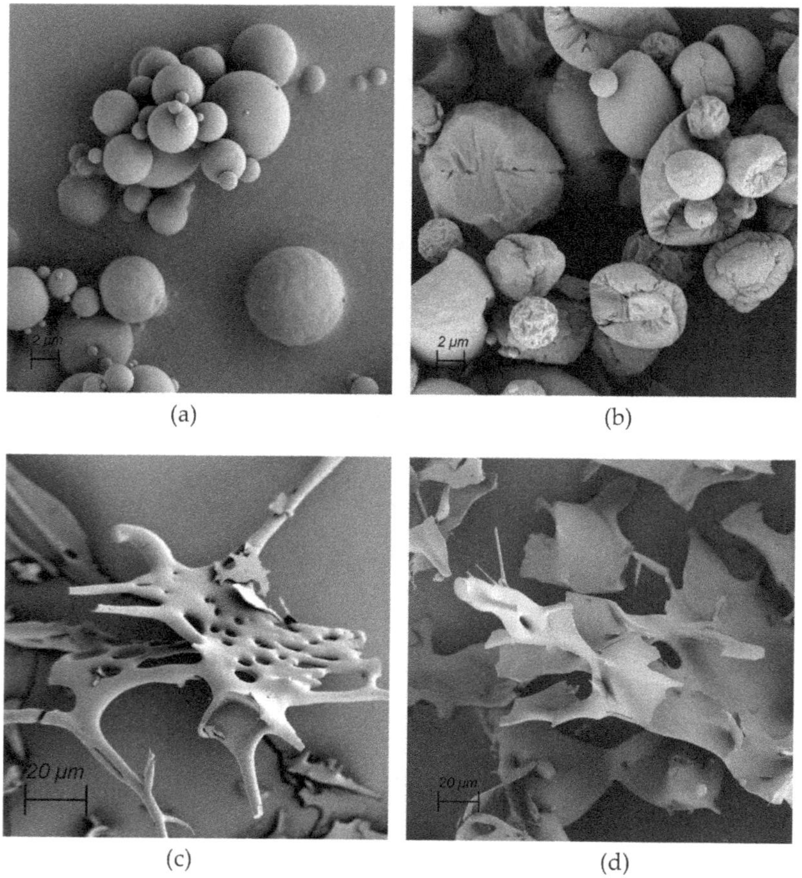

Figure 5. SEM images of dried powders. (**a**) Spray-dried empty archaeosomes. (**b**) Spray-dried archaeosomes loaded with insulin. (**c**) Lyophilized empty archaeosomes. (**d**) Lyophilized archaeosomes loaded with insulin.

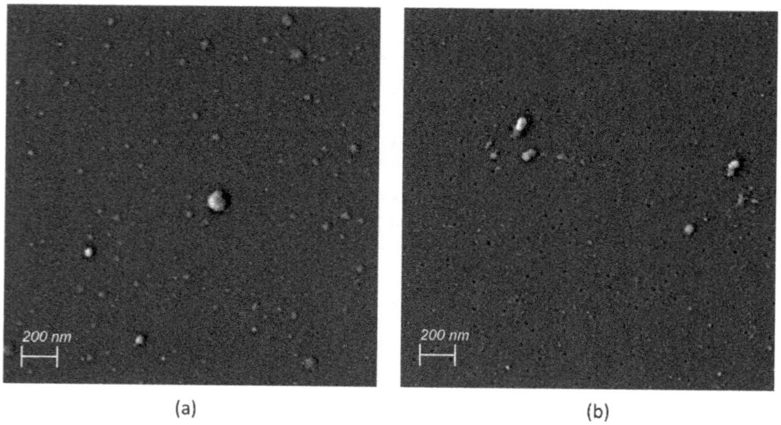

Figure 6. SEM images of redissolved insulin-loaded archaeosomes after spray drying (**a**) and lyophilization (**b**).

3.5. Insulin Loading for Dry Powder Formulations

Insulin was used as a model peptide drug and encapsulated into archaeosomes in the course of the microfluidics-assisted self-assembling process of archaeosomes. The insulin-loaded archaeosomes exhibited an average size of 97.5 nm and a PDI value of 0.285, comparable to empty ones. The samples were then lyophilized and spray dried as described above. The powder formulation was subsequently redissolved with pure water for size measurements. Both the mean particle size and the PDI values slightly increased after rehydration to 105.9 nm and 103.1 nm with PDI values of 0.348 and 0.324 for spray-dried (SD) and lyophilized (LYO) samples (Table 4). It is notable to mention that the archaeosomes have to endure extreme temperature ranges throughout these specific drying processes. For lyophilization, the sample needed to be frozen at −80 °C, while the spray-drying process was performed at elevated temperatures (inlet air 140 °C, head ~80 °C, bottom ~50 °C). Although the particles do not experience the maximum temperature due to the cooling effect of the evaporated solvent, the archaeosomes will experience heating in the laminar flow of the drying gas. Throughout both processes the archaeosomes have demonstrated exceptional stability across all temperature ranges, remaining largely unaffected by the conditions inherent in these processes at least in their size distribution.

Table 4. Mean particle size and polydispersity index (PDI) of insulin-loaded archaeosomes subsequent to preparation (T_ins), after spray drying (SD) and lyophilization (LYO), respectively (T_ins SD, T_ins LYO). Initial encapsulation efficiency % EE and overall recovery % after rehydration are shown (n = 3).

	Insulin	T_ins	T_ins SD *	TEL_ins LYO *
Mean particle size [nm]		97.5 ± 0.5	103.1 ± 1.2	105.9 ± 1.4
PDI		0.285 ± 0.003	0.348 ± 0.009	0.324 ± 0.004
Insulin [µg/mL]	10,261 ± 35	3631 ± 13	2045 ± 17	2120 ± 12
% EE		~35		
Overall recovery %			~20	~21

* Redissolved.

To determine the encapsulation efficiency (% EE) of insulin, the concentration of insulin was determined using the BCA protein assay. The % EE was calculated as

$$\% \text{ EE} = (c_{total}/c_{inc}) \times 100\% \quad (1)$$

where c_{total} is the initial amount of insulin used and c_{inc} is the insulin concentration found after microfluidics preparation and removal of unencapsulated insulin. To determine c_{inc} the archaeosomes were disrupted with Triton X-100 to quantitatively release the entrapped insulin. After preparation, about 35% of the initially used insulin was encapsulated (Table 4). After the drying and rehydration process, the overall recovery of insulin decreased by approximately one-third. It can be assumed that during drying procedures and handling of the powdered material a substantial amount of archaeosomes has been lost. As the protein assay cannot distinguish between archaeosomal entrapped insulin and released free insulin in solution, native gel electrophoresis was performed.

This method not only allowed us to distinguish between the localization of insulin (entrapped or free) but also exhibited a much higher sensitivity compared to conventional protein assays. As seen on the native gels (Figure 7), the insulin standard migrated a defined distance into the gel according to its molecular weight and charge (lane 2). For archaeosomes containing encapsulated insulin no discernible band of free insulin was visible (lane 3), unlike to archaeosomes that were disrupted with detergent prior to gel loading (lane 4), thus confirming successful loading. Comparable results were obtained for the redissolved powdered formulations, where no noticeable release of insulin was detected in the gel neither for the spray-dried (lane 5) nor for the lyophilized (lane 7) formulations. However, upon disruption of the archaeosomes by addition of detergent, a single band corresponding to insulin became evident (lanes 6 and 8) indicating the release of insulin. Notably, no indications of insulin oligomerization or aggregates became visible in the gel. This analysis confirms the successful encapsulation and retention of insulin within the archaeosome formulations throughout the drying processes.

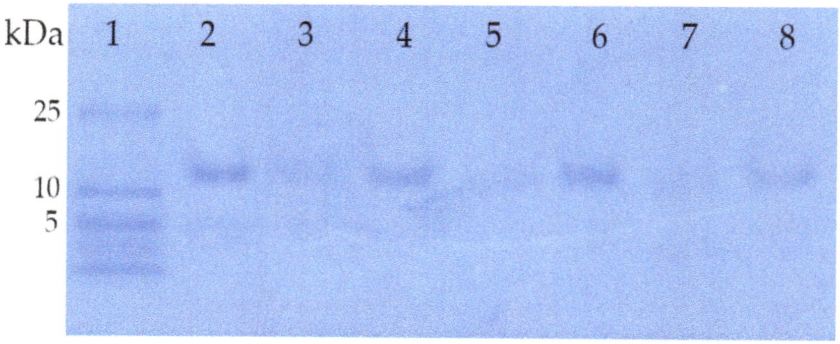

Figure 7. Acrylamide gradient native gel (4–12%) of insulin-loaded archaeosomes. Lane 1 presents the low-molecular-weight marker panel. Lane 2, reference insulin (1 µg) used for the encapsulation process. Lane 3, archaeosome formulation with encapsulated insulin directly after the preparation using microfluidics. The majority of insulin is encapsulated within the archaeosomes, resulting in minimal Coomassie blue staining. Only a faint band is visible due to a portion of non-encapsulated insulin. Lane 4 shows the same formulation mixed with Triton X-100, which disrupts the archaeosomes, leading to the release of encapsulated insulin. Thus, lane 4 corresponds to the amount of initially encapsulated insulin. Lanes 5 and 7 contain insulin-loaded archaeosomes after spray-drying and lyophilization processes, respectively. The powdered formulations were dissolved in water and loaded onto gel. The absence of insulin bands in lanes 5 and 7 suggests negligible insulin release during the drying processes. Lanes 6 and 8 display the same formulations after disruption with Triton X-100, confirming the presence of insulin inside the spray-dried and lyophilized archaeosomes, respectively.

The primary aim of creating powdered formulations was to confirm the stability of archaeosomes during the drying process without releasing their payload. Based on the promising findings we propose drug-loaded archaeosomes as good candidates for oral delivery in tablet form. Accordingly, the dry powders containing insulin-loaded archaeosomes and a lactose matrix as a filler could be transformed into an oral tablet by adding a binder or proceeding with dry granulation by applying pressure to form a pill. Considerations regarding the final dose to be delivered are challenging due to its dependency on various factors including the class of the active ingredient and individual patient-specific needs. In particular, for the delivery of insulin parameters like body weight, insulin sensitivity, and current blood glucose level have to be considered. In this context, a slow-release formulation could offer significant advantages by providing a sustained and constant supply of insulin over a certain time.

4. Discussion

Efficient production of archaeosomes, derived from diether and tetraether lipids isolated from *Sulfolobus acidocaldarius*, was achieved using a microfluidics-based mixing method [33,43]. While batch process synthesis remains the standard in the pharmaceutical industry, flow-based manufacturing processes have emerged over the past decade. With this simple self-assembling synthesis protocol, archaeosomes could be fabricated and loaded with drugs in a single step. This is an important prerequisite for the establishment of a continuous manufacturing process in compliance with good manufacturing practice (GMP) standards, which are a critical requirement for the pharmaceutical industry. Certain parameters must be considered when a microfluidics-assisted manufacturing process is used for the production and simultaneous loading of drugs in archaeosomes. These parameters are generally the same as those for the microfluidic production of liposomes [31]. They include the type and concentration of lipids, kind of organic solvent, and the physicochemical properties of the compounds to be encapsulated. Among these, the key factors influencing the manufacturing process and the characteristics of the final product are the total flow rate (TFR) and the flow rate ratio (FRR) between the aqueous and the organic phases. However, it is equally important to consider the relationship between those parameters, particularly assessing the compatibility between substances dissolved either in the organic or aqueous phase. Keeping in mind that the archaeosomes are intended for drug delivery, the primary objective was to keep the lipid concentration as high as possible to enhance the encapsulation efficiency while minimizing the concentration of the organic solvent within the formulation. The latter point was highly important as an exposure to high concentrations of organic solvents resulted in particle destabilization and aggregation. It is needless to stress that such conditions could also negatively impact the encapsulated compounds (e.g., causing protein aggregation or rapid drug release). Considering all these aspects, the values for TFR, FRR between aqueous and organic phase, lipid concentration, buffer system, and notably salt content were systematically adjusted. However, it has to be mentioned that depending on the individual batches of TEL, the choice of the organic solvent, and the loaded compounds, some variations in the particle size distribution and the PDI values were observed, as shown in Table 1. In this way, archaeosomes of tailored particle sizes exhibiting good encapsulation efficiencies were produced while maintaining remarkable stability over 6 months when stored at 4 °C. Using the hydrophilic model compound insulin, a successful encapsulation within the aqueous core of archaeosomes could be demonstrated in a continuous flow process. Encapsulation of hydrophilic compounds in the absence of any driving force that will stimulate loading efficiency leads to an even distribution of the active ingredient in the inner particle volume and the total liquid preparation volume. One strategy to increase encapsulation efficiency would be to increase the particle size, occupying more space within the same liquid volume. Another option would be to increase the particle concentration in the formulation. Increasing particle concentration necessitates higher lipid solubility within the organic phase, which could be achieved by an exchange of the organic phase. Consequently, improved solubility of tetraether lipids in the organic phase would allow employment of higher flow rate ratios in favor of the aqueous phase. This, in turn, would lead to a lower concentration of organic solvent and an increased concentration of archaeosomes in the final product. Taking all these considerations into account, the maximal solubility of the archaeosomal lipids in both ethanol and DMSO/propanol was limited to approximately 20–21 mg/mL. The optimal process parameters to obtain homogeneous archaeosomes of about 100 nm in size were TFR 1.7 mL/min with an FFR of 2:1 aqueous to organic phase. Despite thorough dialysis against the buffer, it was estimated that about 1–2% of organic solvent remained in the samples. For the experiments presented, this concentration was entirely acceptable. However, for continuous flow production of larger volumes, a tangential flow filtration system could be connected to remove the organic solvent quantitatively.

A detailed study on the stability of archaeosomes in different media has shown an ideal behavior in simulated gastric fluid, suggesting that archaeosomes can easily withstand the stomach content and safely transport the encapsulated drug to the intestine. The pronounced stability of archaeosomes was also retained in simulated intestinal fluid, even in the presence of phospholipases that typically degrade membranes [12]. Given that the target site of the archaeosomes is the small intestine, this finding poses a challenge when the drug is to be released on-site. To address this issue, one option would be to destabilize the structure of the lipid membrane by increasing membrane fluidity and permeability. This could either be achieved by direct modifications of the archaeal lipids, for example, by modifying their typical growth conditions [44] or by alterations of the lipid composition in the archaeosomes e.g., by addition of conventional unsaturated lipids or fatty acids, which are known to have destabilizing effects on membranes [45]. Indeed, even a slight change in the lipid bilayer composition by addition of conventional phospholipids (0.003 mol % DOPE) resulted in a higher drug release rate. Accordingly, most studies published so far use hybrid/mixed vesicular systems or conventional liposomes that are enriched with archaeal lipids for drug delivery [13,46,47].

To allow efficient uptake by intestinal epithelial cells, the archaeosomes need to have a certain size. If they are too large they cannot be taken up by cells and, even more importantly, the particles may not diffuse fast enough into the mucus layer [48]. While the archaeosomes synthesized in this study had an appropriate size, they did not cross the intestinal barrier after 4 h of exposure as evident in the in vitro uptake assay. This could be due to the presence of the mucus layer present in the Caco-2/HT29-MTX culture system. The mucus mesh has hydrophobic regions hampering the free passage of particles that have to penetrate the mucus layer at rates faster than mucus renewal and clearance, which is estimated to be 50–270 min [49,50]. Nevertheless, the archaeosomes revealed a remarkable affinity (about 30%) to the cell membrane. This enhanced adhesion affinity is expected to prolong the timeframe for retarded release of encapsulated drugs, facilitating the absorption through the intestine wall.

So far, first studies have indicated the potential utility of archaeosomes for oral drug delivery, showing corresponding in vivo results [12,13]. For example, an in vivo study using insulin-loaded hybrid archaeosomes composed of a mixture of archaeal lipids and synthetic phospholipids orally applied in diabetic mice revealed that insulin was retained significantly longer in the GI tract when stabilized by archaeosomes. Significant lower levels of blood glucose were found when compared to conventional liposomal formulations [14]. However, similar to our studies, the in vitro transport across Caco-2 cell monolayers was limited. The pronounced stability of archaeosomes is probably due to the unique structure of the lipids, the tight membrane organization, and the negatively charged surface of the archaeosomes [51,52]. These distinct structural characteristics apparently improve the stability of proteins, peptides, and water-insoluble compounds in the GI tract, whereas archaeosomes are not readily taken up in the intestine [15,53]. Parmentier et al. observed the presence of radiolabeled ether lipids in the inner organs of rats and subsequently in the urine after renal excretion following oral administration of liposomes containing specific mixtures of conventional phospholipids and ether lipids. From this, the authors proposed that the hybrid liposomes adsorb to enterocytes, enabling the drug to permeate into the bloodstream after being released, while only a negligible fraction of the hybrid liposomes were taken up [54]. In contrast, Morilla et al. detected a considerable amount of a radiolabeled substance with low intestinal permeability in the blood of rats after oral administration of archaeosomes composed exclusively of archaeols. The authors attributed this finding to the uptake of intact archaeosomes by M cells in Peyer's patches, while drug leakage occurs during transcytosis [55]. Within this context, various types of archaeosomes characterized by different molecular lipid compositions and structural features have been proposed as oral vaccines targeting M cells within Peyer's patches. There, archaeal glycerolipids act as strong adjuvants mediating T-cell immune responses [56,57]. These studies have demonstrated that an enhanced in vivo uptake of archaeosomes by M cells is linked to an increased surface hydrophobicity of the archaeosomes and larger particle sizes exceeding 400 nm [55]. However, the limited number of M cells in the intestine has hindered the effective targeting of M cells and subsequent antigen delivery into mucosa-associated lymphoid tissue. Hence, it is more likely that the archaeosomes interact with goblet cells and the mucus layer that covers the intestinal epithelium. To improve mucus penetration the hydrophobic and electrostatic interactions with the mucus layer may be reduced by modifying the surface properties of the archaeosomes. Another strategy to enhance mucus penetration and cellular uptake could be to modify the surface of archaeosomes with cell-specific targeting ligands. Cell surface binding might be an important step for subsequent internalization of the particles via various non-specific endocytosis pathways for intracellular drug release. Alternatively, upon mucus layer adhesion drug absorption could occur via an adsorption mechanism and/or through passive permeation of the released drug. Thus, the underlying intestinal uptake mechanisms of archaeosomes remain uncertain.

Notably, current literature has not reported any adverse side effects associated with orally administered archaeosomes. In fact, the in vivo studies rather emphasize the remarkable biocompatibility, low toxicity, and the good safety profile of archaeosome formulations [46]. These findings underline the high potential of archaeosomes as safe and effective delivery systems for various applications.

In this study, insulin, a small peptide hormone, was chosen as a model drug for various reasons. First of all, the number of diabetic patients depending on a constant exogenous supply of insulin is steadily increasing and diabetes has emerged as one of the most prevalent non-communicable diseases worldwide [58]. This makes insulin one of the most commonly used peptide therapeutics. Today, insulin is typically administered by subcutaneous injections, which are often associated with injection pain, patient discomfort, and local infections [59]. Consequently, extensive efforts have been made to explore non-invasive methods for insulin administration to improve patient compliance. Among these, the oral route is the most patient-friendly and convenient way for drug administration. However, challenges that impede effective oral delivery of insulin include rapid inactivation by proteolytic enzymes in the GIT and low epithelial permeability due to its large molecular weight, hydrophilicity, and negative net charge at neutral pH [60]. Moreover, the transport of insulin across the mucus layer, which functions as the initial diffusional and enzymatic barrier to intestinal uptake, is probably hindered by electrostatic repulsion due to the negatively charged mucus layer [61]. Thus, to improve intestinal uptake and bioavailability of insulin, various carrier systems have been developed to shield insulin from enzymatic degradation and enhance its intestinal transport [62]. So far, no ideal oral delivery system has been reported to transport insulin at an acceptable level to circulation. While oral delivery of insulin remains an unsolved issue, the field of oral peptide delivery is rapidly emerging as biological macromolecules gain increasing significance. In this regard, lipid-based delivery systems including archaeosomes offer a promising platform for improving the efficacy of therapeutic peptides [63]. Moreover, it is noteworthy to highlight that archaeosomes can serve as delivery vehicles not only for peptides but also for small molecules, oligonucleotides, proteins, or antibodies.

Here, it was shown that archaeosomes can be easily fabricated and loaded with insulin using microfluidics technology, enabling continuous flow large-scale production in the future. The encapsulation efficiency of insulin was satisfying and the archaeosomes could be lyophilized and spray dried without any detectable release of their payload. These findings underscore the pronounced resilience of insulin-loaded archaeosomes, making them a viable option for oral medication as tablets.

5. Conclusions

This study aimed to provide a better understanding of archaeosome-based drug delivery systems from their manufacturing process and physicochemical characterization to their interaction with the intestinal barrier and, finally, the development of a stable solid dosage form. While insulin serves as a model drug, archaeosomes will function as a versatile delivery system for a wide range of pharmaceuticals. However, adapting process parameters and conducting physicochemical tests remain necessary when encapsulating other pharmaceutical substances. Despite this requirement, the selected methodologies, specifically single-step microfluidics-assisted synthesis with constant drug loading alongside the production of dry powder formulations as presented in this paper, effectively address some challenges associated with the formulation and manufacturing process of peptide drugs for oral administration.

Author Contributions: Conceptualization, I.V., K.K., J.Q., O.S. and R.P.; Funding acquisition, O.S.; Methodology, I.V., D.F., J.K., E.F., G.L. and C.H.; Investigation, I.V., K.K., D.F., C.H. and J.Q.; Data acquisition and analysis, I.V., D.F. and C.H.; Project administration, R.P.; Resources, G.L., J.K. and E.F.; Visualization, I.V. and D.F.; Writing—original draft, I.V.; Writing—review and editing, I.V., K.K., D.F., C.H., J.Q., J.K., E.F., G.L., O.S. and R.P. All authors have read and agreed to the published version of the manuscript.

Funding: FFG Spin-off fellowship "NovoSome" Projektnummer: 874250.

Institutional Review Board Statement: Not applicable.

Informed Consent Statement: Not applicable.

Data Availability Statement: The original contributions presented in the study are included in the article, further inquiries can be directed to the corresponding author.

Acknowledgments: The authors would like to thank Markus Absenger-Novak, Robert Reimer, and Gerhard Ledinski for technical assistance and support in experimental work. The authors thank David Wurm from NovoArc GmbH, Vienna, Austria, for providing archaea lipid extracts.

Conflicts of Interest: The co-authors Christina Horn and Julian Quehenberger are currently employed by the company NovoArc GmbH, Vienna, Austria. The remaining authors declare that the research was conducted in the absence of any commercial or financial relationships that could be construed as a potential conflict of interest.

References

1. De Rosa, M.; Gambacorta, A.; Gliozzi, A. Structure, biosynthesis, and physicochemical properties of archaebacterial lipids. *Microbiol. Rev.* **1986**, *50*, 70–80. [CrossRef] [PubMed]
2. Charles-Orszag, A.; Lord, S.J.; Mullins, R.D. High-Temperature Live-Cell Imaging of Cytokinesis, Cell Motility, and Cell-Cell Interactions in the Thermoacidophilic Crenarchaeon *Sulfolobus acidocaldarius*. *Front. Microbiol.* **2021**, *12*, 707124. [CrossRef]
3. Quehenberger, J.; Shen, L.; Albers, S.V.; Siebers, B.; Spadiut, O. Sulfolobus—A Potential Key Organism in Future Biotechnology. *Front. Microbiol.* **2017**, *8*, 2474. [CrossRef]
4. Salvador-Castell, M.; Golub, M.; Erwin, N.; Deme, B.; Brooks, N.J.; Winter, R.; Peters, J.; Oger, P.M. Characterisation of a synthetic Archeal membrane reveals a possible new adaptation route to extreme conditions. *Commun. Biol.* **2021**, *4*, 653. [CrossRef] [PubMed]
5. Jacquemet, A.; Barbeau, J.; Lemiègre, L.; Benvegnu, T. Archaeal tetraether bipolar lipids: Structures, functions and applications. *Biochimie* **2009**, *91*, 711–717. [CrossRef] [PubMed]
6. Gulik, A.; Luzzati, V.; De Rosa, M.; Gambacorta, A. Structure and polymorphism of bipolar isopranyl ether lipids from archaebacteria. *J. Mol. Biol.* **1985**, *182*, 131–149. [CrossRef]
7. Chong, P.L.; Ravindra, R.; Khurana, M.; English, V.; Winter, R. Pressure perturbation and differential scanning calorimetric studies of bipolar tetraether liposomes derived from the thermoacidophilic archaeon *Sulfolobus acidocaldarius*. *Biophys. J.* **2005**, *89*, 1841–1849. [CrossRef]
8. Chong, P.L.; Sulc, M.; Winter, R. Compressibilities and volume fluctuations of archaeal tetraether liposomes. *Biophys. J.* **2010**, *99*, 3319–3326. [CrossRef]
9. De Rosa, M.; Gambacorta, A.; Nicolaus, B. A New type of cell membrane, in thermophilic archaebacteria, based on bipolar ether lipids. *J. Membr. Sci.* **1983**, *16*, 287–294. [CrossRef]
10. Chong, P.L. Archaebacterial bipolar tetraether lipids: Physico-chemical and membrane properties. *Chem. Phys. Lipids* **2010**, *163*, 253–265. [CrossRef]
11. Jeworrek, C.; Evers, F.; Erlkamp, M.; Grobelny, S.; Tolan, M.; Chong, P.L.; Winter, R. Structure and phase behavior of archaeal lipid monolayers. *Langmuir* **2011**, *27*, 13113–13121. [CrossRef]
12. Kaur, G.; Garg, T.; Rath, G.; Goyal, A.K. Archaeosomes: An excellent carrier for drug and cell delivery. *Drug Deliv.* **2016**, *23*, 2497–2512. [CrossRef]
13. Romero, E.L.; Morilla, M.J. Ether lipids from archaeas in nano-drug delivery and vaccination. *Int. J. Pharm.* **2023**, *634*, 122632. [CrossRef]
14. Li, Z.; Chen, J.; Sun, W.; Xu, Y. Investigation of archaeosomes as carriers for oral delivery of peptides. *Biochem. Biophys. Res. Commun.* **2010**, *394*, 412–417. [CrossRef]
15. Uhl, P.; Helm, F.; Hofhaus, G.; Brings, S.; Kaufman, C.; Leotta, K.; Urban, S.; Haberkorn, U.; Mier, W.; Fricker, G. A liposomal formulation for the oral application of the investigational hepatitis B drug Myrcludex B. *Eur. J. Pharm. Biopharm.* **2016**, *103*, 159–166. [CrossRef]
16. Uhl, P.; Pantze, S.; Storck, P.; Parmentier, J.; Witzigmann, D.; Hofhaus, G.; Huwyler, J.; Mier, W.; Fricker, G. Oral delivery of vancomycin by tetraether lipid liposomes. *Eur. J. Pharm. Sci.* **2017**, *108*, 111–118. [CrossRef]

17. Franzé, S.; Selmin, F.; Samaritani, E.; Minghetti, P.; Cilurzo, F. Lyophilization of Liposomal Formulations: Still Necessary, Still Challenging. *Pharmaceutics* **2018**, *10*, 139. [CrossRef]
18. Santonocito, D.; Sarpietro, M.G.; Castelli, F.; Lauro, M.R.; Torrisi, C.; Russo, S.; Puglia, C. Development of Solid Lipid Nanoparticles as Dry Powder: Characterization and Formulation Considerations. *Moleculea* **2023**, *28*, 1545. [CrossRef]
19. Quehenberger, J.; Pittenauer, E.; Allmaier, G.; Spadiut, O. The influence of the specific growth rate on the lipid composition of *Sulfolobus acidocaldarius*. *Extremophiles* **2020**, *24*, 413–420. [CrossRef] [PubMed]
20. Forbes, N.; Hussain, M.T.; Briuglia, M.L.; Edwards, D.P.; ter Horst, J.H.; Szita, N.; Perrie, Y. Rapid and scale-independent microfluidic manufacture of liposomes entrapping protein incorporating in-line purification and at-line size monitoring. *Int. J. Pharm.* **2019**, *556*, 68–81. [CrossRef] [PubMed]
21. Joshi, S.; Hussain, M.T.; Roces, C.B.; Anderluzzi, G.; Kastner, E.; Salmaso, S.; Kirby, D.J.; Perrie, Y. Microfluidics based manufacture of liposomes simultaneously entrapping hydrophilic and lipophilic drugs. *Int. J. Pharm.* **2016**, *514*, 160–168. [CrossRef] [PubMed]
22. Kastner, E.; Kaur, R.; Lowry, D.; Moghaddam, B.; Wilkinson, A.; Perrie, Y. High-throughput manufacturing of size-tuned liposomes by a new microfluidics method using enhanced statistical tools for characterization. *Int. J. Pharm.* **2014**, *477*, 361–368. [CrossRef]
23. Perrie, Y.; Kastner, E.; Khadke, S.; Roces, C.B.; Stone, P. Manufacturing Methods for Liposome Adjuvants. *Methods Mol. Biol.* **2017**, *1494*, 127–144. [CrossRef] [PubMed]
24. Oku, N.; Kendall, D.A.; MacDonald, R.C. A simple procedure for the determination of the trapped volume of liposomes. *Biochim. Biophys. Acta (BBA) Biomembr.* **1982**, *691*, 332–340. [CrossRef]
25. Gradauer, K.; Vonach, C.; Leitinger, G.; Kolb, D.; Frohlich, E.; Roblegg, E.; Bernkop-Schnurch, A.; Prassl, R. Chemical coupling of thiolated chitosan to preformed liposomes improves mucoadhesive properties. *Int. J. Nanomed.* **2012**, *7*, 2523–2534. [CrossRef]
26. Sleigh, S.H. Insulin preparations and analogues: Structure and properties. *J. Diabetes Nurs.* **1998**, *2*, 150.
27. Pabst, G.; Rappolt, M.; Amenitsch, H.; Laggner, P. Structural information from multilamellar liposomes at full hydration: Full q-range fitting with high quality x-ray data. *Phys. Rev. E. Stat. Phys. Plasmas. Fluids Relat. Interdiscip. Top.* **2000**, *62*, 4000–4009. [CrossRef] [PubMed]
28. Pabst, G.; Koschuch, R.; Pozo-Navas, B.; Rappolt, M.; Lohner, K.; Laggner, P. Structural analysis of weakly ordered membrane stacks. *J. Appl. Crystallogr.* **2003**, *63*, 1378–1388. [CrossRef]
29. Kornmueller, K.; Lehofer, B.; Leitinger, G.; Amenitsch, H.; Prassl, R. Peptide self-assembly into lamellar phases and the formation of lipid-peptide nanostructures. *Nano Res.* **2017**, *11*, 913–928. [CrossRef]
30. Schimpel, C.; Teubl, B.; Absenger, M.; Meindl, C.; Frohlich, E.; Leitinger, G.; Zimmer, A.; Roblegg, E. Development of an advanced intestinal in vitro triple culture permeability model to study transport of nanoparticles. *Mol. Pharm.* **2014**, *11*, 808–818. [CrossRef]
31. He, H.; Lu, Y.; Qi, J.; Zhu, Q.; Chen, Z.; Wu, W. Adapting liposomes for oral drug delivery. *Acta Pharm. Sin. B* **2019**, *9*, 36–48. [CrossRef]
32. Tetyczka, C.; Hartl, S.; Jeitler, R.; Absenger-Novak, M.; Meindl, C.; Froehlich, E.; Riedl, S.; Zweytick, D.; Roblegg, E. Cytokine-Mediated Inflammation in the Oral Cavity and Its Effect on Lipid Nanocarriers. *Nanomaterials* **2021**, *11*, 1330. [CrossRef] [PubMed]
33. Jia, Y.; Agbayani, G.; Chandan, V.; Iqbal, U.; Dudani, R.; Qian, H.; Jakubek, Z.; Chan, K.; Harrison, B.; Deschatelets, L.; et al. Evaluation of Adjuvant Activity and Bio-Distribution of Archaeosomes Prepared Using Microfluidic Technology. *Pharmaceutics* **2022**, *14*, 2291. [CrossRef] [PubMed]
34. Shepherd, S.J.; Warzecha, C.C.; Yadavali, S.; El-Mayta, R.; Alameh, M.-G.; Wang, L.; Weissman, D.; Wilson, J.M.; Issadore, D.; Mitchell, M.J. Scalable mRNA and siRNA Lipid Nanoparticle Production Using a Parallelized Microfluidic Device. *Nano Lett.* **2021**, *21*, 5671–5680. [CrossRef] [PubMed]
35. Piunti, C.; Cimetta, E. Microfluidic approaches for producing lipid-based nanoparticles for drug delivery applications. *Biophys. Rev.* **2023**, *4*, 031304. [CrossRef] [PubMed]
36. Polak, A.; Tarek, M.; Tomšič, M.; Valant, J.; Ulrih, N.P.; Jamnik, A.; Kramar, P.; Miklavčič, D. Structural properties of archaeal lipid bilayers: Small-angle X-ray scattering and molecular dynamics simulation study. *Langmuir* **2014**, *30 28*, 8308–8315. [CrossRef]
37. Balgavý, P.; Dubničková, M.; Kučerka, N.; Kiselev, M.A.; Yaradaikin, S.P.; Uhríková, D. Bilayer thickness and lipid interface area in unilamellar extruded 1,2-diacylphosphatidylcholine liposomes: A small-angle neutron scattering study. *Biochim. Biophys. Acta (BBA) Biomembr.* **2001**, *1512*, 40–52. [CrossRef]
38. Minekus, M.; Alminger, M.; Alvito, P.; Ballance, S.; Bohn, T.; Bourlieu, C.; Carrière, F.; Boutrou, R.; Corredig, M.; Dupont, D.; et al. A standardised static in vitro digestion method suitable for food—An international consensus. *Food Funct.* **2014**, *5*, 1113–1124. [CrossRef] [PubMed]
39. Salhi, A.; Amara, S.; Mansuelle, P.; Puppo, R.; Lebrun, R.; Gontero, B.; Aloulou, A.; Carrière, F. Characterization of all the lipolytic activities in pancreatin and comparison with porcine and human pancreatic juices. *Biochimie* **2020**, *169*, 106–120. [CrossRef]
40. Patel, G.B.; Sprott, G.D. Archaeobacterial ether lipid liposomes (archaeosomes) as novel vaccine and drug delivery systems. *Crit. Rev. Biotechnol.* **1999**, *19*, 317–357. [CrossRef]
41. Guldiken, B.; Linke, A.; Capanoglu, E.; Boyacioglu, D.; Kohlus, R.; Weiss, J.; Gibis, M. Formation and characterization of spray dried coated and uncoated liposomes with encapsulated black carrot extract. *J. Food Eng.* **2019**, *246*, 42–50. [CrossRef]
42. Sun-Waterhouse, D.; Wadhwa, S.S.; Waterhouse, G.I.N. Spray-Drying Microencapsulation of Polyphenol Bioactives: A Comparative Study Using Different Natural Fibre Polymers as Encapsulants. *Food Bioprocess. Technol.* **2013**, *6*, 2376–2388. [CrossRef]

43. Sedlmayr, V.; Horn, C.; Wurm, D.J.; Spadiut, O.; Quehenberger, J. Archaeosomes facilitate storage and oral delivery of cannabidiol. *Int. J. Pharm.* **2023**, *645*, 123434. [CrossRef] [PubMed]
44. Rastädter, K.; Wurm, D.J.; Spadiut, O.; Quehenberger, J. The Cell Membrane of Sulfolobus spp.-Homeoviscous Adaption and Biotechnological Applications. *Int. J. Mol. Sci.* **2020**, *21*, 3935. [CrossRef] [PubMed]
45. Bramkamp, M. Fluidity is the way to life: Lipid phase separation in bacterial membranes. *EMBO J.* **2022**, *41*, e110737. [CrossRef] [PubMed]
46. Santhosh, P.B.; Genova, J. Archaeosomes: New Generation of Liposomes Based on Archaeal Lipids for Drug Delivery and Biomedical Applications. *ACS Omega* **2023**, *8*, 1–9. [CrossRef] [PubMed]
47. Kejžar, J.; Osojnik Črnivec, I.G.; Poklar Ulrih, N. Advances in Physicochemical and Biochemical Characterization of Archaeosomes from Polar Lipids of Aeropyrum pernix K1 and Stability in Biological Systems. *ACS Omega* **2023**, *8*, 2861–2870. [CrossRef] [PubMed]
48. Lai, S.K.; Wang, Y.Y.; Hanes, J. Mucus-penetrating nanoparticles for drug and gene delivery to mucosal tissues. *Adv. Drug Deliv. Rev.* **2009**, *61*, 158–171. [CrossRef] [PubMed]
49. Fröhlich, E.; Roblegg, E. Mucus as barrier for drug delivery by nanoparticles. *J. Nanosci. Nanotechnol.* **2014**, *14*, 126–136. [CrossRef]
50. Lehr, C.-M.; Poelma, F.G.J.; Junginger, H.E.; Tukker, J.J. An estimate of turnover time of intestinal mucus gel layer in the rat in situ loop. *Int. J. Pharm.* **1991**, *70*, 235–240. [CrossRef]
51. Patel, G.B.; Agnew, B.J.; Deschatelets, L.; Fleming, L.P.; Sprott, G.D. In vitro assessment of archaeosome stability for developing oral delivery systems. *Int. J. Pharm.* **2000**, *194*, 39–49. [CrossRef] [PubMed]
52. Sprott, G.D. Structures of archaebacterial membrane lipids. *J. Bioenerg. Biomembr.* **1992**, *24*, 555–566. [CrossRef] [PubMed]
53. Parmentier, J.; Hofhaus, G.; Thomas, S.; Cuesta, L.C.; Gropp, F.; Schröder, R.; Hartmann, K.; Fricker, G. Improved Oral Bioavailability of Human Growth Hormone by a Combination of Liposomes Containing Bio-Enhancers and Tetraether Lipids and Omeprazole. *J. Pharm. Sci.* **2014**, *103*, 3985–3993. [CrossRef] [PubMed]
54. Parmentier, J.; Thewes, B.; Gropp, F.; Fricker, G. Oral peptide delivery by tetraether lipid liposomes. *Int. J. Pharm.* **2011**, *415*, 150–157. [CrossRef] [PubMed]
55. Morilla, M.J.; Gomez, D.M.; Cabral, P.; Cabrera, M.; Balter, H.; Tesoriero, M.V.; Higa, L.; Roncaglia, D.; Romero, E.L. M cells prefer archaeosomes: An in vitro/in vivo snapshot upon oral gavage in rats. *Curr. Drug Deliv.* **2011**, *8*, 320–329. [CrossRef] [PubMed]
56. Krishnan, L.; Dicaire, C.J.; Patel, G.B.; Sprott, G.D. Archaeosome vaccine adjuvants induce strong humoral, cell-mediated, and memory responses: Comparison to conventional liposomes and alum. *Infect. Immun.* **2000**, *68*, 54–63. [CrossRef] [PubMed]
57. Patel, G.B.; Zhou, H.; KuoLee, R.; Chen, W. Archaeosomes as adjuvants for combination vaccines. *J. Liposome Res.* **2004**, *14*, 191–202. [CrossRef] [PubMed]
58. Brayden, D.J. The Centenary of the Discovery of Insulin: An Update on the Quest for Oral Delivery. *Front. Drug Deliv.* **2021**, *1*, 726675. [CrossRef]
59. Gedawy, A.; Martinez, J.; Al-Salami, H.; Dass, C.R. Oral insulin delivery: Existing barriers and current counter-strategies. *J. Pharm. Pharmacol.* **2018**, *70*, 197–213. [CrossRef]
60. Drucker, D.J. Advances in oral peptide therapeutics. *Nat. Rev. Drug Discov.* **2020**, *19*, 277–289. [CrossRef]
61. Limenh, L.W. A review on oral novel delivery systems of insulin through the novel delivery system formulations: A review. *SAGE Open Med.* **2024**, *12*, 1–11. [CrossRef] [PubMed]
62. Pinelo, R.; Roque, L.; Reis, C.P. Oral insulin delivery: Utopia, currently possible or a near reality? *Ther. Deliv.* **2021**, *12*, 477–488. [CrossRef] [PubMed]
63. Haddadzadegan, S.; Dorkoosh, F.; Bernkop-Schnürch, A. Oral delivery of therapeutic peptides and proteins: Technology landscape of lipid-based nanocarriers. *Adv. Drug Deliv. Rev.* **2022**, *182*, 114097. [CrossRef] [PubMed]

pharmaceutics
MDPI

Article

Cryo-Milled β-Glucan Nanoparticles for Oral Drug Delivery

Guanyu Chen [1], Yi Liu [1], Darren Svirskis [2], Hongyu Li [3], Man Ying [4], Weiyue Lu [4,*] and Jingyuan Wen [2,*]

1 School of Pharmaceutical Sciences (Shenzhen), Shenzhen Campus of Sun Yat-sen University, Shenzhen 518107, China
2 School of Pharmacy, Faculty of Medical and Health Sciences, University of Auckland, 95 Park Road, Grafton, Auckland 1142, New Zealand
3 School of Medicine, University of Texas Health San Antonio & College of Pharmacy, University of Texas, Austin, TX 78759, USA
4 Department of Pharmaceutics, School of Pharmacy, Zhangjiang Campus of Fudan University, 826 Zhangheng Road, Pudong New Area, Shanghai 200433, China
* Correspondence: wylu@shmu.edu.cn (W.L.); j.wen@auckland.ac.nz (J.W.)

Abstract: Gemcitabine is a nucleoside analog effective against a number of cancers. However, it has an oral bioavailability of less than 10%, due to its high hydrophilicity and low permeability through the intestinal epithelium. Therefore, the aim of this project was to develop a novel nanoparticulate drug delivery system for the oral delivery of gemcitabine to improve its oral bioavailability. In this study, gemcitabine-loaded β-glucan NPs were fabricated using a film-casting method followed by a freezer-milling technique. As a result, the NPs showed a small particle size of 447.6 ± 14.2 nm, and a high drug entrapment efficiency of 64.3 ± 2.1%. By encapsulating gemcitabine into β-glucan NPs, a sustained drug release profile was obtained, and the anomalous diffusion release mechanism was analyzed, indicating that the drug release was governed by diffusion through the NP matrix as well as matrix erosion. The drug-loaded NPs had a greater ex vivo drug permeation through the porcine intestinal epithelial membrane compared to the plain drug solution. Cytotoxicity studies showed a safety profile of the β-glucan polymers, and the IC_{50s} of drug solution and drug-loaded β-glucan NPs were calculated as 228.8 ± 31.2 ng·mL^{-1} and 306.1 ± 46.3 ng·mL^{-1}, respectively. Additionally, the LD_{50} of BALB/c nude mice was determined as 204.17 mg/kg in the acute toxicity studies. Notably, pharmacokinetic studies showed that drug-loaded β-glucan NPs could achieve a 7.4-fold longer $T_{1/2}$ and a 5.1-fold increase in oral bioavailability compared with plain drug solution. Finally, in vivo pharmacodynamic studies showed the promising capability of gemcitabine-loaded β-glucan NPs to inhibit the 4T1 breast tumor growth, with a 3.04- and 1.74-fold reduction compared to the untreated control and drug solution groups, respectively. In conclusion, the presented freezer-milled β-glucan NP system is a suitable drug delivery method for the oral delivery of gemcitabine and demonstrates a promising potential platform for oral chemotherapy.

Keywords: β-glucan; cryo-mill; cryogenic; nanoparticle; sustained release

1. Introduction

Cancer is still one of the major causes of death, and its incidence is continuously increasing. Most anticancer drugs are generally administered through intravenous (*i.v.*) injection or infusions, and this often causes the administered drug to exceed the maximum tolerable concentration, which leads to serious side effects and subsequent fast excretion from the circulation system, resulting in low oral drug bioavailability [1].

Among all the drug administration routes, the oral route is the most preferred for most drug delivery due to greater patient compliance, lower production costs, and higher therapeutic efficacy [2,3]. Oral chemotherapy is usually designed with a sustained drug release form and thus is able to maintain a moderate plasma drug concentration over a period of time to achieve a prolonged exposure of tumors to the drug as well as to avoid a drug dose over the maximum tolerable dosage, resulting in much higher drug efficacy without side effects [4]. However, a large number of orally administered anticancer/cytosine drugs have difficulties entering the systemic circulation due to the poor solubility, permeability, and stability of the drugs. In addition, other associated challenges include hepatic first-pass metabolism, intestinal enzymatic degradation, and P-glycoprotein (P-gp) efflux [5].

Polymeric nanoparticles (NPs) with a small particle size of less than 1 μm have raised interest as a drug carrier system for a wide range of drug candidates. It offers advantages over other colloidal carriers in terms of greater drug stability in the gastrointestinal (G.I.) tract and greater ability to minimize its intestinal enzymatic degradation and P-gp efflux in general [6,7]. It has the potential to improve drug permeability, with its sustained drug release manner, resulting in higher oral drug bioavailability, thus promoting the therapeutic effect [8,9]. In addition, NPs have a smaller particle size than microparticles, which allows for enhanced extravasation into tumor sites by the enhanced permeability and retention (EPR) effect [10].

β-Glucans are linear, unbranched polysaccharides containing monomeric β-D-glucopyranosyl residues with linkages of (1-3)-O-linked-β-D-glucopyranosyl units and (1-4)-O-linked β-D-glucopyranosyl units [11]. They have attracted scientists' attention and have been utilized to fabricate oral pharmaceutical formulations since formulations using β-glucans can ensure (1) the prolonged release of the drug candidate; (2) great protection from hydrolytic and enzymatic degradation, thus resulting in longer drug half-life; and (3) the stimulation of the immune response, which is beneficial for some immune-related drugs [12]. Cyclodextrins have been recently receiving growing attention since they have complex-forming ability with drug candidates and are able to enhance the solubility of hardly soluble drugs. However, the rigid structure and poor water solubility of cyclodextrins limit their further application. Compared with cyclodextrins, the advantages of β-glucans over cyclodextrins mainly involve their higher water solubility; additionally, β-glucans also exhibit high viscosities at very low concentrations (1%) and are stable with a wide range of pH levels [13]. Peter et al. reported that the oral delivery of β-glucan was bound by intestinal epithelial and gut-associated lymphoid tissue (GALT) cells and pointed to the promotion of the systemic levels of the drug candidate [14]. Huong et al. encapsulated curcumin into β-glucan NPs (Cur–Glu) and found them to be much more soluble in water not only compared with free curcumin but also compared with other biodegradable polymer-encapsulated curcumin NPs [15].

Milling is a common mechanical process to reduce the particle size of NPs, and it has been frequently used in the pharmaceutical industry [16]. However, the high levels of mechanical energy used during milling may cause particle fracture and changes in crystal structure of drugs, including polymorphic transformations, as well as localized heating, which may result in drug degradation [17]. In contrast, cryo-milling is a high-energy milling process operated at a very low temperature using cryogenic media such as liquid nitrogen [18]. This method represents an effective technique for reducing the risk of the recrystallization of the amorphous material due to reduced heat production compared to conventional continuous milling. Freezer mills consist of a compartment containing liquid nitrogen (−195.5 °C) that cools down the entire internal assembly, which consists a polycarbonate tube containing the sample and a steel impactor for milling the sample. The sample is embrittled with liquid nitrogen and then milled with the steel impactor, which is magnetically driven back and forth against the stationary end plugs. According to the machine specification, the procedure includes precooling, milling, and cooling in between each cycle, and the impact rate can be adjusted. In this study, the optimal milling settings of the program were investigated. The advantage of this technique is its low cost, easy fabrication, and great availability for scale-up production.

Gemcitabine (2′, 2′difluorodeoxycytidine), is a well-known anticancer drug that is currently in clinical use for the treatment of several types of cancers. Unfortunately, it is rapidly metabolized with a short plasma half-life of 8–17 min via intravenous infusion [19], and its cytostatic action is strongly exposure-time-dependent. It is rapidly deaminated by cytidine deaminase in the blood, kidney, and liver [20]. Thus, in order to maintain a required plasma concentration over a sufficient period, repeated administration of relatively high doses is required. However, this will lead to severe systemic toxicity [21].

To date, there has been no oral formulation of gemcitabine in the market. Additionally, this is the first time to report this novel health-beneficial carrier system for oral gemcitabine delivery. β-Glucan is a well-known nutrient that is beneficial for gastrointestinal health as well as the overall immune system. Therefore, this is an environmentally friendly oral delivery system and a promising oral drug carrier as well as a nutrient beneficial for human health. Secondly, the freezer-milled technique is of benefit to pharmaceutical researchers, since it has significant advantages such as ease in processing capable of scale-up and low cost, thus demonstrating its great potential in future applications involving the development of nanomedicines [22].

2. Materials and Methods

2.1. Materials

Gemcitabine hydrochloride, MW 299.66, β-glucan, (hydroxypropyl)methyl cellulose (HPMC), ethylcellulose (with 48% ethoxy content) (EC), acetic acid, 3-(4, 5-dimethyl-thiazol-2-yl)-2, and 5-diphenyl tetrazolium bromide (MTT) were purchased from Sigma-Aldrich (St. Louise, MO, USA). Methylcellulose LR was purchased from Chem-Supply (Gillman, South Australia). Chitosan (MW 150,000, DD 70%), was purchased from Comwin Fine Chemicals Co. (Changzhou, China). Methylcellulose (MC) was purchased from ICN Biomedical, Inc. (Santa Ana, CA, USA). Polypropylene glycol was purchased from Midwest Pharmaceutics (Hawke's Bay, New Zealand). Dimethyl sulfoxide (DMSO) was purchased from Labpartner (Shanghai, China). The 4T1breast cancer cell line was purchased from the American Type Culture Collection (ATCC; Rockville, MD, USA). The Roswell Park Memorial Institute (RPMI) medium 1640 basic was purchased from Gibco (Grand Island, NE, USA), and fetal calf serum was purchased from Hyclone (Logan, UT, USA). Penicillin–streptomycin–glutamine and nonessential amino acids were purchased from Life Technology (Grand Island, NY, USA). All other chemicals used were of reagent grade. Milli-Q water was obtained through reverse osmosis using a Millipak® system (Millipore, Burlington, MA, USA, 0.22 μm).

2.2. Methods

The selected polymers and gemcitabine were mixed with various concentrations, and the films were developed using the conventional casting method [23]. Briefly, 15 mL of different concentrations of water-soluble mucoadhesive polymers (MC, HPMC, EC, β-glucan, and chitosan) were individually mixed with gemcitabine (0.5% *w*/*v*), and 5 mL of 5% *v*/*v* polypropylene glycol was added as a plasticizer. The solution was mixed well and the resulting gel-like solution was then cast on a Petri dish and dried in an oven at 37 °C for 48 h. Once the films had formed, they were trimmed into small pieces and loaded into the milling vials containing an impactor. Subsequently, an intensive milling process was carried out via a freezer mill (6970EFM Freezer/Mill®, Metuchen, NJ, USA) with optimized settings to generate pulverized drug-loaded NPs. The optimal formulation was selected from characterization and carried out for cellular uptake and transport studies, in vivo pharmacokinetic studies, and pharmacodynamic studies.

3. Characterization

3.1. Optimization of Polymeric Films and Freezer Mill Process Settings

MC, HPMC, EC, β-glucan, and chitosan were selected for forming the polymeric films. The first step of this process involved finding suitable polymers to form the films using the casting method. Meanwhile, suitable concentrations of the polymers to produce the films with the ideal physical appearance and stability were investigated. The optimal films were selected to carry out the milling process. Different settings of precooling time, milling period, operating cycles, and impact rate were trialed. The optimal setting was predicted from the resultant NPs with the optimal physical appearance and relatively smaller particle size.

3.2. Particle Size, Zeta Potential, Surface Morphology, and Entrapment Efficiency

The particle size, Polydispersity Index (PDI), and zeta potential of the cyro-milled NPs were determined using a Malvern Zetasizer Nano-ZS (Malvern Instruments Ltd., Malvern, UK). The surface morphology of the NPs was observed by using scanning electron microscopy (SEM, Phillips XL305 Field Emission Gun, Eindhoven, The Netherlands). The obtained NPs in powder form were sputter-coated with a thin layer of platinum on the surface, and images were captured using SEM. The drug entrapment efficiency (EE) was determined using a reverse-phase high-performance liquid chromatography (HPLC) method indirectly [24]. A GraceSmart C18 column (250 × 4.6 mm, 5 μm; GraceSmart, India) was used, in which acetonitrile and 1.38% *w*/*v* pH 6.5 sodium dihydrogen phosphate buffer at the volume ratio of 7:93 were added in the mobile phase, and the parameters were set as 1 mL/min flow rate and 270 nm UV detection [25].

3.3. In Vitro Drug Release Studies

The in vitro release of gemcitabine from NPs was studied using a Franz diffusion apparatus (FDC-6, Logan, NJ, USA). The gemcitabine solution (1% *w*/*v*) and an equivalent amount of the drug comprising gemcitabine-loaded NP samples were added to the donor chamber, with a cellulose membrane (MW 12,000, Membra-Cel®, Viskase, Loudon, TN, USA) sandwiched between the donor and receptor chambers, maintaining the sink condition. PBS with pH 7.4 was used as the medium, and the temperature was kept at 37 ± 1 °C. Then, aliquots of 500 μL each were withdrawn at various time intervals, and 500 μL of fresh PBS was replaced. The release drug amount over time was determined with HPLC.

The release kinetics were evaluated using four different models, namely zero order, first order, Higuchi equation, and Korsmeyer–Peppas equation, to characterize the mechanism of drug release from the NPs. For the different models, the obtained data were plotted in the following manner: the zero-order model as the cumulative percentage of drug release versus time, the first-order model as the log cumulative percentage of drug remaining versus time, Higuchi's model as the cumulative percentage of drug released versus square root of time, and the Korsmeyer–Peppas model as log the cumulative percentage of drug released versus log time.

3.4. Ex Vivo Permeation Studies

The ex vivo permeation study of gemcitabine-loaded NPs was also conducted using Franz diffusion cells with the same method as that used in the drug release study. Here, the cellulose membrane was replaced with the porcine intestinal epithelial membrane. Porcine mucosal tissue was previously soaked in pH 7.4 PBS overnight. After the accumulative drug amount was determined using HPLC, the apparent permeation coefficient (P_{app}) was calculated. P_{app} is the rate at which a drug will permeate over the intestinal wall and enter the portal circulation [26], and it is calculated using Equation (1):

$$P_{app} = \frac{dXr}{dt} \times \frac{1}{A \cdot Co} \quad (1)$$

where Xr is the cumulative drug amount (μg), A is the area of the permeation membrane (cm^2), C_0 is the initial concentration in the donor compartment (μg/mL), and dX_r/dt is the flux, which is the gradient of the best-fit line when the cumulative amount of drug permeated over time [27].

3.5. Cell Culture and Cytotoxicity Studies

Briefly, 4T1, a breast cancer cell line derived from a BALB/c mammary tumor, was cultured in an RPMI medium 1640 basic containing 10% fetal calf serum, 1% penicillin–

streptomycin–glutamine, and 1% nonessential amino acids. The cells were cultured as a monolayer at 37 °C in a 98% humidified atmosphere containing 5% CO_2.

The cytotoxicity of the NP materials was evaluated using an MTT assay. The cells were cultured on 96-well microtiter plates (0.1 mL, containing approximately 5×10^3 cells/well) for 24 h at 37 °C to allow cell attachment to the plates. Briefly, 100 µL of the drug solution and drug-loaded NPs with various concentrations (established via serial dilution) were added to the growth medium and incubated for another 72 h under the same conditions. To evaluate cell survival, 20 µL of the 5 mg/mL MTT solution was added to each well and incubated for 4 h. Subsequently, the MTT solution was withdrawn, and 200 µL of dimethyl sulfoxide (DMSO) was added to dissolve formazan crystals; then, the absorbance was measured with a microtiter plate reader (SpectraMax® Plus, Molecular Devices, San Jose, CA, USA) at 596 nm. The percentage cell viability was calculated using the absorbance test, and the values of treated cells were compared with the control (untreated cells) and expressed in percentage. The IC_{50} was then determined from the cell viability profile [28].

3.6. In Vivo Pharmacokinetic Studies Using Sprague Dawley Rats

Male Sprague Dawley (SD) rats (200 ± 20 g) were purchased from the BK Lab Animal, Ltd. (Shanghai, China) and housed at a temperature of 25 ± 1 °C and humidity of 50 ± 10% with free access to food and water. Three groups of SD rats (n = 6) were subjected to a single dose for oral bioavailability tests. The first group was intravenously injected with the gemcitabine solution at a dose of 80 mg/kg. The second group was administered the gemcitabine solution by oral gavage, while the third group received the drug-loaded NPs orally at the same dose [29]. Blood samples were drawn via retro-orbital venous plexus puncture with the aid of capillary tubes at predetermined intervals post-oral dose. The blood samples were collected in heparinized Eppendorf tubes, which were rinsed using 20 µm of tetrahydrouridine and then centrifuged at 42,018× *g* for 5 min; the plasma was then stored at −70 °C until analysis. An organic solvent was needed to extract gemcitabine from the plasma; to prepare the solvent, 1 mL of acetonitrile was added, vortexed for 1 min, and centrifuged at 101,890× *g* for 15 min. The supernatant was filtered and determined using HPLC. Prior to the animal studies, ethical approval was obtained by the Ethics Committee of Fudan University (Approval Number 04-YJ-LWY-01).

3.7. In Vivo Acute Toxicity Studies

BALB/c nude mice were used for in vivo pharmacodynamic studies. In order to determine a suitable oral drug dose in this model, the LD_{50} had to be determined, as no data were available in the literature. Acute toxicity studies were conducted under ethics approval 04-YJ-LWY-01. Male BALB/c nude mice weighing 23 ± 2 g were purchased from BK Lab Animal, Ltd. (Shanghai, China) and housed in the same conditions as the SD rats. Five different doses of 60, 120, 240, 480, and 960 mg/kg were administered via oral gavage to each group (n = 10). Their motion behaviors were observed, weight loss and the number of deaths were recorded over 10 days, and the LD_{50} of BALB/c nude mice was determined [30].

3.8. In Vivo Pharmacodynamic Studies Using BALB/c Nude Mice

Three groups of BALB/c nude mice (n = 6) were used for in vivo pharmacodynamic studies. Prior to the study, 4T1 tumor cells were cultured at the same mentioned condition, and then the cells were collected and injected subcutaneously into the prep axillary (armpit) area of each mouse. Until the solid tumors were developed, the first group was orally administrated a saline solution, while the second and the third group were orally administrated the gemcitabine solution and gemcitabine-loaded NPs, respectively, at a dose of 30 mg/kg on days 0, 2, and 4. Tumor size and body weight were measured every 2 days throughout the study. The study was terminated after 12 days; the mice were euthanized, and the tumors were harvested.

3.9. Statistical Analysis

Statistical data analysis was performed using the Microsoft Excel 2020 software (Redmond, WA, USA). Data comparisons were conducted using regression analysis and two-tailed *t*-tests. A *p*-value of $\leq$0.05 was considered statistically significant.

4. Results and Discussion

4.1. Optimization of Polymeric Films, and Freezer Mill Settings

Polymeric films were formed with different polymer concentrations of 2%, 4%, 6%, and 8% *w*/*v*. As a result, the optimal films of MC, HPMC, and chitosan were more likely formed at lower concentrations, while EC and β-glucan with higher polymer concentrations formed more physically stable films. The water-soluble polymers MC, HPMC, β-glucan, and chitosan have high water absorbing and swelling properties; thus, they easily produce more viscous and gel-like forms, which allows for faster and better casting of the films [31,32]. Chitosan, β-glucan, and EC films generated fine and pulverized nanoparticulate powder after milling. However, for MC and HPMC formulations, the films were brittle and difficult to remove from the Petri dishes. This brittleness of MC and HPMC films is caused by their high intermolecular bonds between polymer chains [33]. Therefore, a small amount of polyethylene glycol (2% *w*/*v*) was added as a plasticizer. Plasticizer facilitates ease in film removal by reducing intermolecular interactions between these chains. The reduced inter-chain interaction also increases chain mobility and chain flexibility [31,33]. In contrast, the particles generated from the HPMC films did not produce pulverized powders as the HPMC NPs removed from the milling tubes were slightly moist and easily aggregated. This could be due to the high moisture retention properties of HPMC. HPMC films are known to have a poor water vapor barrier, which prevents water loss [34]. Due to clumping, characterization tests were not performed with HPMC NPs. The NPs generated from the other polymers were used in the next stage of characterization studies.

Although a previous study reported that extended milling times, normally over 10 min, resulted in progressively larger particle size, this study was performed using ball milling at room temperature. Physical milling is a high-energy process that may generate excess heat and can therefore cause alterations to the surface of the particles forming amorphous particle morphology. These areas are more likely to recrystallize, which may result in particle–particle fusion, thus increasing the particle size [35]. However, as our freezer mill operated at cryogenic temperatures, the effects of the high energy processes associated with milling may be less pronounced, thus leading to less particle aggregation. The optimal freezer mill settings were predicted based on the evaluation of the particles' physical appearance and their particle size. The settings were 20 min precooling time, five operating cycles, and 10 min running/milling time with 14 CPS impact rate, followed by 5 min cooling time prior to the next milling cycle.

4.2. Particle Size, Zeta Potential, Surface Morphology, and Entrapment Efficiency

A smaller particle size is more desirable, as there is a greater surface area of the NPs to adhere to the lining of the gut for drug absorption. Generally, there are three absorption mechanisms for NPs to permeate over the GI epithelial membrane [5]. Firstly, very small-sized particles of less than 50 nm often permeate the epithelial cells through tight junctions via the paracellular route. Particles of less than 500 nm are small enough to undergo endocytosis as a result of intestinal enterocytes lining the GI tract; the smaller the particles, the more efficient for the particles to undergo uptake through this route [5,36]. Particles less than 5 μm can be absorbed by the intestinal microfold cells of Peyer's patches through the lymphatic system [37]. According to the results, β-glucan and EC NPs showed relatively smaller particle sizes of 447.6 ± 14.2 and 472.6 ± 21.7, respectively. Considering these sizes, it can be deduced that they are absorbed via the endocytosis pathway.

Zeta potential is a measure of the magnitude of charge repulsion or attraction between particles, which is closely related to particle stability [38]. Good stability is important in preventing the aggregation of particles. In addition, zeta potential is an important parameter for investigating the interactive binding of NPs with the intestinal mucosal layer for absorption. NPs with zeta potential values of greater than +15 mV or less than −15 mV are considered to be stable, as they will repel each other and reduce the extent of aggregation [39]. The zeta potential results of the formulations are shown in Table 1. Although β-glucan is a cationic polymer, the zeta potential of the β-glucan NPs was −1.2 ± 0.5 mV. At low pH, it has a positive zeta potential, whereas at neutral or high pH, the zeta potential becomes negative. Since gemcitabine is negatively charged, it may have contributed to the negative zeta potential due to the adsorption of gemcitabine to the outer surface of the β-glucan NPs [40]. EC and MC NPs both exhibited negative zeta potentials, and EC NPs showed a desirable zeta potential of −20.1 mV. In contrast, chitosan NPs showed a positive surface charge. Through visual observation, some aggregation of β-glucan nanoparticles was observed, especially when resuspended in water. This was because the zeta potential results did not fall in the ideal range. This is one of the limitations that should be considered in future studies.

In the EE study, β-glucan showed the highest drug EE of 64.3 ± 2.1%, while EC had the lowest EE of 56.3 ± 1.8%. The reasons for the differences in drug EE between these formulations may be related to different interactions and the levels of these interactions between gemcitabine and the polymer chains [37]. The EE of NPs prepared using traditional methods such as solvent evaporation or solvent displacement is influenced by various factors such as the concentration of the polymer and emulsifier, drug-to-polymer ratio, and chemical interaction between the drug and polymers [37]. In contrast, the film casting method followed by cryogenic milling results in much higher EE than traditional methods, as the drug is fully dissolved into the polymer solution, and after the films are formed, it is directly ground into NPs. Thus, the drug is assumed to be greatly encapsulated due to being chemically bound to the polymer chains or physically embedded within the polymeric network of the particles.

Based on the results, β-glucan NPs were selected as the optimal formulation for further studies since they had relatively a smaller particle size, more promising zeta potential, and higher EE. As shown in the SEM images (Figure 1), β-glucan NPs have rough surfaces and irregular shapes; this is expected for particles fabricated using the freezer-milling method.

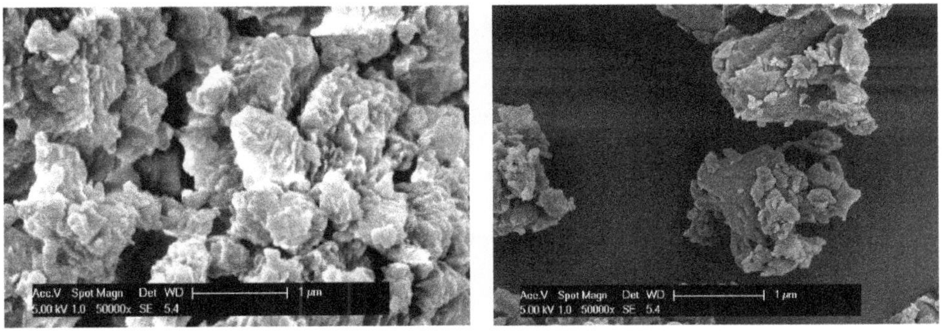

Figure 1. SEM images (50,000× magnification) of the optimal formulation of β-glucan NPs prepared via freezer milling.

Table 1. Particle size, PDI, zeta potential, and EE of drug-loaded freezer-milled NPs (n = 3, mean ± SD).

	Particle Size (d.nm)	PdI	Zeta Potential (mV)	Entrapment Efficiency (%)
MC NPs	555.0 ± 32.2	0.24 ± 0.13	−0.6 ± 0.7	63.9 ± 1.8
β-Glucan NPs	447.6 ± 14.2	0.18 ± 0.07	−1.2 ± 0.5	64.3 ± 2.1
EC NPs	472.6 ± 21.7	0.32 ± 0.11	−20.1 ± 1.2	56.3 ± 1.8
Chitosan NPs	643 ± 52.4	0.13 ± 0.11	+6.9 ± 1.4	60.2 ± 1.3

4.3. In Vitro Drug Release Studies

Through diffusion, the gemcitabine solution permeated the cellulose membrane with 95.4 ± 3.2% of the drug diffused into the receptor chamber within 15 min, while β-glucan NPs showed sustained release over 10 h (Figure 2). In fact, β-glucan NPs exhibited a biphasic drug release profile [41]. The first phase of the profile involved the release of unentrapped gemcitabine, which was adsorbed on the outer surface of the NPs, this was also considered to be an initial burst release. After this phase, a sustained release occurred, resulting from the slow diffusion of gemcitabine out of the polymer matrix [41]. The biphasic release profile suggested that the majority of the drug was entrapped within the polymer network rather than being adsorbed at the surface of the NPs [41]. Finally, the data obtained from the drug release were fitted to different kinetic models to investigate the kinetic drug release mechanisms. The modeled kinetic parameters are reported in Table 2. The release data were subjected to goodness-of-fit test (r^2) using linear regression analysis according to the selected release kinetic models.

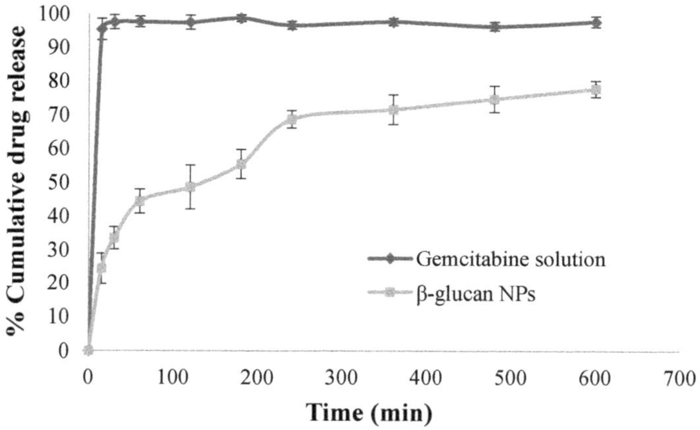

Figure 2. In vitro drug release of gemcitabine solution and gemcitabine loaded β-glucan NPs (mean ± SD, n = 3).

Table 2. Release kinetic parameters of β-glucan NPs subjected to different drug release models.

	Zero Order		First Order		Higuchi Model		Korsmeyer–Peppas Model		
β-Glucan NPs	r^2	k_0	r^2	k_1	r^2	k_h	r^2	n	k_k
	0.73	28.45	0.88	1.86	0.94	20.75	0.96	0.52	1.04

From the results, we can see that the Korsmeyer–Peppas model shows the highest r^2 of 0.96, indicating that the gemcitabine release from β-glucan NPs complies with this model well. The diffusional release exponent (n) in the model can reflect the diffusion mechanism. When $n = 0.45$, Fickian diffusion is expected, in which diffusion is affected by the permeation of a solvent with constant velocity into the drug carriers. If $n = 1.0$, it demonstrates zero-order release kinetics, with release occurring independently of concentration. If $0.45 < n < 1$, then it is non-Fickian or anomalous diffusion as a combination of Higuchi and zero-order diffusion methods [42]. The release exponent n was 0.52, indicating that the drug release was governed by diffusion through the NP matrix as well as matrix erosion, hence considered the so-called anomalous diffusion. This anomalous diffusion is evidence that the gemcitabine released from β-glucan NPs was controlled by more than one process.

This release profile demonstrates the benefit of β-glucan NPs in minimizing enzymatic degradation in the GI tract, ensuring the transition of most of the entrapped drug to the small intestinal membrane, where the main drug absorption occurs [43]. Moreover, the sustained release profile allows the intact drug-loaded NPs to retain in the systemic circulation for sufficient time, promoting the NPs to accumulate at the tumor site due to the EPR effect [44].

4.4. Ex Vivo Permeation Studies

The ex vivo permeation studies on the porcine intestinal epithelial membrane showed that the drug-loaded β-glucan NPs had a higher permeation rate than the plain drug solution (Figure 3). A total of 45.1 ± 3.8% gemcitabine was permeated through the epithelial membrane from the β-glucan NPs compared to 28.1 ± 4.2% from the drug solution over 24 h. The results also showed that the flux of drug-loaded β-glucan NPs across the epithelial membrane was significantly higher than that of the control. The apparent partition coefficients (P_{app}) were calculated using Equation (1). The flux (dX_r/dt), which is the gradient of the best-fit line, was determined, and the results showed that drug-loaded β-glucan NPs and the drug solution had flux values of 31.74 and 19.14, respectively. The linear part of the permeation curve from time 0 to 12 h indicates that the main permeation process occurred during this period. The surface area A was 1.77 cm^2, and C_0 was 5000 μg/mL. The P_{app} of the drug solution and drug-loaded β-glucan NPs were determined as $(2.17 \pm 0.26) \times 10^{-3}$ cm/s and $(3.59 \pm 0.22) \times 10^{-3}$ cm/s, respectively ($p < 0.05$). The larger the P_{app} values, the higher the drug absorption, and thus the higher the oral bioavailability expected [45]; these results correspond to the results from the later pharmacokinetic studies.

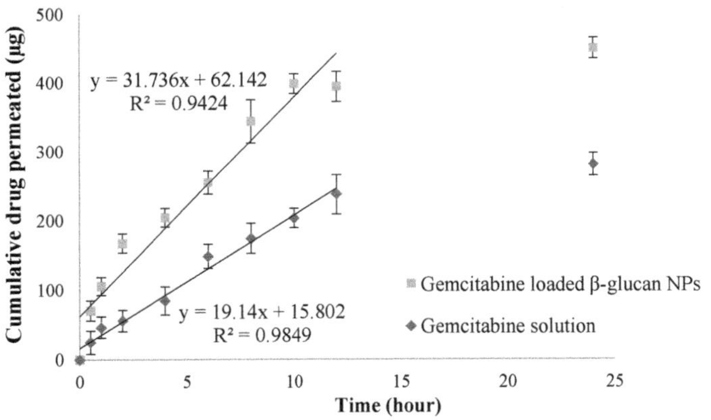

Figure 3. Ex vivo permeation studies of gemcitabine loaded β-glucan NPs and gemcitabine solution through the porcine intestinal epithelial membrane (mean ± SD, n = 3).

4.5. Cell Culture and Cytotoxicity Studies

Cytotoxicity studies for the gemcitabine solution and gemcitabine-loaded β-glucan NPs in 4T1 breast cancer cells were assessed based on mitochondrial activity (MTT) assay. As 4T1 tumor cells were used in the later pharacodynamic studies, the toxicity profiles of the formulations were evaluated before conducting the studies. The β-glucan polymer showed no significant cytotoxicity after 3 h of incubation with 4T1 cells, demonstrating the biocompatibility of the polymer with the tumor cells. Subsequently, the cytotoxicity studies of the drug solution and drug-loaded β-glucan NPs on 4T1 cells were performed for 72 h, and a dose-dependent cytotoxicity profile was observed (Figure 4). The IC_{50} values were then determined for the drug solution and drug-loaded β-glucan NPs, which were 228.8 ± 31.2 ng·mL^{-1} and 306.1 ± 46.3 ng·mL^{-1}, respectively. Both the drug solution and the drug-loaded β-glucan NPs showed similar cytotoxicity profiles and similar IC_{50} values. In contrast, β-glucan NPs had slightly higher IC_{50} than the plain drug solution, which may be attributed to the fact that most of the drug was retained within the nanocarrier system with gradual drug release over time.

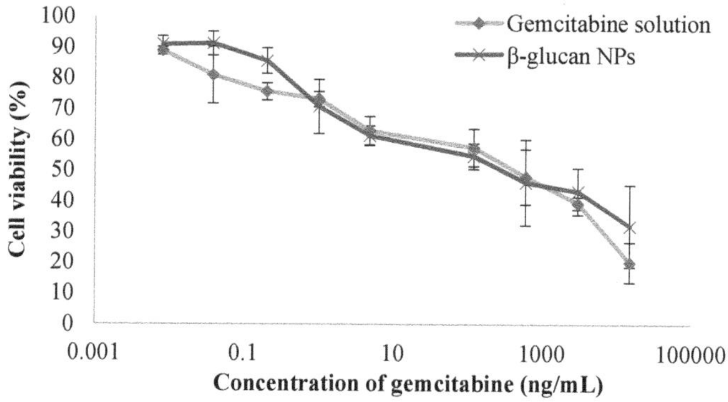

Figure 4. Cytotoxicity of gemcitabine solution and drug-loaded β-glucan NPs on 4T1 breast cancer cells at the tested concentrations (mean ± SD, n = 3).

4.6. In Vivo Pharmacokinetic Studies Using Sprague Dawley Rats

In the pharmacokinetic study, the plasma drug concentration-versus-time profiles were plotted for the orally administered drug solution, drug-loaded β-glucan NPs, and intravenously (*i.v.*) administered drug solution in SD rats (n = 6), which are shown in Figure 5. Table 3 shows all the resulting pharmacokinetic parameters that were analyzed using GraphPad Prism Software (version 6.0). Veltkamp et al. (2008) found that the oral bioavailability of a pure gemcitabine solution was very low due to an extensive first-pass effect, but it was well tolerable at lower doses [46]. In our study, the maximum drug concentration (C_{max}) of gemcitabine-loaded β-glucan NPs was 761.04 ± 214.32 ng/mL, which was higher than the plain drug solution of 577.11 ± 98.23 ng/mL. A higher C_{max} demonstrated the drug-loaded NPs were capable of bypassing hepatic first-pass metabolism and directly reaching the systemic circulation by virtue of the size and surface properties of the nanocarrier system [47]. The time at which C_{max} was reached (T_{max}) for the drug solution and β-glucan NPs were 8 and 30 h, respectively. The delayed T_{max} indicated that, after intestinal transit, the majority of the drug was released while circulating in the systemic circulation. The area under the curve (AUC) value of drug-loaded β-glucan NPs was 46,457 ± 2124 ng·h/mL, significantly greater than that of the plain drug solution, which was only 9176 ± 785 ng·h/mL. The higher AUC of the drug-loaded β-glucan NPs indicated the sustained release of the drug candidate from NPs, which would avoid the drug being rapidly metabolised. Hao et al. reported a self-micro-emulsifying drug delivery system for the oral delivery of gemcitabine. Their developed carrier system enhanced the C_{max} significantly, but its half-life ($T_{1/2}$) was not improved [48]. In this study, the $T_{1/2}$ of drug-loaded β-glucan NPs was 69.98 ± 20.50 h, which was significantly improved compared with that of the pure drug solution at 9.40 ± 2.13 h. Finally, the absolute oral bioavailability of drug-loaded β-glucan NPs (49.92%) was 5.1-fold higher than that of the drug solution (9.86%).

Table 3. Pharmacokinetic parameters of gemcitabine in SD rats following the oral administration of drug solution, drug-loaded β-glucan NPs, and *i.v.* administration of drug solution (mean ± SD, n = 6).

PK Parameters	Gemcitabine (*i.v.*)	Gemcitabine Solution (Oral)	β-Glucan NPs (Oral)
C_{max} (ng/mL)	94,152 ± 3435	577.11 ± 98.23	761.04 ± 214.32
T_{max} (h)	0.25	8	30
$AUC_{0\text{-}inf}$ (ng·h/mL)	93,050 ± 1459	9176 ± 785	46,457 ± 2124
$T_{1/2}$ (h)	1.18 ± 0.85	9.40 ± 2.13	69.98 ± 20.50
Oral bioavailability	100%	9.86%	49.92%

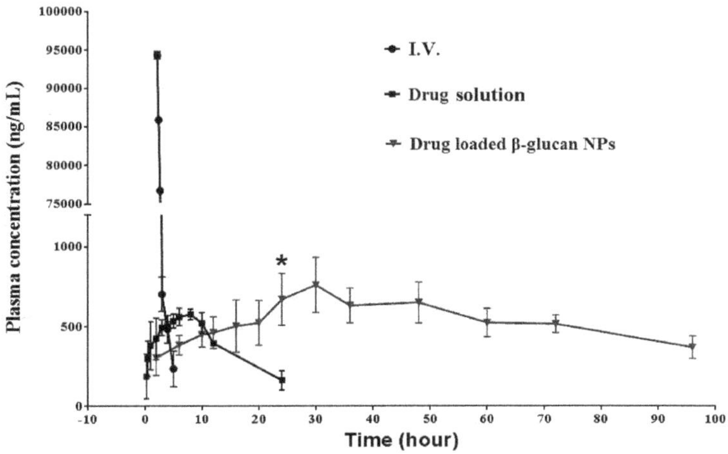

Figure 5. Plasma concentrations of the drug in SD rats following the oral administration of drug solution, drug-loaded β-glucan NPs, and *i.v.* injection of drug solution (mean ± SD, n = 6). The oral administration group results were significantly different from the results obtained with the *i.v.* administration of gemcitabine ($p < 0.001$) and the oral administration of gemcitabine solution; (*), $p < 0.01$.

4.7. In Vivo Acute Toxicity Studies

An in vivo acute toxicity study was required to determine a suitable oral dosage of gemcitabine for BALB/c nude mice prior to in vivo pharmacodynamic studies. Figure 6A displays the changes in the body weight of mice orally administered one of the five different dosages over 10 days. At doses above 60 mg/kg, gemcitabine caused a decline in body weight, and the higher the dosage, the larger the decrease in weight. At the highest dosage of 960 mg/kg, all mice died after 4 days, while 3, 6, 9, and 10 mice survived through to 10 days at 480 mg/kg, 240 mg/kg, 120 mg/kg, and 60 mg/kg dosages, respectively. Furthermore, over the 10 days of observation, the groups that received doses above 60 mg/kg suffered from diarrhea, with slower movement. Symptoms were more severe in groups administrated with higher doses of gemcitabine. Figure 6B shows the number of deaths plotted against log concentration. The LD_{50} was 204.17 mg/kg.

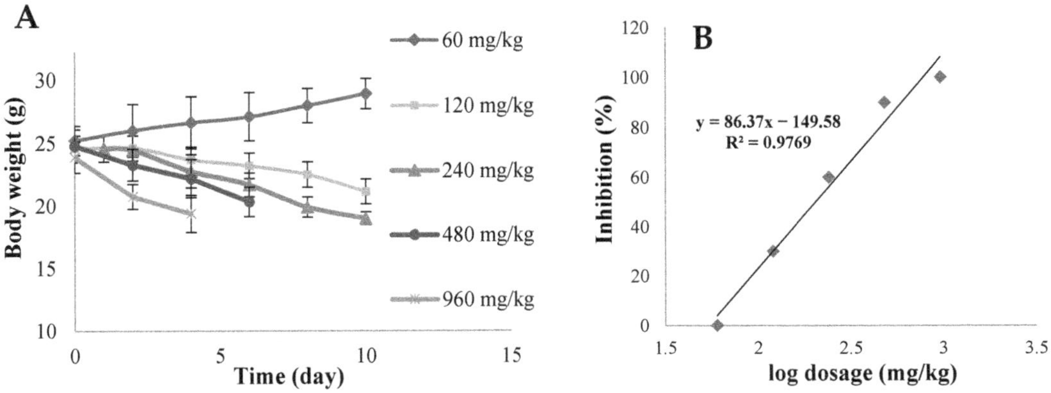

Figure 6. (**A**) Changes in the body weight of BALB/c nude mice after the oral administration of various dosages over 10 days (mean ± SD, n = 10); (**B**) percentage inhibition versus logarithm of dosages to determine LD_{50} of gemcitabine in BALB/c nude mice.

4.8. In Vivo Pharmacodynamic Studies Using BALB/c Nude Mice

The size of 4T1 breast tumors in the control group with no treatment markedly increased over the study period, while the tumor growth rate significantly reduced ($p < 0.01$) in the drug-loaded β-glucan NP group, with 3.04-fold and 1.74-fold reduction compared to the untreated control group and the drug solution group, respectively. This result corresponds to the in vivo pharmacokinetic studies indicating greater oral bioavailability and longer plasma half-life of drug-loaded β-glucan NP group compared to the plain drug solution group. Figure 7B shows a significant reduction in body weight of nude mice in both the drug solution group and the drug-loaded β-glucan NP group. The drug solution group had the greatest body weight loss, which demonstrated the high toxicity in this group. This phenomenon also corresponds to the acute toxicity study, which revealed that the mice in the drug solution group had severe diarrhea, reflecting the serious local side effects induced in the GI tract [49]. Interestingly, despite the greatly elevated oral bioavailability of the drug-loaded β-glucan NPs, a lesser reduction in body weight was observed. This may suggest that β-glucan NPs are absorbed into the systemic circulation as intact NPs [43,47,50], as well as limited drug exposure to nontarget organs.

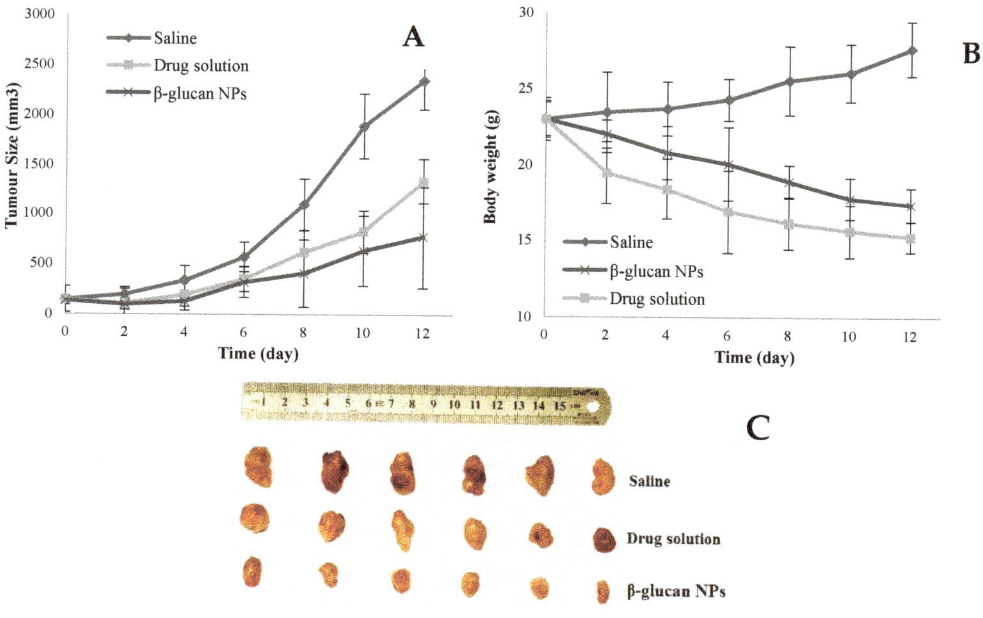

Figure 7. (**A**) The time course of tumor size in BALB/c nude mice recorded during the period of treatment with drug solution and drug-loaded β-glucan NPs, as well as in those without treatment (saline group) over 12 days (mean ± SD, n = 6, $p < 0.01$ at day 12); (**B**) the body weight change in BALB/c nude mice during the period of treatment over 12 days (mean ± SD, n = 6, $p < 0.01$ at day 12); (**C**) photography of the solid tumors with saline, 3 doses of 30 mg/kg drug solution, and an equivalent dose of drug-loaded β-glucan NPs, given on days 0, 2, and 4, and harvested on day 12 (n = 6).

5. Conclusions

Gemcitabine-loaded polymeric films were prepared using the conventional casting method, and then pulverized NPs were obtained via the freezer-milling technique. The NPs showed promising characteristics of a relatively small particle size of 447.6 ± 14.2 nm, a relatively high entrapment efficiency of 64.3 ± 2.1%, a sustained in vitro drug release profile, and greater ex vivo permeation through the porcine intestinal epithelial membrane compared to the plain drug solution. Cytotoxicity studies highlighted the safety of the β-glucan polymers, and the IC_{50} values of the gemcitabine solution and gemcitabine-loaded β-glucan NPs were also determined. Pharmacokinetic studies in SD rats showed that gemcitabine-loaded β-glucan NPs achieved a 7.4-fold longer $T_{1/2}$, and a 5.1-fold increase in absolute oral bioavailability was observed compared with plain drug solution. Furthermore, in vivo pharmacodynamic studies showed the promising capability of gemcitabine-loaded β-glucan NPs to inhibit 4T1 breast tumor growth, suggesting that this novel freezer-milled β-glucan NP system is a suitable drug delivery strategy for the oral delivery of gemcitabine and a promising potential platform for oral chemotherapy.

Author Contributions: Conceptualization, G.C., H.L. and J.W.; Methodology, G.C., Y.L. and M.Y.; Software, G.C. and Y.L.; Validation, G.C., Y.L., D.S. and M.Y.; Formal analysis, G.C. and J.W.; Investigation, G.C. and M.Y.; Resources, G.C., D.S. and H.L.; Data curation, G.C., M.Y. and J.W.; Writing—original draft, G.C.; Writing—review & editing, G.C. and J.W.; Visualization, G.C. and J.W.; Supervision, D.S., H.L., W.L. and J.W.; Project administration, D.S., W.L. and J.W.; Funding acquisition, G.C., W.L. and J.W. All authors have read and agreed to the published version of the manuscript.

Funding: The authors are grateful to the School of Pharmacy, University of Auckland, for the foundational support throughout this project. The authors acknowledge the Senior Visiting Collaboration Scholarship from the Department of Pharmaceutics, School of Pharmacy, Fudan University. This work was also supported by grants from the National Natural Science Foundation of China (82273871), the Guangdong Basic and Applied Basic Research Foundation (2021A1515110006), and the Fundamental Research Funds for the Central Universities, Sun Yat-sen University (23qnpy122).

Institutional Review Board Statement: The animal study protocol was approved by the Ethics Committee of the Sun Yat-sen University (SYSU-YXYSZ-20210304) on 1 March 2021.

Informed Consent Statement: Not applicable.

Data Availability Statement: All the data is contained within the article.

Conflicts of Interest: The authors declare no conflicts of interest.

References

1. Mei, L.; Zhang, Z.; Zhao, L.; Huang, L.; Yang, X.-L.; Tang, J.; Feng, S.-S. Pharmaceutical nanotechnology for oral delivery of anticancer drugs. *Adv. Drug Deliv. Rev.* **2013**, *65*, 880–890. [CrossRef] [PubMed]
2. Chen, G.; Kang, W.; Li, W.; Chen, S.; Gao, Y. Oral delivery of protein and peptide drugs: From non-specific formulation approaches to intestinal cell targeting strategies. *Theranostics* **2022**, *12*, 1419. [CrossRef] [PubMed]
3. Yun, Y.; Cho, Y.W.; Park, K. Nanoparticles for oral delivery: Targeted nanoparticles with peptidic ligands for oral protein delivery. *Adv. Drug Deliv. Rev.* **2013**, *65*, 822–832. [CrossRef]
4. Al, G.M.; Liu, M.; Wen, J. Ligands for oral delivery of peptides across the blood-brain-barrier. *Acta Mater. Medica* **2022**, *1*, 106–123.
5. Win, K.Y.; Feng, S.-S. Effects of particle size and surface coating on cellular uptake of polymeric nanoparticles for oral delivery of anticancer drugs. *Biomaterials* **2005**, *26*, 2713–2722. [CrossRef] [PubMed]
6. Galindo-Rodriguez, S.A.; Allemann, E.; Fessi, H.; Doelker, E. Polymeric nanoparticles for oral delivery of drugs and vaccines: A critical evaluation of in vivo studies. *Crit. Rev. Ther. Drug Carr. Syst.* **2005**, *22*, 419–464. [CrossRef]
7. Spleis, H.; Sandmeier, M.; Claus, V.; Schnürch, A.B. Surface design of nanocarriers: Key to more efficient oral drug delivery systems. *Adv. Colloid Interface Sci.* **2023**, *313*, 102848. [CrossRef]
8. Song, N.; Liu, W.; Tu, Q.; Liu, R.; Zhang, Y.; Wang, J. Preparation and in vitro properties of redox-responsive polymeric nanoparticles for paclitaxel delivery. *Colloids Surf. B Biointerfaces* **2011**, *87*, 454–463. [CrossRef]
9. Pradhan, R.; Poudel, B.K.; Ramasamy, T.; Choi, H.-G.; Yong, C.S.; Kim, J.O. Docetaxel-loaded polylactic acid-co-glycolic acid nanoparticles: Formulation, physicochemical characterization and cytotoxicity studies. *J. Nanosci. Nanotechnol.* **2013**, *13*, 5948–5956. [CrossRef]
10. Bensaid, F.; Boullay, O.T.D.; Amgoune, A.; Pradel, C.; Reddy, L.H.; Didier, E.; Sablé, S.; Louit, G.; Bazile, D.; Bourissou, D. Y-Shaped mPEG-PLA Cabazitaxel Conjugates: Well-Controlled Synthesis by Organocatalytic Approach and Self-Assembly into Interface Drug-Loaded Core–Corona Nanoparticles. *Biomacromolecules* **2013**, *14*, 1189–1198. [CrossRef]
11. Ajithkumar, A.; Andersson, R.; Siika-aho, M.; Tenkanen, M.; Åman, P. Isolation of cellotriosyl blocks from barley β-glucan with endo-1, 4-β-glucanase from *Trichoderma reesei*. *Carbohydr. Polym.* **2006**, *64*, 233–238. [CrossRef]
12. Wu, Y.; Li, P.Y.; Jiang, Z.Z.; Sun, X.L.; He, H.Q.; Yan, P.J.; Xu, Y.; Liu, Y. Bioinspired yeast-based β-glucan system for oral drug delivery. *Carbohydr. Polym.* **2023**, *319*, 121163. [CrossRef] [PubMed]

13. Min, C.J.; Jeong, D.; Piao, J.; Kim, K.; Nguyen, A.B.L.; Kwon, N.J.; Lee, M.K.; Yu, J.H.; Jung, S. Hydroxypropyl cyclic β-(1→2)-d-glucans and epichlorohydrin β-cyclodextrin dimers as effective carbohydrate-solubilizers for polycyclic aromatic hydrocarbons. *Carbohydr. Res.* **2015**, *401*, 82–88.
14. Li, S.; Li, W.; Yang, X.; Gao, Y.; Chen, G. Dietary-polysaccharide-modified fish-oil-based double emulsion as a functional colloidal formulation for oral drug delivery. *Pharmaceutics* **2022**, *14*, 2844. [CrossRef] [PubMed]
15. Huong, L.M.; Thu, H.P.; Thuy, N.T.B.; Ha, T.T.H.; Thi, H.T.M.; Trang, M.T.; Hang, T.T.N.; Nghi, D.H.; Phuc, N.X.; Quang, D.T. Preparation and Antitumor-promoting Activity of Curcumin Encapsulated by 1,3-β-Glucan Isolated from Vietnam Medicinal Mushroom *Hericium erinaceum*. *Chem. Lett.* **2011**, *40*, 846–848. [CrossRef]
16. Qi, S.; Weuts, I.; De Cort, S.; Stokbroekx, S.; Leemans, R.; Reading, M.; Belton, P.; Craig, D.Q.M. An investigation into the crystallisation behaviour of an amorphous cryomilled pharmaceutical material above and below the glass transition temperature. *J. Pharm. Sci.* **2010**, *99*, 196–208. [CrossRef] [PubMed]
17. Chieng, N.; Zujovic, Z.; Bowmaker, G.; Rades, T.; Saville, D. Effect of milling conditions on the solid-state conversion of ranitidine hydrochloride form 1. *Int. J. Pharm.* **2006**, *327*, 36–44. [CrossRef] [PubMed]
18. Pérez, C.R.; González, M.D.A.; Sarria, F.R.; López, M.C.H.; Gallego, J.M.C. Investigating the room-and cryo-milling impact in lignocellulosic biomass and its consequence over pyrolysis and oxidative treatments. *J. Clean. Prod.* **2024**, *437*, 140761. [CrossRef]
19. Derakhshandeh, K.; Fathi, S. Role of chitosan nanoparticles in the oral absorption of Gemcitabine. *Int. J. Pharm.* **2012**, *437*, 172–177. [CrossRef]
20. Vandana, M.; Sahoo, S.K. Long circulation and cytotoxicity of PEGylated gemcitabine and its potential for the treatment of pancreatic cancer. *Biomaterials* **2010**, *31*, 9340–9356. [CrossRef]
21. Trickler, W.J.; Khurana, J.; Nagvekar, A.A.; Dash, A.K. Chitosan and glyceryl monooleate nanostructures containing gemcitabine: Potential delivery system for pancreatic cancer treatment. *AAPS Pharm. Sci. Technol.* **2010**, *11*, 392–401. [CrossRef]
22. Zhou, L.J.; Du, K.X.; Dai, Y.H.; Zeng, Y.M.; Luo, Y.B.; Ren, M.D.; Pan, W.B.; Liu, Y.; Zhang, L.; Zhu, R.; et al. Metabolic reprogramming based on RNA sequencing of gemcitabine-resistant cells reveals the FASN gene as a therapeutic for bladder cancer. *J. Transl. Med.* **2024**, *22*, 55. [CrossRef]
23. Semalty, M.; Semalty, A.; Kumar, G. Formulation and characterization of mucoadhesive buccal films of glipizide. *Indian J. Pharm. Sci.* **2008**, *70*, 43. [CrossRef]
24. Chen, G.; Svirskis, D.; Lu, W.; Ying, M.; Huang, Y.; Wen, J. N-trimethyl chitosan nanoparticles and CSKSSDYQC peptide: N-trimethyl chitosan conjugates enhance the oral bioavailability of gemcitabine to treat breast cancer. *J. Control. Release* **2018**, *10*, 142–153. [CrossRef]
25. Nabil, W.N.N.; Xi, Z.; Liu, M.; Li, Y.; Yao, M.; Liu, T.; Dong, Q.; Xu, H. Advances in therapeutic agents targeting quiescent cancer cells. *Acta Mater. Medica* **2022**, *8*, 56–71. [CrossRef]
26. Youdim, K.A.; Avdeef, A.; Abbott, N.J. In vitro trans-monolayer permeability calculations: Often forgotten assumptions. *Drug Discov. Today* **2003**, *8*, 997–1003. [CrossRef] [PubMed]
27. Chen, G.; Svirskis, D.; Lu, W.; Ying, M.; Li, H.; Liu, M.; Wen, J. N-trimethyl chitosan coated nano-complexes enhance the oral bioavailability and chemotherapeutic effects of gemcitabine. *Carbohydr. Polym.* **2021**, *273*, 118592. [CrossRef]
28. Fotakis, G.; Timbrell, J.A. In vitro cytotoxicity assays: Comparison of LDH, neutral red, MTT and protein assay in hepatoma cell lines following exposure to cadmium chloride. *Toxicol. Lett.* **2006**, *160*, 171–177. [CrossRef]
29. Hussain, A.; Sasidharan, S.; Ahmed, T.; Ahmed, M.; Sharma, C. Clove (*Syzygium aromaticum*) extract potentiates gemcitabine cytotoxic effect on human cervical cancer cell line. *Int. J. Cancer Res.* **2009**, *5*, 95–104. [CrossRef]
30. Wolz, E.; Pfannkuch, F.; Straub, J.; van Huygevoort, A. *Assessment of Acute Oral Toxicity with Ro 26-7624/000 (EGCG) in the Rat (Acute Toxic Class Method)*; Report; Roche Vitamins Ltd.: Basel, Switzerland, 2001.
31. Rehman, U.; Shoaib, M.; Raza, Z.A.; Rehan, Z.A.; Bakhtiyar, M.J.; Sharif, F.; Yousaf, M. Citric acid crosslinked biocompatible silk fibroin-mediated porous chitosan films for sustained drug release application. *Mater. Today Commun.* **2023**, *34*, 105373. [CrossRef]
32. Kowalczuk, J.; Tritt-Goc, J.; Piślewski, N. The swelling properties of hydroxypropyl methyl cellulose loaded with tetracycline hydrochloride: Magnetic resonance imaging study. *Solid State Nucl. Magn. Reson.* **2004**, *25*, 35–41. [CrossRef]
33. Bourtoom, T. Plasticizer effect on the properties of biodegradable blend film from rice starch-chitosan. *Sonklanakarin J. Sci. Technol.* **2008**, *30*, 149.
34. Dhanapal, A.; Sasikala, P.; Rajamani, L.; Kavitha, V.; Yazhini, G.; Banu, M.S. Edible films from polysaccharides. *Food Sci. Qual. Manag.* **2012**, *3*, 9–18.
35. Gaisford, S.; Dennison, M.; Tawfik, M.; Jones, M.D. Following mechanical activation of salbutamol sulphate during ball-milling with isothermal calorimetry. *Int. J. Pharm.* **2010**, *393*, 75–79. [CrossRef]
36. Yang, X.; Li, W.Q.; Li, S.Z.; Chen, S.M.; Hu, Z.; He, Z.Y.; Zhu, X.Q.; Niu, X.S.; Zhou, X.M.; Li, H.H.; et al. Fish oil-based microemulsion can efficiently deliver oral peptide blocking PD-1/PD-L1 and simultaneously induce ferroptosis for cancer immunotherapy. *J. Control. Release* **2024**, *365*, 654–667. [CrossRef]
37. Oliveira, M.B.; Mano, J.F. Polymer-based microparticles in tissue engineering and regenerative medicine. *Biotechnol. Prog.* **2011**, *27*, 897–912. [CrossRef] [PubMed]
38. Lotina, A.S.; Portela, R.; Baeza, P.; Rodriguez, V.A.; Villarroel, M.; Ávila, P. Zeta potential as a tool for functional materials development. *Catal. Today* **2023**, *423*, 113862. [CrossRef]

39. Zhao, W.; Li, M.; Zhang, Z.; Peng, H.-X. EMI shielding effectiveness of silver nanoparticle-decorated multi-walled carbon nanotube sheets. *Int. J. Smart Nano Mater.* **2010**, *1*, 249–260. [CrossRef]
40. Lash, L.H. Mitochondrial glutathione in toxicology and disease of the kidneys. *Toxicol. Res.* **2012**, *1*, 39–46. [CrossRef]
41. Arias, J.L.; López-Viota, M.; López-Viota, J.; Delgado, Á.V. Development of iron/ethylcellulose (core/shell) nanoparticles loaded with diclofenac sodium for arthritis treatment. *Int. J. Pharm.* **2009**, *382*, 270–276. [CrossRef] [PubMed]
42. Pragnesh, D.; Pradip, N.; Macwan, M.; Kamaliya, B. Biodegradable Gg-cl-poly (NIPAm-co-AA)/-o-MWCNT based hydrogel for combined drug delivery system of metformin and sodium diclofenac: In vitro studies. *RSC Adv.* **2023**, *13*, 22875–22885.
43. Esquivel, S.V.; Himanshu, N.; Bhatt, N.; Diwan, R.; Habib, A.; Lee, W.Y.; Khatun, Z.; Nurunnabi, M. β-Glucan and Fatty Acid Based Mucoadhesive Carrier for Gastrointestinal Tract Specific Local and Sustained Drug Delivery. *Biomolecules* **2023**, *13*, 768. [CrossRef] [PubMed]
44. Natarajan, J.V.; Nugraha, C.; Ng, X.W.; Venkatraman, S. Sustained-release from nanocarriers: A review. *J. Control. Release* **2014**, *193*, 122–138. [CrossRef]
45. Rezvanjou, S.N.; Niavand, M.R.; Shayesteh, O.H.; Yeganeh, E.M.; Moghadam, D.A.; Derakhshandeh, K.; Mahjub, R. Preparation and characterisation of self-emulsifying drug delivery system (SEDDS) for enhancing oral bioavailability of metformin hydrochloride using hydrophobic ion pairing complexation. *J. Microencapsul.* **2023**, *40*, 53–66. [CrossRef]
46. Veltkamp, S.A.; Pluim, D.; van Tellingen, O.; Beijnen, J.H.; Schellens, J.H.M. Extensive metabolism and hepatic accumulation of gemcitabine after multiple oral and intravenous administration in mice. *Drug Metab. Dispos.* **2008**, *36*, 1606–1615. [CrossRef]
47. Joshi, G.; Kumar, A.; Sawant, K. Enhanced bioavailability and intestinal uptake of Gemcitabine HCl loaded PLGA nanoparticles after oral delivery. *Eur. J. Pharm. Sci.* **2014**, *60*, 80–89. [CrossRef]
48. Hao, W.-H.; Wang, J.-J.; Hsueh, S.-P.; Hsu, P.-J.; Chang, L.-C.; Hsu, C.-S.; Hsu, K.-Y. In vitro and in vivo studies of pharmacokinetics and antitumor efficacy of D07001-F4, an oral gemcitabine formulation. *Cancer Chemother. Pharmacol.* **2013**, *71*, 379–388. [CrossRef] [PubMed]
49. Ejeh, S.A.; Abu, H.A.; Onyeyili, P.A.; Abenga, J.N.; Ogbe, R.J.; Abalaka, S.E. Acute and sub-acute toxicological evaluation of ethanol extract of Alchornea cordifolia leaves in Wistar rats. *Sci. Afr.* **2023**, *19*, e01575. [CrossRef]
50. Sonaje, K.; Lin, Y.-H.; Juang, J.-H.; Wey, S.-P.; Chen, C.-T.; Sung, H.-W. In vivo evaluation of safety and efficacy of self-assembled nanoparticles for oral insulin delivery. *Biomaterials* **2009**, *30*, 2329–2339. [CrossRef]

pharmaceutics

MDPI

Article

Cellular Uptake and Transport Mechanism Investigations of PEGylated Niosomes for Improving the Oral Delivery of Thymopentin

Mengyang Liu [1], Darren Svirskis [1], Thomas Proft [2,3], Jacelyn Loh [2,3], Yuan Huang [4] and Jingyuan Wen [1,3,*]

[1] School of Pharmacy, Faculty of Medical and Health Sciences, The University of Auckland, 95 Park Road, Grafton, Auckland 1010, New Zealand; m.liu@auckland.ac.nz (M.L.); d.svirskis@auckland.ac.nz (D.S.)
[2] Department of Molecular Medicine and Pathology, Faculty of Medical and Health Sciences, The University of Auckland, Auckland 1010, New Zealand; t.proft@auckland.ac.nz (T.P.); mj.loh@auckland.ac.nz (J.L.)
[3] Maurice Wilkins Centre for Molecular Biodiscovery, The University of Auckland, Auckland 1010, New Zealand
[4] Key Laboratory of Drug Targeting and Drug Delivery, West China School of Pharmacy, Sichuan University, Chengdu 610017, China; huangyuan@scu.edu.cn
* Correspondence: j.wen@auckland.ac.nz

Abstract: Background: Although its immunomodulatory properties make thymopentin (TP5) appealing, its rapid metabolism and inactivation in the digestive system pose significant challenges for global scientists. PEGylated niosomal nanocarriers are hypothesized to improve the physicochemical stability of TP5, and to enhance its intestinal permeability for oral administration. Methods: TP5-loaded PEGylated niosomes were fabricated using the thin film hydration method. Co-cultured Caco-2 and HT29 cells with different ratios were screened as in vitro intestinal models. The cytotoxicity of TP5 and its formulations were evaluated using an MTT assay. The cellular uptake and transport studies were investigated in the absence or presence of variable inhibitors or enhancers, and their mechanisms were explored. Results and Discussion: All TP5 solutions and their niosomal formulations were nontoxic to Caco-2 and HT-29 cells. The uptake of TP5-PEG-niosomes by cells relied on active endocytosis, exhibiting dependence on time, energy, and concentration, which has the potential to significantly enhance its cellular uptake compared to TP5 in solution. Nevertheless, cellular transport rates were similar between TP5 in solution and its niosomal groups. The cellular transport of TP5 in solution was carried out mainly through MRP5 endocytosis and a passive pathway and effluxed by MRP5 transporters, while that of TP5-niosomes and TP5-PEG-niosomes was carried out through adsorptive- and clathrin-mediated endocytosis requiring energy. The permeability and transport rate was further enhanced when EDTA and sodium taurocholate were used as the penetration enhancers. Conclusions: This research has illustrated that PEG-niosomes were able to enhance the cellular uptake and maintain the cellular transport of TP5. This study also shows this formulation's potential to serve as an effective carrier for improving the oral delivery of peptides.

Keywords: cellular uptake; cellular transport; niosome; PEGylation; thymopentin; oral delivery

1. Introduction

The peptide thymopentin (TP5) has recently attracted significant attention owing to its immunomodulatory properties and its potential application in the treatment of immunological diseases in both humans and animals [1,2]. TP5, illustrated in Figure 1, is a compact pentapeptide with therapeutic properties, consisting of the amino acids Arginine, Lysine, Aspartic Acid, Valine, and Tyrosine, and possessing a molecular weight of 679 g/mol. Initially extracted from the bovine thymus, it was later identified at the molecular level as a single-peptide chain named thymopoietin II, consisting of 49 amino acids, as depicted in Figure 1 [3]. Early in 1985, Rinaldi Garaci et al. revealed that TP5 is able to stimulate dendritic cells to provide resistance against fungal infections through the activation of antifungal T-cell helper 1 (Th1) responses, with the involvement of Toll-like receptor (TLR) 2 signaling being its potential immunomodulatory mechanism [4]. TP5 has shown to have pleiotropic effects in immunomodulation including T cell and B cell differentiation, IgG production, T cell proliferation, and Interleukin-2 production [5]. Therefore, TP5 has been investigated for its potential efficacy in treating ailments such as severe acute respiratory syndrome (SARS) by ameliorating clinical symptoms, enhancing immune function recovery, reducing lung inflammation, minimizing hormone dosage, and shortening treatment duration [6].

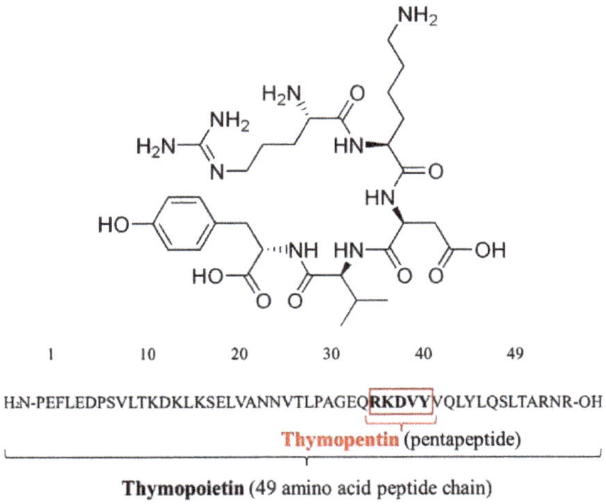

Figure 1. The chemical structure of TP5 and the amino acid sequences of thymopoietin and thymopentin.

Similar to other peptide and protein medications, the only currently accessible form of TP5 is a lyophilized powder designed for intramuscular or intravenous administration [3]. This limitation is attributed to the instability and rapid metabolism (degradation) experienced when administered through alternative routes. Several factors contribute to the inadequate oral absorption of TP5, such as high degradation in the gastrointestinal (GI) tract, a low log P, and a high molecular weight [7–9]. Transdermal and alternative non-invasive administration routes pose challenges for the absorption of TP5, including issues related to low skin or tissue permeability [10–14]. The physicochemical properties of TP5 limit its efficacy as an immunomodulator for immune-related diseases in both humans and animals [15]. Employing formulation strategies may be useful to surmount the inherent constraints of TP5, thereby facilitating its oral delivery [16,17].

PEGylation, which involves the attachment of PEGs to a protein or nucleic acid molecule, can increase its aqueous solubility, prolong its circulation time, protect it from in vivo biological inactivation via proteolysis, and reduce its immunogenicity in some cases [18]. The primary purpose of using PEGylation technology to improve drug stability in vivo is to prolong the half-life of the drug, which can reduce its clearance via the kidneys [19]. PEGylating a drug delivery system like niosome can improve systemic circulation time and decrease immunogenicity to obtain higher stability [20]. Niosomes offer several advantages in oral delivery, including possessing a (1) nanometer-sized particle to enhance the bioactive absorption; (2) a spherical shape to expand contact area for drug absorption; (3) an encapsulation structure to improve the stability of drug; and (4) a controlled and sustained drug release profile to reduce the frequency of drug administration [20].

The human adenocarcinoma cell lines Caco-2 and HT-29 have been developed as a co-cultured model for the intestinal epithelium. Caco-2 and HT-29 cells were originally isolated from the human colon adenocarcinoma by Fogh et al. [21]. The co-cultured Caco-2 and HT-29 cell system is commonly employed in an in vitro intestinal absorption model in both industry and academia for assessing the permeability of various compounds in the intestine [21,22]. These cells also showcase the presence of nutrient and drug transporters, enabling the investigations of carrier-mediated uptake and efflux mechanisms [21–23].

In this study, a series of in vitro cell assays were used to explore the oral delivery of TP5. In specific, the cytotoxicity of both niosomes and TP5 were investigated. The cellular uptake studies were also assessed for TP5 with and without niosome and PEGylation technologies. Various absorption inhibitors and enhancers were employed to investigate the transport mechanisms of TP5-PEG-niosomes, which may be affected by interactions between the drugs or formulations and intestinal cellular transporters. The main aim of this project is to illustrate enhanced cellular uptake and gain insights into the transport of TP5-PEG-niosomes, to achieve an enhance the oral delivery of TP5. This research contributes to the field by providing insights into the novel approach of employing TP5-PEG-niosomes for improved oral delivery, potentially offering beneficial therapeutic outcomes for TP5-based treatments.

2. Materials and Methods

2.1. Materials

TP5 (≥95% LC-MS validated) was purchased from Wuhan DanGang Biological Technology company (DGpeptide, Wuhan, China). Soybean trypsin and chymotrypsin inhibitors (SBTCI), PEG600-cholesterol, cholesterol (CH), stearic acid, sorbitan monostearate (Span® 60), polyoxyethylenesorbitan monooleate (Tween® 80), and dihexadecyl phosphate (DCP) were obtained from Merck (Merck, Darmstadt, Germany). Methanol and acetonitrile (ACN) of analytical reagent grade were ordered from Sigma-Aldrich (Sigma, San Jose, CA, USA). Phosphoric acid (PPA), trifluoroacetic acid (TFA), and ethylenediaminetetraacetic acid (EDTA) were obtained from Honeywell Fluka (Honeywell Fluka, Seelze, Germany). Dulbecco's Modified Eagle Medium (DMEM) with high glucose and L-glutamine, Hank's Balanced Salt Solution (HBSS), phosphate-buffered saline (PBS), non-essential amino acid solution (NEAA), heat-inactivated Fetal Bovine Serum (FBS), penicillin-streptomycin, and trypsin-EDTA were obtained from Invitrogen (Auckland, New Zealand). 3-(4,5-dimethylthiazol-2-yl)-2,5-diphenyltetrazolium bromide (MTT) was purchased from Sigma-Aldrich (Sigma, San Jose, CA, USA). All other reagents were of analytical grade.

2.2. Analytical Method of TP5

The RP-HPLC analytical method for TP5 was developed in a prior study [10]. In brief, TP5 peak separation was accomplished using a Gemini C18 column (250 × 4.60 mm, 5 μm; Phenomenex, Torrance, CA, USA) equipped with a C18 guard column (10 × 3.0 mm; Phenomenex, Torrance, CA, USA) and maintained at 25 ± 1 °C. The RP-HPLC-UV conditions included a wavelength of 210 nm, a flow rate of 1.0 mL/min, and a mobile phase consisting of 0.1% phosphoric acid (pH 2.6)/methanol with a ratio of 80:20 (*v*/*v*).

2.3. In Vitro Cell Culture Investigation

2.3.1. Cell Co-Culture

Caco-2 or HT-29 cells were cultured in DMEM media, which is composed of 10% FBS, 1% non-essential amino acid (NEAA) and 1% penicillin-streptomycin (antibiotics) with pH values maintained at 7.4 ± 0.2. The cells were incubated in an incubator at 37 °C in the presence of 5% CO_2. Caco-2 or HT-29 cells were fed fresh DMEM every 3 days until the confluence value reached 80% for the subculture. In brief, the DMEM medium was removed, and the Caco-2 or HT-29 cells were washed with pre-warmed PBS (37 °C) to remove traces of the serum, which may inhibit the action of trypsin. These cells were subsequently incubated with a 0.25% trypsin-EDTA (0.2 mL/cm^2) mixture for about 3 min to guarantee all the cells were floating and detached. Later, an equal amount of FBS was added to the cell culture to deactivate trypsin. The Caco-2 or HT-29 cell suspension was then centrifuged at 300× *g* for 10 min. The supernatant was discarded, and the cells were re-suspended in the fresh DMEM medium. The secondary suspension was then divided into two parts and cultured separately using DMEM medium. The newly cultured Caoco-2 and HT-29 cells were used as co-cultured models in the following sections.

2.3.2. Cell Line Integrity

The Caco-2 and HT-29 cells were co-cultured in ratios of 1:0, 0:1, 1:1, 1:2, 1:3, 3:1, 5:1, 7:1, and 9:1. This co-cultured cell line was evaluated by transepithelial electrical resistance (TEER) values to determine the tissue integrity. The TEER measurements were performed at 3-day intervals until the confluence reached 80%. TEER = (Rm − Rb) × A, where Rm, Rb, and A were the measured TEER values, TEER value of the blank transwell, and the membrane surface area of the transwell, respectively. The ratio with the best TEER value was selected as the final ratio for further experiments.

2.3.3. Preparation of TP5 Stock Solution and TP5-PEG-Niosomes

TP5 stock solution was prepared by dissolving TP5 in a cell culture medium, resulting in a final concentration of 10 mg/mL. TP5-PEG-niosomes were prepared and fabricated in two parts based on our previous research with particle size at 156 ± 36 nm [24]. In brief, it started with the conjugation of PEG600 and cholesterol. In the second part, TP5-PEG-niosomes were fabricated using a thin film hydration method [24]. In short, a 10 mL blend of methanol and chloroform (1:4, *v*/*v*) comprising 2 μmoL DCP, 30 μmol cholesterol (including 22.5 μmol PEG600-cholesterol), and 120 μmol Span 60 was prepared. The mixture was rotary evaporated (Laborota 4000, Buchi, Switzerland) at 45 °C to generate a thin, dry lipid film. This film was subsequently purified under a nitrogen flow until the residual organic solvent was eliminated. The final lipid film was hydrated with 10 mL cell DMEM medium, containing 10 mg of TP5, at 60 °C for 60 min to produce the TP5-PEG-niosomes. The TP5 concentration in the final formulation was prepared as 1 mg/mL.

2.3.4. Cytotoxicity Study

MTT assay was used for the cytotoxicity study. The Caco-2 and HT-29 co-cultured cell lines were cultured in 96-well plates (BD Falcon™, Auckland, New Zealand) at a seeding density of 5000 cells per well for 24 h at 37 °C to promote cell adhesion. The DMEM was discarded, and the Caco-2 and HT-29 co-cultured cells were washed with PBS before introducing TP5 test samples. The cells were then treated with filtered TP5 solutions (0.005 to 10 mg/mL) or TP5-PEG-niosomes (niosome numbers 0.01 to 10.00 × 10^{12}/mL) and cultured for 24, 48, and 72 h. The cells were examined using a microscope (EvosTM XL Core microscope with a magnification of 10× (eyepiece lens) and 10× (objective lens) from Thermo Fisher Scientific® (Thermo Fisher, Waltham, MA, USA). Subsequently, 20 μL of MTT (5 mg/mL) was added, and the cells were incubated for an additional 4 h. Dimethyl sulfoxide (DMSO) was introduced to dissolve the formazan crystals, and the absorbance at 570 nm was measured using a microplate UV-Vis spectrophotometer (SpectraMax® Plus, Molecular Devices, San Jose, CA, USA). The percentage of cell viability was calculated in comparison to the untreated control group.

For each test sample group and at every time point over the course of three days, cell viability was computed. The outcomes were consolidated using the SoftMax Pro v5 software system through Equation (1).

$$V = \frac{A}{A_0} \times 100\% \tag{1}$$

where V is the cell viability, A is sample absorbance, and A_0 is control absorbance.

2.3.5. Cellular Uptake

Fluorescence and Confocal Microscopy Analysis

First, TP5 was labeled with fluorescein isothiocyanate (FITC) [25]. Briefly, 25 mg of TP5 and 2.5 mg of FITC were dissolved in 5 mL of 0.1 M carbonate buffer, pH 8.5, and stirred in the dark for 8 h at 4 °C. The mixtures underwent fractionation through gel permeation chromatography utilizing a Sephadex G-25M column (Sigma Aldrich, St. Louis, MO, USA). In a concise procedure, 1 mL of the mixture was loaded onto the top of the column gel bed, and the column was eluted with 10 mL of PBS (0.01, pH 7.4). Fractions of 1 mL each were collected, and the absorbance of each fraction was assessed at 280 nm. During elution, two bands were discernible. The conjugates were identified in the first band (fractions 3–5, with absorbance > 0.4). Fractionated FITC-TP5 conjugates were dehydrated by freeze drying (Labconco, Kansas City, MO, USA), and loaded into PEG-niosomes as described previously.

Caco-2 and HT-29 co-cultured cells were transferred into 8-well chamber slides (BD Falcon, Fort Pierce, FL, USA) at a density of 10^4 cells/cm^2 and grown in a complete DMEM culture medium. On the following day (24 h culture), cell monolayers were pre-incubated with 1 mL of HBSS for 15 min at 37 °C. After equilibrating, the medium was replaced with 1 mL suspensions of FITC-TP5, FITC-TP5-loaded PEG-niosomes (1 mg TP5 per mL in HBSS) followed by incubation for 1 h at 37 °C (513). Then, the cells were washed eight times with cold sterile PBS (7.4) and fixed with freshly prepared 4% (weight per volume) (*w*/*v*) p-formaldehyde (PFA, pH 7.4) for 20 min, followed by cell nuclei staining with DAPI (100 nm in PBS) for 10 min. Sample time points were set as 0.5, 1, 2, and 3 h for the TP5 solution, and 0.5, 1, 2, 3, 4 and 5 h for the TP5 formulation. After removing the culture chambers, the slides were thoroughly washed with PBS and mounted with CITI-Fluor (a medium used to decrease photobleaching during observation under microscopy). Coverslips were placed on top of the slides and sealed with nail polish.

Prior to the experiment, the slides were stored at 4 °C and protected from the light. The slides were visualized by fluorescence microscope (Nikon TE2000E, Nikon, Tokyo, Japan) first before using the laser scanning confocal microscope. Cell nuclear was stained with 0.1% Hoechst 33342 in 0.01M PBS containing 0.1% tween (PBST) for 15 min. To prevent photobleaching, a drop of mounting solution was added to the specimens before observation using a Zeiss™ LSM 710 inverted confocal microscope (Carl Zeiss Ltd., München, Germany). The excitation wavelength was set at 405 nm for Hoechst, 560 nm for Nile red and 488 nm for FITC-TP5. The samples were also investigated using a laser scanning confocal microscope (Leica TCS SP2, Bio-strategy, Rosedale, NZ, USA).

The fluorescence images were evaluated with Leica Confocal Software (LCS) version 2.61 (Bio-strategy, Rosedale, NZ) and ImageJ™ software, version 1.5 (National Institutes of Health, Bethesda, MD, USA).

Quantitative Analysis of the Cellular Uptake of TP5 and TP5-PEG-Niosomes

Briefly, 5 mL of Caco-2 and HT-29 co-cultured cells' suspension at a density of 10^5 cells/cm^2 was seeded onto 60 mm plastic dishes (Corning, New York, NY, USA), fed complete DMEM every 3 days and incubated at 37 °C in an atmosphere of 5% CO_2 and 95% relative humidity. On reaching 80% confluence, the culture medium was replaced with HBSS (2 mL). After 30 min of incubation at 37 °C, the medium was replaced with 1 mL TP5 solution with different concentrations (5, 10, 50, 100, 200, 500, and 1000 μg/mL in HBSS) and TP5-PEG-niosomes (1 mg TP5 in 0.01, 0.05, 0.10, 1.00, 2.00, and 5.00 × 10^{12} numbers niosomes per mL in HBSS) and incubated for 4 h at 37 °C to investigate the effect of drug and niosome concentration on TP5 cellular uptake. For time-dependent cellular uptake experiments, the cells were incubated for 0.5, 1, 2, 3, 4 and 5 h at 37 °C, respectively. Then, the cells were washed with cold sterile PBS (pH 7.4) eight times and solubilized in 1 mL 10% Triton X-100 in methanol followed by the extraction of TP5. Then, 25 μL of the cell lysates from each well were subjected to a BCA protein assay (Thermo Scientific, Waltham, MA, USA) to determine the amount of cell protein. The entire protein concentration in each group was calculated based on the linearity equation obtained from the BSA standard curve. Then, cell lysates were centrifuged for 15 min at 14,000 rpm, and the supernatants were analyzed for the amount of uptake TP5 using the RP-HPLC method mentioned earlier. The uptake of TP5 by Caco-2 and HT-29 co-cultured cells was calculated and expressed as the amount of drug (ng) uptake per μg cell protein.

Cellular Uptake Mechanisms of TP5 and TP5-PEG-Niosomes

One of the mechanisms for cellular uptake depends on concentration. To carry out a drug-concentration-dependent cellular uptake study, aliquots of 2 mL TP5 of different concentrations (10, 50, 100, 200, 500 and 1000 μg/mL) in HBSS were added into the dish and incubated for 60 min in triplicate. To carry out a noisome-concentration-dependent cellular uptake study, 2 mL TP5-PEG-niosomes of different niosome numbers (0.01, 0.05, 0.10, 1.00, 2.00, and 5.00 × 10^{12} /mL measured by NanoSight NS300 (Malvern Instruments Ltd., Worcestershire, UK) and prepared by series dilution) in HBSS was added into the dish and incubated for 4 h in triplicate. The treated Caco-2 and HT-29 co-cultured cells were then scraped off into a 2 mL microcentrifuge tube containing 1.0 mL extraction solution (10% Triton X-100) and sonicated to accelerate cell lysis. Then, 25 μL of the cell lysates from each well were subjected to a BCA protein assay (Thermo Scientific, Waltham, MA, USA) to determine the amount of cell protein as mentioned above. Then, cell lysates were centrifuged for 15 min at 14,000 rpm, and the supernatants were analyzed for the amount of uptake TP5 using the RP-HPLC method mentioned above. The uptake of TP5 by Caco-2 and HT-29 co-cultured cells was calculated and expressed as the amount of drug (ng) uptake per μg cell protein.

To investigate other cellular uptake mechanisms, Caco-2 and HT-29 co-cultured cell monolayers were treated with different inhibitors and different conditions for 1 h before cellular uptake started. The inhibitors used in this study include an active transport inhibitor (sodium azide, 100 mM), an adsorptive-mediated endocytosis inhibitor (protamine sulphate, 1 mM), a clathrin-mediated endocytosis inhibitor (chlorpromazine, 10 μg/mL), and a caveolae-mediated endocytosis inhibitor (filipin, 5 μg/mL) [23]. The incubation temperature of 4 °C was also tested. After the removal of the drug solution and formulation (4 h incubation), the dishes were immediately rinsed twice with ice-cold HBSS solution (5 mL). The treated Caco-2 and HT-29 co-cultured cells were then scraped off into a 2 mL microcentrifuge tube containing 1.0 mL extraction solution (10% Triton X-100) and sonicated to accelerate cell lysis. Furthermore, 25 μL of the cell lysates from each well were subjected to a BCA protein assay (Thermo Scientific, Waltham, MA, USA) to determine the amount of cell protein mentioned above. Then, cell lysates were centrifuged for 15 min at 14,000 rpm, and the supernatants were analyzed for the amount of cellular uptake TP5 using the RP-HPLC method mentioned above. The uptake of TP5 by Caco-2 and HT-29 co-cultured cells was calculated and expressed as the amount of drug (ng) uptake per μg cell protein.

2.3.6. Cellular Transport

Transwell Culture

Caco-2 and HT-29 co-cultured cells at a density of 10^5 cells/cm^2 were seeded on 12-well Insert Transwell® inserts (0.4 μm pore diameter, 1.1 cm^2 area, Corning, New York, NY, USA). Caco-2 and HT-29 co-cultured cells were incubated at 37 °C in an atmosphere of 5% CO_2 and 95% relative humidity in complete DMEM. The medium was replaced every 3 days with 0.5 mL medium on the apical (AP) side and 1.5 mL on the basolateral (BL) side, as shown in Figure 2. The integrity of the co-cultured cell monolayer was assessed by monitoring transepithelial electrical resistance (TEER). TEER measurements were conducted using a Millicell-ERS Volt-Ohm meter connected to a pair of chopstick electrodes (Millipore Corp, Boston, MA, USA). The electrodes, sterilized with 70% ethanol for 15 min and air-dried for 15 s, were immersed in a manner where the shorter electrode was on the AP side, and the more extended electrode was on the BL side, ensuring they did not come into contact with the cell monolayer. TEER measurements were taken at 3-day intervals until the TEER values surpassed 350 Ω·cm^2 (around 24 days post-seeding in this study). The TEER calculation utilized the formula TEER = (Rm − Rb) × A, where Rm, Rb, and A represent the measured TEER values, TEER values of the blank transwell, and the membrane surface area of the transwell (1.13 cm^2), respectively. Caco-2 monolayers with TEER values exceeding 350 $\Omega \cdot cm^2$ were deemed to have acceptable integrity and were considered suitable for the transport study.

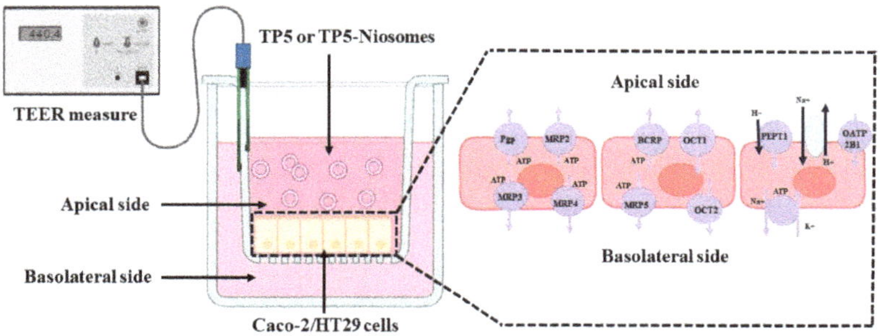

Figure 2. Schematic diagrams of transcellular transport and different transporters in Caco-2 and HT-29 co-cultured cell monolayers.

Transepithelial Transport of TP5 and TP5-PEG-Niosomes

Before the transport experiments, Caco-2 and HT-29 co-cultured cell monolayers underwent equilibration with HBSS for 30 min and were subsequently aspirated. All transport studies were carried out at 37 °C. A 0.5 mL solution of TP5 and TP5-PEG-niosomes (0.1 mg TP5 per mL in HBSS) was introduced on the AP side, while the BL side of the inserts contained 1.5 mL of HBSS, as depicted in Figure 2. At 0, 60, 120, 240, and 360 min of incubation, 200 μL was withdrawn from the BL-receiving chamber and immediately replaced with an equal volume of pre-warmed HBSS (37 °C). The concentration of TP5 in the transport medium was analyzed using RP-HPLC.

Cellular Transport Mechanism of TP5 and TP5-PEG-Niosomes

TP5 transport mechanisms were investigated in the absence or presence of variable inhibitors or enhancers. As shown in Figure 2, there were numerous transporters in Caco-2 cell transport. By considering both apical and basolateral sides, active transport inhibitor (10 to 20 mM sodium azide, Adenosine triphosphate (ATP) inhibitor), clathrin-mediated endocytosis inhibitor (10 to 20 μg/mL chlorpromazine), permeability glycoprotein (P-gp) inhibitor (50 to 100 μM verapamil), multidrug-resistance-associated protein 2 (MRP2) inhibitor (100–150 μM MK-571), multidrug-resistance-associated protein 5 (MRP5) inhibitor (20–40 μM Silymarin), tight junction opener (10–20 mM Sodium taurocholate) and absorption enhancer (5–10 mM EDTA) were selected to investigate the cellular transport mechanism, as shown in Table 1.

The concentration of these selected inhibitors and enhancers was screened by cytotoxicity using Caco-2 and HT-29 co-cultured cells by MTT assay. Then, these inhibitors and enhancers with safe concentrations were added to the AP side with a 0.5 mL 1 mg/mL solution of TP5 and TP5-PEG-niosomes, respectively. All inhibitors were dissolved in dimethyl sulfoxide and diluted with HBSS. The transport characteristics of TP5 and TP5-PEG-niosomes through Caco-2 and HT-29 co-cultured cell monolayers were expressed as the cumulative transported drug and transport rate. The transport rate (Flux) was denoted in μg/min/cm^2 and computed using the formula Flux = (dM/dt)/A, where dM/dt represents the cumulative amount of TP5 in the BL side per unit time (μg/min), and A is the surface area of the insert membrane (1.1 cm^2). The apparent permeability (Papp) coefficient was expressed in cm/s and calculated as $Papp$ = (dM/dt)/(60 × A × C), where C represents the initial concentration (1 mg/mL). The TEER values of the monolayers were assessed at 1 h intervals throughout the experimental duration, guaranteeing the integrity of the monolayers.

Table 1. Transporters and inhibitors in Caco-2 and HT-29 co-cultured cell monolayers.

Transporters	Inhibitors	Function	Refs.
Active transport	Sodium azide (10–20 mM)	Adenosine triphosphate (ATP) inhibitor	[26,27]
Clathrin-mediated endocytosis	Chlorpromazine (10–20 μg/mL)	Clathrin-mediated endocytosis efflux inhibitor	[28]
Caveolae-Permeability glycoprotein (P-gp)	Verapamil (50–100 μM)	Caveolae-mediated endocytosis efflux inhibitor	[29,30]
Multidrug resistance-associated protein 2 (MRP2)	MK-571 (100–150 μM)	Protein and peptide transport	[31]
Multidrug resistance-associated protein 5 (MRP5)	Silymarin (20–40 μM)	Protein and peptide transport	[32]
Transport enhancer	EDTA (5–10 mM)	Penetration enhancement	[33]
Transport enhancer	Sodium taurocholate (10–20 mM)	Open tight junction and enhance penetration	[34]

2.4. Data Analysis

Statistical analysis of in vitro cell studies was carried out using GraphPad Prism® version 8.0 software, while significance was determined using two-way ANOVA (p value < 0.05).

3. Results and Discussion

3.1. Analytical Method of TP5

Using the previously established analytical method to quantify the amount of TP5 in cell assays, a distinct peak with an adequate retention time was achieved [10]. The calibration curve, with an r^2 value exceeding 0.999, was established, and the corresponding standard equation (Equation (2)) applicable to the working concentration range of 5 to 100 μg/mL is provided below:

$$Y = 12.48X + 0.2054 \quad (2)$$

(Y represents the area under the curve of the HPLC chromatogram, and X signifies the concentration of the drug. This equation is utilized for the quantification of TP5 in subsequent investigations).

3.2. In Vitro Cell Culture Investigation

3.2.1. Cell Line Integrity

Caco-2 and HT-29 cells co-cultured at ratios of 1:0, 0:1, 1:1, 1:2, 1:3, 3:1, 5:1, 7:1, and 9:1 all displayed similar growth characteristics, reaching 80% confluence in x days (Figure 3). Layer integrity was assessed by TEER measurements every 3 days, and only TEER values exceeding 350 $\Omega\cdot cm^2$ were considered suitable for further study [35–37]. The TEER values of newly cultured Caco-2 and HT-29 cells in different ratios are shown in Table 2. It can be seen that Caco-2 and HT-29 cells with ratios of 1:0, 7:1, and 9:1 met the requirement of tissue integrity. Because of the benefits of the co-culture of Caco-2 and HT-29 cells, it provides the presence of both absorptive and goblet cells, both of which have different culture requirements for optimal growth and function to mimic intestine tissue in vivo [38–42]. Therefore, the ratio of 9:1 was selected based on the presence of both cell types and highest TEER value for subsequent uptake and transport studies.

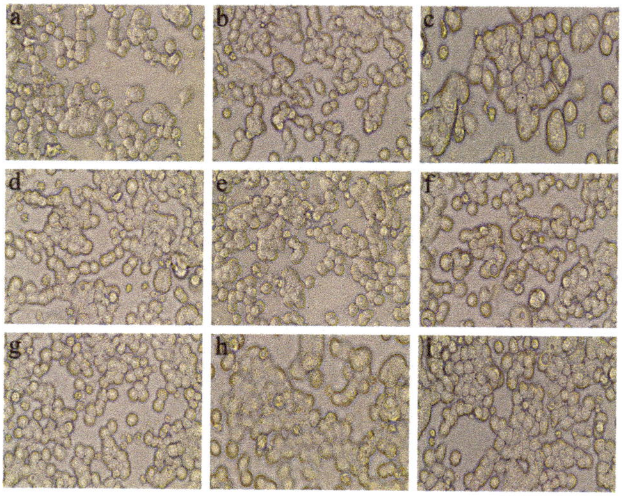

Figure 3. The micrographs of Caco-2 and HT-29 cells after 80% confluence with ratios of (**a**) 1:0, (**b**) 0:1, (**c**) 1:1, (**d**) 1:2, (**e**) 1:3, (**f**) 3:1, (**g**) 5:1, (**h**) 7:1, and (**i**) 9:1.

Table 2. The TEER values of Caco-2 and HT-29 cells after 2 weeks with ratios of (a) 1:0, (b) 0:1, (c) 1:1, (d) 1:2, (e) 1:3, (f) 3:1, (g) 5:1, (h) 7:1, and (i) 9:1 (Mean ± S.D. $n = 6$).

Caco-2/HT29 Ratio	TEER Values (Ω cm^2)
a: 1:0	480.8 ± 45.8
b: 0:1	172.5 ± 18.7
c: 1:1	341.7 ± 37.5
d: 1:2	180.9 ± 21.8
e: 1:3	228.4 ± 28.9
f: 3:1	288.2 ± 22.8
g: 5:1	335.5 ± 36.5
h: 7:1	361.4 ± 39.7
i: 9:1	457.3 ± 40.2

3.2.2. Cytotoxicity Study

Cytotoxicity studies were conducted to investigate the effect of drug and formulation composition on the cell viability of Caco-2 and HT-29 cells in the presence of each TP5 (1 mg/mL) formulation (TP5 solution and TP5-PEG-niosomes) and their respective controls for 72 h (Figure 4). It can be seen that the morphology of Caco-2 and HT-29 cells was similar in all conditions, indicating less cytotoxicity of TP5 formulations [43,44]. However, a quantitative measure was required, in which the MTT assay was also used to determine the cell viability with a wide range of concentrations of the drug and formulation.

As shown in Figure 5a, TP5 was not toxic at all in the tested concentrations. As the concentration increased, there was an increase in proliferation until reaching 5.000 mg/mL, followed by similar cell viability when the concentration reached 10.000 mg/mL. This indicates that non-cytotoxicity can be observed in all TP5 solutions at three different time intervals (24, 48, and 72 h). This is in correspondence with the results from the literature that TP5 is able to promote cell growth because TP5 can provide nutrition to Caco-2 and HT-29 cells due to its amino acid nature [43,44]. Cytotoxicity studies were also conducted to investigate the effect of formulation concentration on the cell viability of Caco-2 and HT-29 cells in the presence of TP5. Caco-2 and HT-29 cells were incubated with PEG-TP5-niosome of niosome numbers ranging from 0.01 to 10.00 × 10^{12} /mL for 24, 48, and 72 h, respectively. As shown in Figure 5b, PEG-niosomes were not toxic in most concentrations from 0.01 to

2.00×10^{12} /mL for 24, 48, and 72 h. As the niosome numbers increased, there was a light increase in cell growth until the niosomes' number reached 2.000×10^{12} /mL, followed by a decreased cell viability after the concentration reached 5.00×10^{12} /mL. It may be due to the weak toxicity of surfactants used in PEG-niosomes [45,46]. Because the higher numbers of niosomes contain a higher drug loading, the cellular uptake and transport of TP5 can be increased. Therefore, PEG-niosomes with a concentration under 2.00×10^{12} /mL provide a safety profile when treated on human Caco-2 and HT-29 cells according to the increased cell viability compared to the blank control group.

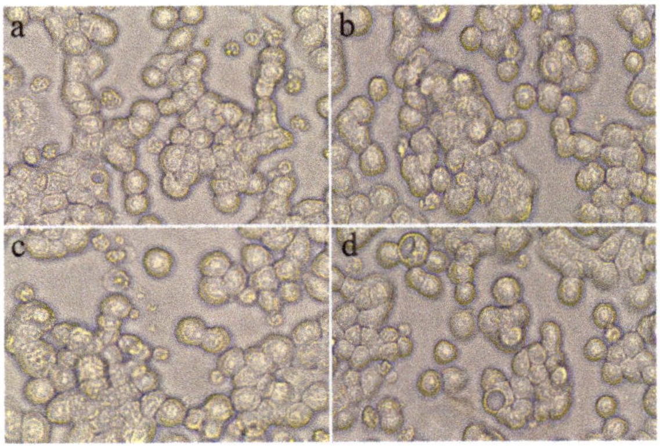

Figure 4. The micrographs of Caco-2 and HT-29 cells after 72 h, (**a**) Caco-2 and HT-29 cells without any TP5 formulations; (**b**) Caco-2 and HT-29 cells treated with TP5 solution; (**c**) Caco-2 and HT-29 cells treated with blank PEG-niosomes suspension; (**d**) Caco-2 and HT-29 cells treated with TP5-PEG-niosomes.

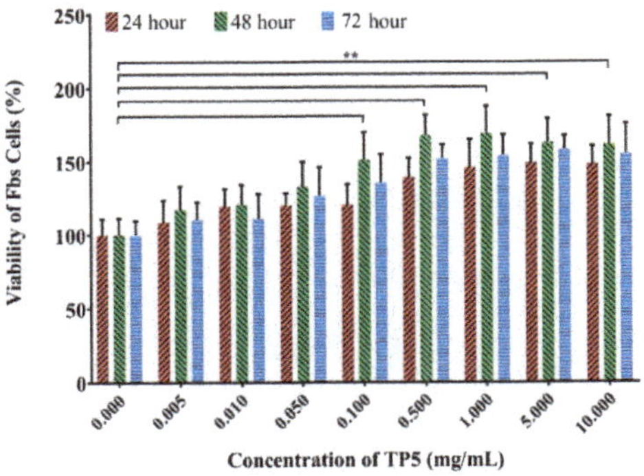

(**a**)

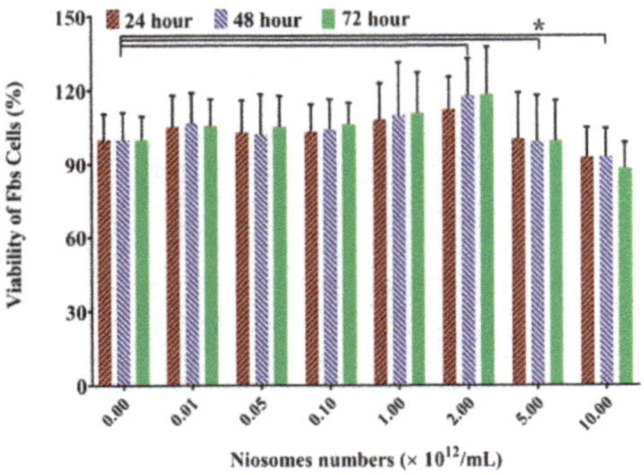

(**b**)

Figure 5. MTT viability assay showing the effect of TP5 formulations on co-cultured Caco-2 and HT-29 cells. (**a**) Effect of increasing TP5 concentrations in solution; (**b**) effect of increasing PEG-TP5-niosome concentrations. Cells were incubated with drug at 37 °C for 24, 48, and 72 h (p value < 0.05 * and 0.01 ** to control) (Mean ± S.D., n = 6).

3.2.3. Cellular Uptake

Fluorescence and Confocal Microscopy Analysis

TP5 was labeled with fluorescein isothiocyanate (FITC) [25]. The cellular uptake of FITC-TP5 by Caco-2 and HT-29 co-cultured cells after 0.5, 1, 2, and 3 h was visualized by fluorescence and confocal microscopy. As shown in Figures 6 and 7, the green fluorescence of FITC-TP5 was observed within cells after 0.5 h incubation at 37 °C, and continued to increase in cells until at least 3 h. Overlaying images of cell nuclei (blue) and cytoplasm (red) indicated that TP5 was found in the cytoplasm.

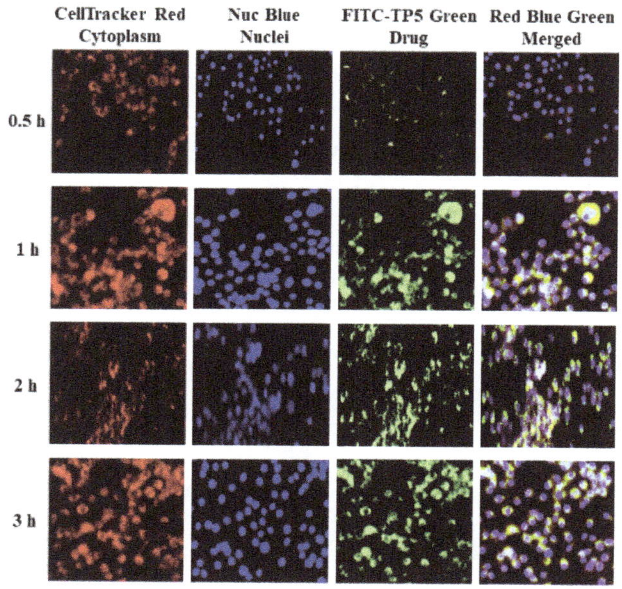

Figure 6. Fluorescence microscopy images of Caco-2 and HT-29 cells treated with FITC-TP5 (green) at 0.5, 1, 2, and 3 h in contrast to cell nuclei (blue), cytoplasm (red), and merged (green, blue, and red) (magnification = 500×).

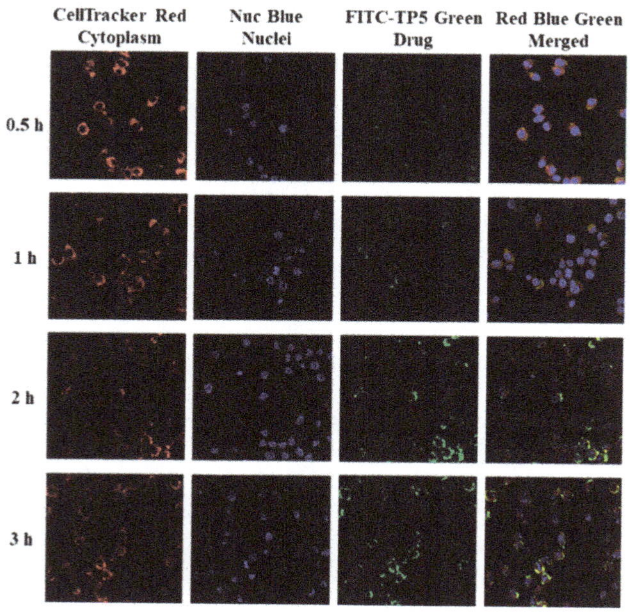

Figure 7. Confocal laser scanning microscopy 3D cross-section images of Caco-2 and HT-29 cells treated with FITC-TP5 (green) at 0.5, 1, 2, and 3 h in contrast to cell nuclei (blue), cytoplasm (red), and merged (green, blue, and red) (magnification = 500×).

The cellular uptake of FITC-TP5-PEG-niosomes by Caco-2 and HT-29 co-cultured cells was explored over a more extended period because of the controlled release profile of TP5 from PEG-niosomes. The cellular uptake at 0.5, 1, 2, 3, 4, and 5 h was visualized by fluorescence microscopy first and then by confocal microscopy analysis. As shown in Figures 8 and 9, the green fluorescence of FITC-TP5-PEG-niosomes was observed within cells after 0.5 h incubation at 37 °C in contrast to cell nuclei (blue) and cytoplasm (red), which, indicating TP5 from FITC-TP5-PEG-niosomes, were internalized into cells within 0.5 h and reached the highest concentration at 3 to 5 h because of the highest fluorescence intensity observed at this time point.

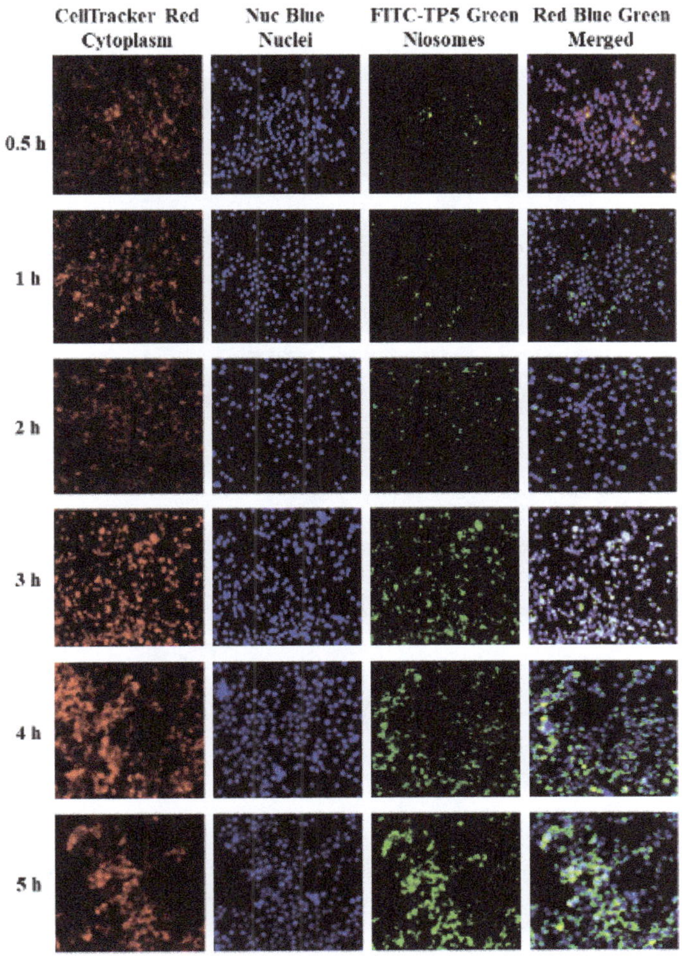

Figure 8. Fluorescence microscopy images of Caco-2 and HT-29 cells treated with FITC-TP5-PEG-niosomes (green) at 0.5, 1, 2, 3, 4, and 5 h in contrast to cell nuclei (blue), cytoplasm (red), and merged (green, blue, and red) (magnification = 500×).

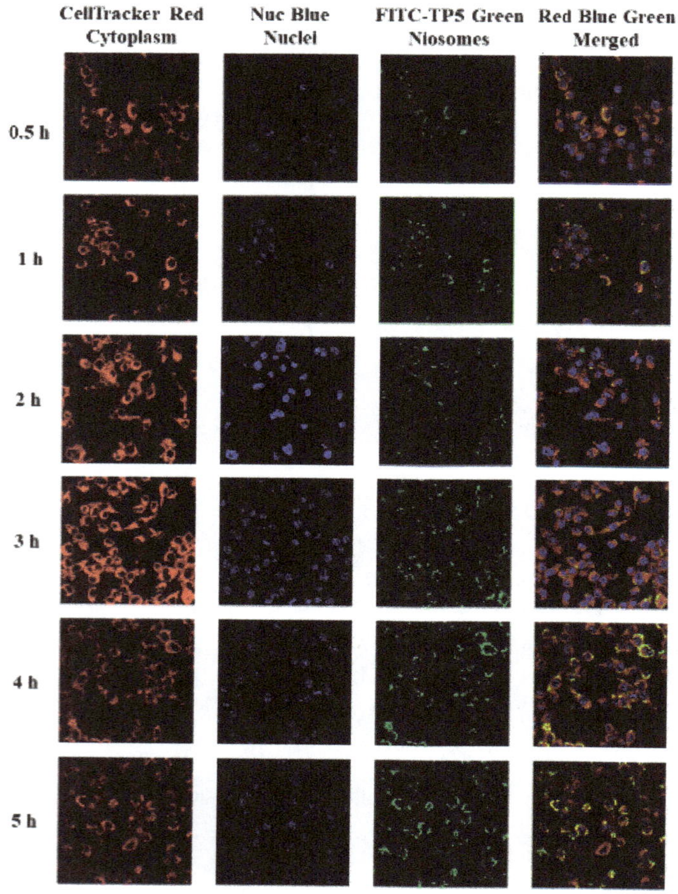

Figure 9. Confocal laser scanning microscopy 3D cross-section images of Caco-2 and HT-29 cells treated with FITC-TP5-PEG-niosomes (green) at 0.5, 1, 2, 3, 4, and 5 h in contrast to cell nuclei (blue), cytoplasm (red), and merged (green, blue, and red) (magnification = 500×).

It can be seen that the resolution and pixels improved when confocal laser scanning microscopy was used compared to fluorescence microscopy. Therefore, the intensity data from confocal laser scanning microscopy were selected to be analyzed by ImageJ™ software, version 1.5 (National Institutes of Health, Bethesda, MD, USA). As shown in Figure 10a, the cellular uptakes of FITC-TP5 solution and FITC-TP5-PEG-niosomes suspension were quantified by their fluorescence intensity obtained from the data of confocal laser scanning microscopy. The pure drug exhibited the highest intensity of cellular uptake at 2 h, whilst that of the niosomal formulation was observed at 4 h. This confirmed the controlled release profile of the designed formulation. Furthermore, there was also no significant difference after 3 h, indicating the optimized formulation has drug absorption in the intestine similar to that of a pure drug. This behavior emphasized the possibility of high intestinal permeability and effective drug absorption in the human digestive system [47].

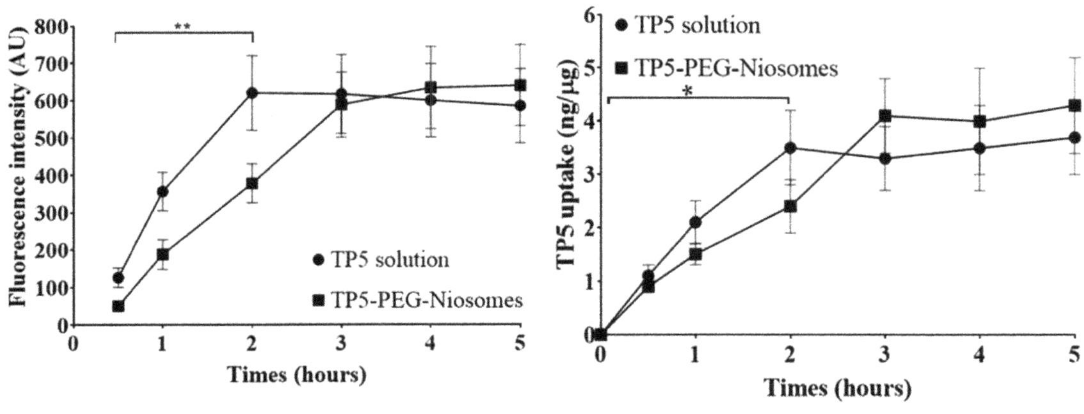

(a) (b)

Figure 10. (**a**) Fluorescence-intensity-derived cellular uptake of Caco-2 and HT-29 cells treated with FITC-TP5-PEG-niosomes (green) at 0.5, 1, 2, 3, 4, and 5 h; (**b**) HPLC and BCA quantitative cellular uptake of Caco-2 and HT-29 cells treated with FITC-TP5-PEG-niosomes (green) at 0.5, 1, 2, 3, 4, and 5 h (Mean ± S.D., $n = 3$) (0.05 * and 0.01 ** < 0.05).

Quantitative Analysis of the Cellular Uptake of TP5 and TP5-PEG-Niosomes

The cellular uptake was further investigated quantitatively by HPLC and BCA assay (Figure 10b). These results corresponded to the fluorescence-intensity-derived data, in which TP5 exhibited the highest amount of cellular uptake drug at 2 h, whilst that of the niosomal formulation was observed at 3 to 5 h. This further confirmed the time-dependent uptake of TP5 and TP5-PEG-niosomes by Caco-2 and HT-29 co-cultured cells. TP5 reached saturation/equilibrium after 2 h, whereas TP5-PEG-niosome uptake was slower. In detail, for pure drug solution, the cellular uptake value was increased to 3.56 ± 1.13 ng/µg in 2 h and maintained at this amount for the remaining hours. In the group of TP5-PEG-niosomes with the equivalent amount of 1 mg/mL TP5, the cellular uptake value steadily increased to 4.05 ± 0.94 ng/µg, and slightly increased to 4.58 ± 1.21 ng/µg. This longer cellular uptake of TP5-PEG-niosomes indicates the long circulating ability to reach the target area and therefore enhances the therapeutic effect on site [48].

Cellular Uptake Mechanisms of TP5 and TP5-PEG-Niosomes

As shown in Figure 11, the cellular uptake of TP5 was drug concentration and noisome concentration dependent from up to 1000 µg/mL TP5 and 5.00×10^{12} /mL the number of niosomes. Specifically, the TP5 cellular uptake value can reach 41.32 ± 10.33 ng/µg maximum when a dose of 1 mg/mL TP5 is given, whereas the TP5 cellular uptake value can be improved to 6.87 ± 1.23 ng/µg maximum when there are higher numbers of niosomes used for drug delivery. However, considering the safety issues (cytotoxicity studies of PEG-niosomes), a niosome number lower than 2.00×10^{12} /mL should be used for TP5 oral delivery.

To investigate whether active cellular uptake mechanisms were involved for TP5 and its formulation, inhibitors that block adsorptive-mediated endocytosis, clathrin-mediated endocytosis and caveolae-mediated endocytosis or a reduction in temperature were used. The results are shown in Figure 12.

The cellular uptake amount of TP5 was significantly reduced by using 1 mM protamine sulphate, in which the adsorptive-mediated endocytosis pathway was blocked ($p < 0.005$). This indicated that TP5 cellular uptake occurred primarily through adsorptive-mediated endocytosis. Interestingly, when the treatment was changed to a temperature of 4 °C, the cellular uptake amount of TP5 was also significantly decreased. It can be hypothesized that the cellular uptake of the TP5 solution is partially energy dependent, and both passive and active pathways were available for the pure drug of TP5. The results also suggested that TP5-PEG-niosomes were primarily taken up via the caveolae-mediated endocytosis pathways because the cellular uptake values significantly decreased when the pathways were blocked by 5 µg/mL filipin. Cellular uptake was also partially blocked by 10 µg/mL Chlorpromazine, indicating the involvement of clathrin-mediated endocytosis. This corresponds to the results of other studies in which lipid-based nanocarriers mainly follow caveolae- or clathrin-mediated endocytosis for cellular uptake in intestinal epithelial membranes [49–52].

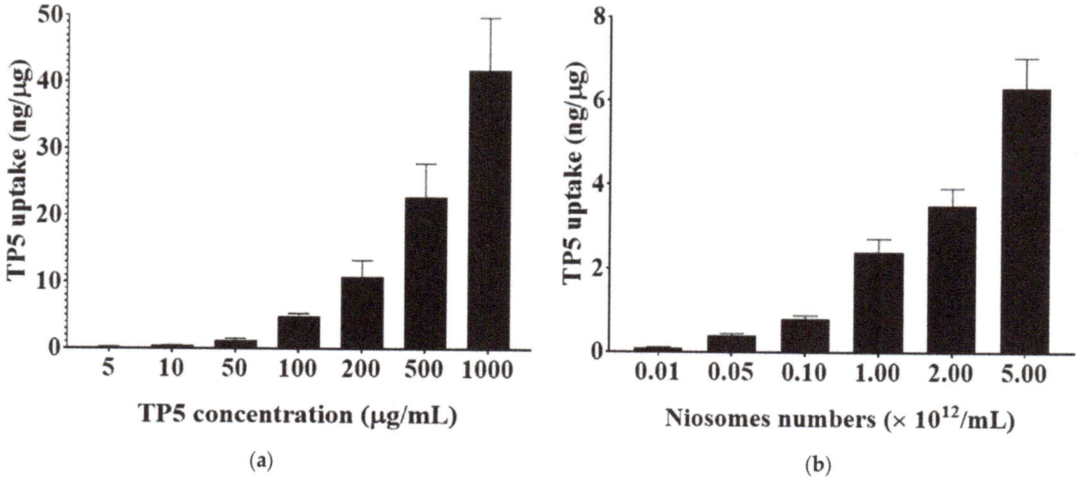

Figure 11. (**a**) The effect of TP5 concentration on TP5 cellular uptake values; (**b**) the effect of niosomes' concentration on TP5 cellular uptake values (mean ± S.D., n = 5).

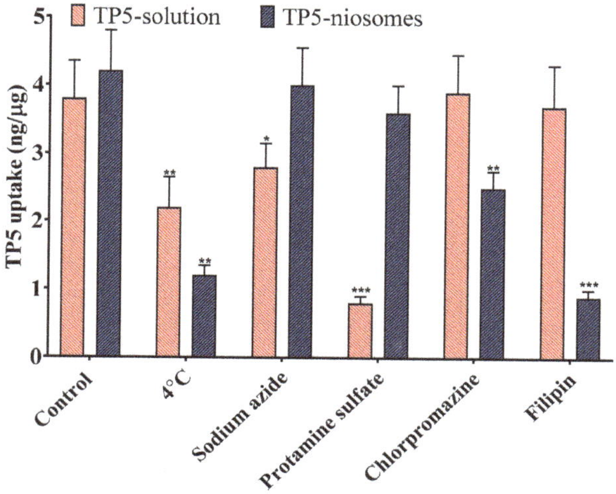

Figure 12. The effect of inhibitors and low temperature on TP5 and its formulation cellular uptake for 4 h on Caco-2 and HT-29 co-cultured cell monolayers (Mean ± S.D., n = 5; *** $p < 0.005$, ** $p < 0.01$, * $p < 0.05$ comparing to control).

In summary, the cellular uptake of the TP5 solution by Caco-2 and HT-29 co-cultured cells is concentration, time, and temperature dependent, and mainly follows adsorptive-mediated endocytosis and a partial passive pathway. The cellular uptake mechanism of TP5-PEG-niosomes is also concentration, time, and temperature dependent, but follows caveolae- or clathrin-mediated endocytosis pathways.

3.2.4. Cellular Transport

Transwell Culture and Cell Line Integrity

Caco-2 and HT-29 were co-cultured at a density of 10^5 cells/cm^2 onto 12-Well Insert Transwell® inserts (0.4 μm pore diameter, 1.1 cm^2 area, Corning, New York, NY, USA) with a ratio of 9:1. In order to determine the integrity of cell monolayers, the TEER measurements were performed at daily intervals for 3 days until the TEER values exceeded 350 Ω·cm^2 (after ~24 days post seeding in this study). As shown in Table 3, Caco-2 and HT-29 monolayers displayed the TEER values 408.2 ± 36.5 Ω cm^2 at testing day 1, 466.8 ± 29.8 Ω cm^2 at testing day 2, and 485.7 ± 66.8 Ω cm^2 at testing day 3, which were all above the 350 Ω·cm^2 required to meet intestinal integrity for transport studies [35–37].

Table 3. The TEER values of Caco-2 and HT-29 cells at 3-day intervals until the TEER values exceeded 350 Ω·cm^2 (Mean ± S.D. n = 6).

Caco-2 and HT-29	Test Day 1	Test Day 2	Test Day 3
TEER (Ω cm^2)	408.2 ± 36.5	466.8 ± 29.8	485.7 ± 66.8

Transepithelial Transport of TP5 and TP5-PEG-Niosomes

Prior to the cellular transport experiments, cumulative amount, flux, and the apparent permeability coefficient (*Papp*) values were investigated for pure drug solution, traditional niosome without PEGylation, and PEG-niosomes. As shown in Figure 13a, there is no significant difference in the cumulative amount of TP5 amongst the TP5 solution, TP5-niosomes, and TP5-PEG-niosomes. This indicates that TP5 niosomal formulation could reach the same cellular transport effect as the drug solution. The result of flux is shown in Figure 13b, in which all three groups reached the highest speed of 30×10^{-4} μg/min/cm^2 at 120 min, and the speed became stable for 6 h. As listed in Table 4, there is also no difference in *Papp* values between the TP5 solution and TP5-niosomes or TP5-PEG-niosomes. All three groups displayed high *Papp* values around 5×10^{-8} cm/s for transport compared with other peptides such as insulin [53–56]. This also emphasizes that TP5 formulations have a similar apparent permeability coefficient compared with the drug itself. Employing niosomal technology ensures equivalent drug transport rates as free drug solutions while safeguarding the drug against enzymatic degradation. This is attributed to the small molecular weight of TP5, which facilitates easier traversal across epithelial membranes, alongside its delicate fragile nature.

Table 4. *Papp* values of TP5 solution, TP5-niosomes, and TP5-PEG-niosomes from the apical to the basolateral chamber with 6 h transport study (Mean ± S.D., n = 6).

Formulations	TP5	TP5-Niosomes	TP5-PEG-Niosomes
Papp values (10^{-8} cm/s)	5.39 ± 0.46	4.69 ± 0.52	4.81 ± 0.19

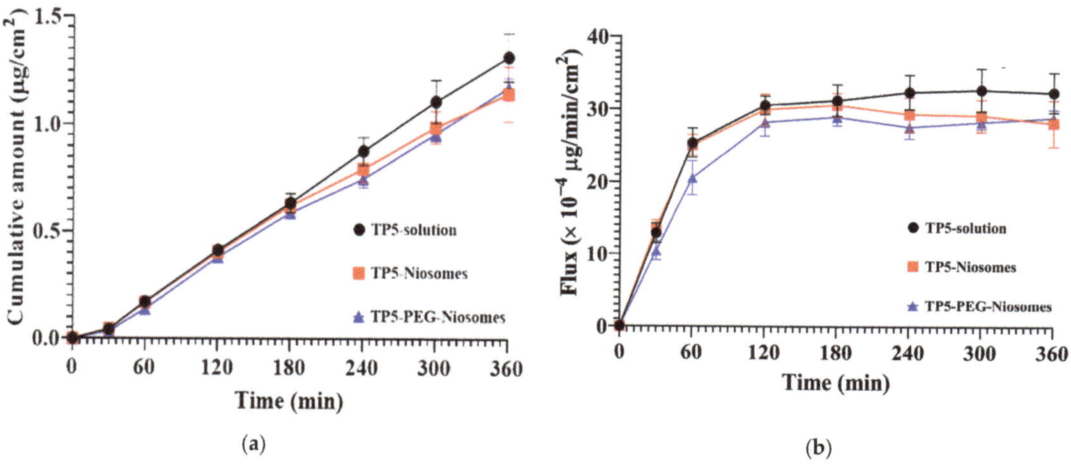

Figure 13. (**a**) Transepithelial transport of cumulative amount of TP5 from TP5 solution, TP5-niosomes, and TP5-PEG-niosomes; (**b**) transepithelial transport of flux rate of TP5 from TP5 solution, TP5-niosomes, and TP5-PEG-niosomes (Mean ± S.D., $n = 6$).

Cellular Transport Mechanism of TP5 and TP5-PEG-Niosomes

The effects of absorption inhibitors or enhancers on transport were investigated in this experiment to explore the TP5 cellular transport. In brief, active transport inhibitor (10–20 mM sodium azide), clathrin-mediated endocytosis inhibitor (10 to 20 µg/mL chlorpromazine), permeability glycoprotein (P-gp) inhibitor (50 to 100 µM verapamil), multidrug-resistance-associated protein 2 (MRP2) inhibitor (100–150 µM MK-571), multidrug-resistance-associated protein 5 (MRP5) inhibitor (20–40 µM Silymarin), tight junction opener (10–20 mM Sodium taurocholate), and absorption enhancer (5–10 mM EDTA) were selected to investigate cellular transport mechanism. However, the safety of these treatments should be investigated. The cytotoxicity of these inhibitors, transporters, and enhancers was evaluated before the transport studies. The result of cytotoxicity is shown in Figure 14a. It can be seen that the safe but still effective range concentrations for treatments were 20 mM sodium azide, 100 µM verapamil, 10 µg/mL chlorpromazine, 100 µM MK-571, 20 µM Silymarin, 10 mM EDTA, and 20 mM Sodium taurocholate. These concentrations were used for the cellular transport studies to investigate the cellular transport mechanism of TP5, TP5-niosomes, and TP5-PEG-niosomes.

The influence of absorption enhancers or inhibitors on the cumulative amount of TP5 drug solution is shown in Figure 14b. At the first 60 min, the TP5 cumulative amount was displayed similarly in all treatment groups. After that, both parameters tended to increase sharply in the EDTA and sodium taurocholate groups and a slight increase was observed in other groups. This indicates that EDTA and sodium taurocholate can work as transport enhancers to improve the TP5 cellular transport. Compared to the control group (drug solution only), when ATP inhibitor (20 mM sodium azide), MRP2 inhibitor (100 µM MK-571), and MRP5 inhibitor (silymarin) were added, the drug cumulative amount of TP5 was reduced. This indicates that TP5 cellular transport partially requires energy, and TP5 may have its own transporters or other peptide transporters on the apical and basolateral membranes of intestinal epithelial cells.

Compared to the drug solution, niosome displayed a lower cumulative amount and cellular transport results in the treatment of sodium azide and verapamil, as shown in Figure 15a. This indicates the cellular transport of niosome was based on caveolae-mediated endocytosis with the energy required. Similar to the drug solution, the cellular transport rate was significantly increased when EDTA and sodium taurocholate were used, showing a 2.8-fold and 2.4-fold enhancement, respectively.

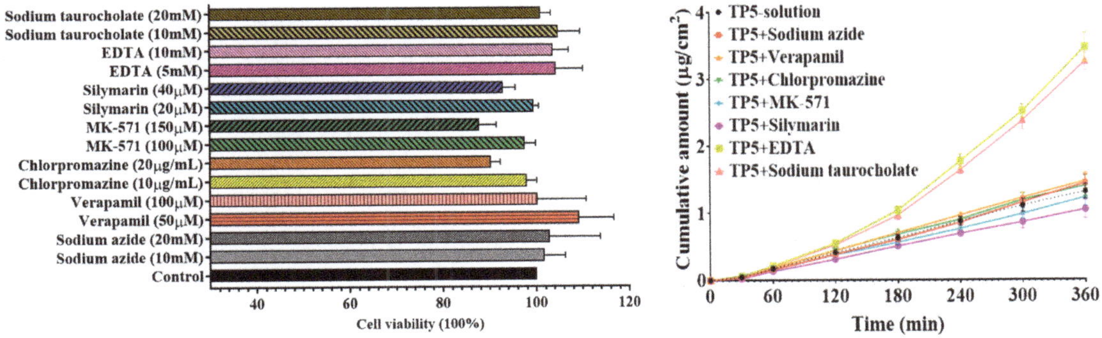

(a) (b)

Figure 14. (**a**) Effect of treatment concentrations on the Caco-2 and HT-29 cells' viability. Cells were incubated with different transporters, inhibitors, and enhancers at 37 °C for 72 h (Mean ± S.D., n = 6); (**b**) TP5 cumulative amount in the absence or presence of variable inhibitors and penetration enhancers for 6 h transport study at 37 °C (Mean ± S.D., n = 6).

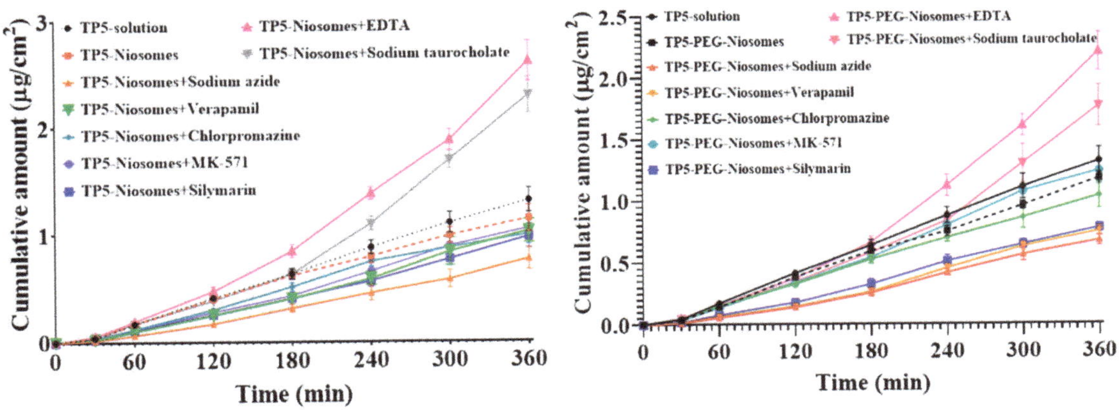

(a) (b)

Figure 15. (**a**) TP5 cumulative amount with or without niosomes in the absence or presence of variable inhibitors and penetration enhancers for 6 h transport study at 37 °C (Mean ± S.D., n = 6); (**b**) TP5 cumulative amount with or without PEG-niosomes in the absence or presence of variable inhibitors and penetration enhancers for 6 h transport study at 37 °C (Mean ± S.D., n = 6).

The influence of absorption enhancers or inhibitors on the cumulative amount of the TP5-PEG-niosome formulation was shown in Figure 15b. Compared to the drug solution, PEGylated niosome displayed a reduced cumulative amount and transport in the treatment of sodium azide, silymarin, and verapamil. This indicates the cellular transport of niosome was still based on caveolae-mediated endocytosis with the energy required. However, there is no significant difference amongst drug solution, niosomes, and PEG-niosomes without any treatments, which shows that the niosome formulation can reach the same cellular transport rate as the TP5 solution. Similar to previous findings, the TP5 cumulative amount can be enhanced by 2.6-fold and 2.1-fold when EDTA and sodium taurocholate are used, respectively.

The *Papp* values of TP5 in all conditions are shown in Table 5. It can be seen that the rank order of *Papp* values of TP5 solution is EDTA > sodium taurocholate >> verapamil > sodium azide > chlorpromazine > no treatment > MK571 > silymarin, and the values range from $4.30 \pm 0.55 \times 10^{-8}$ to $13.36 \pm 0.52 \times 10^{-8}$ cm/s. This shows that the main cellular transport mechanism of the pure drug solution is partially via multidrug-resistance-associated protein 5 transporter, an active endocytosis, and partially via passive transport. The rank order of *Papp* values of TP5-niosomes without PEGylation is EDTA > sodium taurocholate >> no treatment > MK571 > verapamil > chlorpromazine > silymarin > sodium azide, and the values range from $3.15 \pm 0.41 \times 10^{-8}$ to $10.73 \pm 0.77 \times 10^{-8}$ cm/s. This indicates that active cellular transport and clathrin-mediated endocytosis are the main cellular transport mechanisms, and using EDTA can largely improve drug transport efficacy. The rank order of *Papp* values of TP5-PEG-niosomes is EDTA > sodium taurocholate >> MK571 > no treatment > chlorpromazine > silymarin > verapamil > sodium azide, and the values range from $2.76 \pm 0.18 \times 10^{-8}$ to $9.05 \pm 0.64 \times 10^{-8}$ cm/s. Because of the controlled release profile, the *Papp* values in PEG-niosome group were reduced in most treatments compared to traditional niosomes and drug solutions. The lowest Papp value of $2.76 \pm 0.18 \times 10^{-8}$ cm/s in the sodium azide group emphasized that the PEG-niosome cellular transport required energy and may follow clathrin-mediated endocytosis for cellular uptake and cellular transport.

Table 5. *Papp* values of TP5, TP5-niosomes, and TP5-PEG-niosomes from the apical to the basolateral side after 6 h with different treatments (Mean ± S.D., $n = 6$) ($p < 0.01$ ** to no treatment control).

***Papp* Values**		**Formulations**	
(10^{-8} cm/s)	TP5	TP5-Niosomes	TP5-PEG-Niosomes
No treatment	5.39 ± 0.46	4.69 ± 0.52	4.81 ± 0.19
Sodium azide	5.90 ± 0.52	3.15 ± 0.41	2.76 ± 0.18 **
Verapamil	6.03 ± 0.51	4.21 ± 0.45	3.06 ± 0.16 **
Chlorpromazine	5.73 ± 0.63	4.09 ± 0.39	4.25 ± 0.43
MK571	5.04 ± 0.51	4.32 ± 0.51	5.07 ± 0.34
Silymarin	4.30 ± 0.55	4.00 ± 0.45	3.18 ± 0.15
EDTA	14.22 ± 0.89 **	10.73 ± 0.77 **	9.05 ± 0.64 **
Sodium taurocholate	13.36 ± 0.52 **	9.43 ± 0.69 **	7.24 ± 0.69 **

The transporters, namely clathrin-mediated transporter, P-gp, MRP2, and MRP5, are predominantly present on the apical and basolateral membranes of the intestinal epithelia [57–60]. These transporters play essential roles in impeding the absorption of drugs by facilitating their efflux from the gut epithelial cells back into the intestinal lumen, thus preventing their uptake into the bloodstream [61–63]. Hence, inhibiting the efflux pump could potentially augment the cellular transport of drugs into the cells. The primary mechanism leading to an increased concentration of TP5 in cellular transport studies was observed with the inhibition of MRP5. These results, in conjunction with research conducted by others, indicate that MRP5 predominantly influences the regulation of plasma concentrations for various peptide and protein drugs [64]. These results indicate that the penetration across Caco-2 and HT-29 monolayer was energy dependent, and an active cellular transport mechanism was involved. Compared with blank control (drug solution without niosomal formulations), the addition of P-gp inhibitor (100 μM verapamil) or active transport inhibitor (20 Mm sodium azide) caused a significant decrease in the Papp of PEG-niosomes from $5.39 \pm 0.46 \times 10^{-8}$ cm/s to $3.06 \pm 0.16 \times 10^{-8}$ cm/s and $2.76 \pm 0.18 \times 10^{-8}$ cm/s, respectively. This suggested that P-gp might play a significant role in the cellular transport of TP5-niosomes and TP5-PEG-niosomes on the Caco-2 and HT-29 cell membranes and showed energy dependence. The *Papp* values from AP to BL direction in all groups across Caco-2 and HT-29 monolayers exhibited a notable increase in the presence of sodium taurocholate or EDTA. This effect is typically presumed to impact tight junctions between adjacent epithelial cells by modulating paracellular permeability [65]. The process of enhancing the absorption of lipid particles may be elucidated by potentially reducing the extracellular calcium concentration (via the addition of EDTA) or by opening tight junctions of cell monolayers (in the presence of sodium taurocholate) [66–68]. This could result in increased fluidity of cell membranes, disturbance in protein structure across the membranes, and enhancement of the endocytosis pathway.

4. Conclusions

In this article, in vitro studies were conducted to investigate the cell cytotoxicity, cellular uptake, and cellular transport of TP5 solution, TP5-niosomes, and TP5-PEG-niosomes. This study showed a significant improvement regarding using a formulation strategy compared with a pure drug solution towards the cellular uptake and transport of TP5. The cytotoxicity of TP5 pure solution, TP5-niosomes, and TP5-PEG-niosomes on the growth of Caco-2 and HT-29 co-cultured cell lines was investigated using MTT assay. None of the three formulations showed any toxic effects (TP5 concentration: 0 to 10 mg/mL, and niosome numbers: 0 to 2.00×10^{12} /mL) on intestinal Caco-2 and HT-29 cells over three days. The cellular uptake of TP5-PEG-niosomes was based on active endocytosis, and was time, energy, and concentration dependent, which could remarkably improve the cell uptake of TP5. The cellular transport rate was similar in the TP5 solution, TP5-niosomes, and TP5-PEG-niosomes, indicating the formulation has no effect on the drug cellular transport rate. The cellular transport of TP5 occurs mainly through MRP5 endocytosis and a passive pathway and is effluxed by MRP5 transporters, while that of TP5-niosomes and TP5-PEG-niosomes is carried out through adsorptive- and clathrin-mediated endocytosis requiring energy. The permeability and cellular transport rate can be further enhanced when EDTA and sodium taurocholate are used as the penetration enhancers. Overall, the data obtained highlight the safety and feasibility of using PEGylated niosomes as a drug delivery system. This innovative formulation is expected to improve the stability of TP5 and enhance its permeability across intestinal epithelial membranes. Therefore, further studies are warranted to investigate its in vivo efficacy when administered orally for the treatment of immunodeficiency.

Author Contributions: Conceptualization, M.L. and J.W.; methodology, M.L. and J.W.; software, M.L. and J.W.; validation, M.L. and J.W.; formal analysis, M.L.; investigation, M.L. and J.W.; resources, D.S., T.P., J.L., Y.H. and J.W.; data curation, M.L. and J.W.; writing—original draft preparation, M.L. and J.W.; writing—review and editing, M.L., D.S., T.P., J.L., Y.H. and J.W.; visualization, M.L. and J.W.; supervision, D.S., T.P., J.L., Y.H. and J.W.; project administration, D.S., T.P., J.L., Y.H. and J.W.; funding acquisition, M.L., D.S., T.P., Y.H. and J.W. All authors have read and agreed to the published version of the manuscript.

Funding: This research was funded by the New Zealand Pharmacy and Education grant, grant number 332, and the Health Research Council of New Zealand (New Zealand-China Biomedical Research Alliance grant), grant number 21/815. The authors are thankful to the University of Auckland for awarding a Full Doctoral Scholarship to support this research work.

Institutional Review Board Statement: Not applicable.

Informed Consent Statement: Not applicable.

Data Availability Statement: Data are contained within the article.

Conflicts of Interest: The authors declare no conflicts of interest.

References

1. Ferreira, S.A.; Gama, F.M.; Vilanova, M. Polymeric Nanogels as Vaccine Delivery Systems. *Nanomed. Nanotechnol. Biol. Med.* **2013**, *9*, 159–173. [CrossRef]
2. Kim, Y.; Thapa, M.; Hua, D.H.; Chang, K. Biodegradable Nanogels for Oral Delivery of Interferon for Norovirus Infection. *Antivir. Res.* **2011**, *89*, 165–173. [CrossRef]
3. Tischio, J.P.; Patrick, J.E.; Weintraub, H.S.; Chasin, M.; Goldstein, G. Short in Vitro Half-Life of Thymopoietin 32-36 Pentapeptide in Human Plasma. *Int. J. Pept. Protein Res.* **1979**, *14*, 479–484. [CrossRef]
4. Garaci, C.R.; Torrisi, M.R.; Jezzi, T.; Frati, L.; Goldstein, A.L.; Garaci, E. Receptors for Thymosin Alpha 1 on Mouse Thymocytes. *Cell. Immunol.* **1985**, *91*, 289–293. [CrossRef]
5. Singh, V.K.; Biswas, S.; Mathur, K.B.; Haq, W.; Garg, S.K.; Agarwal, S.S. Thymopentin and Splenopentin as Immunomodulators—Current Status. *Immunol. Res.* **1998**, *17*, 345–368. [CrossRef]

6. Zhang, R.; Jiao, Q.; Wang, B. Controlled Clinical Study on 49 Patients of SARS Treated by Integrative Chinese and Western Medicine. *Zhongguo Zhong Xi Yi Jie He Za Zhi Chin. J. Integr. Tradit. West. Med.* **2003**, *23*, 654–657.
7. Ahlstrom, L.A.; Cross, S.E.; Mills, P.C. The Effects of Freezing Skin on Transdermal Drug Penetration Kinetics. *J. Vet. Pharmacol. Ther.* **2007**, *30*, 456–463. [CrossRef]
8. Shah, A.K.; Wei, G.; Lanman, R.C.; Bhargava, V.O.; Weir, S.J. Percutaneous Absorption of Ketoprofen from Different Anatomical Sites in Man. *Pharm. Res.* **1996**, *13*, 168–172. [CrossRef] [PubMed]
9. Nielsen, J.B.; Plasencia, I.; Sørensen, J.A.; Bagatolli, L.A. Storage Conditions of Skin Affect Tissue Structure and Subsequent in Vitro Percutaneous Penetration. *Skin. Pharmacol. Physiol.* **2011**, *24*, 93–102. [CrossRef] [PubMed]
10. Liu, M.; Svirskis, D.; Proft, T.; Loh, J.M.S.; Wen, J. Preformulation Studies of Thymopentin: Analytical Method Development, Physicochemical Properties, Kinetic Degradation Investigations and Formulation Perspective. *Drug Dev. Ind. Pharm.* **2022**, *47*, 1680–1692. [CrossRef] [PubMed]
11. Liu, M.; Sharma, M.; Lu, G.; Zhang, Z.; Yin, N.; Wen, J. Full Factorial Design, Physicochemical Characterization, Ex Vivo Investigation, and Biological Assessment of Glutathione-Loaded Solid Lipid Nanoparticles for Topical Application. *Int. J. Pharm.* **2023**, *630*, 122381. [CrossRef]
12. Liu, M.; Wen, J.; Sharma, M. Solid Lipid Nanoparticles for Topical Drug Delivery: Mechanisms, Dosage Form Perspectives, and Translational Status. *Curr. Pharm. Des.* **2020**, *26*, 3203–3217. [CrossRef] [PubMed]
13. Liu, M.; Chen, S.; Zhang, Z.; Li, H.; Sun, G.; Yin, N.; Wen, J. Anti-Ageing Peptides and Proteins for Topical Applications: A Review. *Pharm. Dev. Technol.* **2022**, *27*, 108–125. [CrossRef] [PubMed]
14. Li, D.; Martini, N.; Liu, M.; Falconer, J.R.; Locke, M.; Wu, Z.; Wen, J. Non-Ionic Surfactant Vesicles as a Carrier System for Dermal Delivery of (+)-Catechin and their Antioxidant Effects. *J. Drug Target.* **2021**, *29*, 310–322. [CrossRef] [PubMed]
15. Wang, L.; Zhang, Y.; Tang, X. Characterization of a New Inhalable Thymopentin Formulation. *Int. J. Pharm.* **2009**, *375*, 1–7. [CrossRef] [PubMed]
16. Wei, T.; Thakur, S.S.; Liu, M.; Wen, J. Oral Delivery of Glutathione: Antioxidant Function, Barriers and Strategies. *Acta Mater. Medica* **2022**, *1*, 177–192. [CrossRef]
17. Al Gailani, M.; Liu, M.; Wen, J. Ligands for Oral Delivery of Peptides Across the Blood-Brain-Barrier. *Acta Mater. Med.* **2022**, *1*, 106–123. [CrossRef]
18. Diwan, M.; Park, T.G. Pegylation Enhances Protein Stability during Encapsulation in PLGA Microspheres. *J. Control. Release* **2001**, *73*, 233–244. [CrossRef]
19. Perry, J.L.; Reuter, K.G.; Kai, M.P.; Herlihy, K.P.; Jones, S.W.; Luft, J.C.; Napier, M.; Bear, J.E.; DeSimone, J.M. PEGylated PRINT Nanoparticles: The Impact of PEG Density on Protein Binding, Macrophage Association, Biodistribution, and Pharmacokinetics. *Nano Lett.* **2012**, *12*, 5304–5310. [CrossRef]
20. Firozian, F.; Karami, S.; Ranjbar, A.; Azandaryani, M.T.; Nili-Ahmadabadi, A. Improvement of Therapeutic Potential N-Acetylcysteine in Acetaminophen Hepatotoxicity by Encapsulation in PEGylated Nano-Niosomes. *Life Sci.* **2020**, *255*, 117832. [CrossRef]
21. Ruhnau, J.; Parczyk, J.; Danker, K.; Eickholt, B.; Klein, A. Synergisms of Genome and Metabolism Stabilizing Antitumor Therapy (GMSAT) in Human Breast and Colon Cancer Cell Lines: A Novel Approach to Screen for Synergism. *BMC Cancer* **2020**, *20*, 617. [CrossRef]
22. Volpe, D.A. Advances in Cell-Based Permeability Assays to Screen Drugs for Intestinal Absorption. *Expert Opin. Drug Discov.* **2020**, *15*, 539–549. [CrossRef] [PubMed]
23. Yao, X.; Bunt, C.; Liu, M.; Quek, S.; Shaw, J.; Cornish, J.; Wen, J. Enhanced Cellular Uptake and Transport of Bovine Lactoferrin using Pectin- and Chitosan-Modified Solid Lipid Nanoparticles. *Pharmaceutics* **2023**, *15*, 2168. [CrossRef] [PubMed]
24. Liu, M.; Svirskis, D.; Proft, T.; Loh, J.; Chen, S.; Kang, D.; Wen, J. Exploring Ex Vivo Peptideolysis of Thymopentin and Lipid-Based Nanocarriers Towards Oral Formulations. *Int. J. Pharm.* **2022**, *625*, 122123. [CrossRef] [PubMed]
25. Zhang, L.; Wei, X.; Zhang, R.; Petitte, J.N.; Si, D.; Li, Z.; Cheng, J.; Du, M. Design and Development of a Novel Peptide for Treating Intestinal Inflammation. *Front. Immunol.* **2019**, *10*, 1841. [CrossRef]
26. Brunkard, J.O.; Xu, M.; Scarpin, M.R.; Chatterjee, S.; Shemyakina, E.A.; Goodman, H.M.; Zambryski, P. TOR Dynamically Regulates Plant Cell–cell Transport. *Proc. Natl. Acad. Sci. USA* **2020**, *117*, 5049–5058. [CrossRef]
27. Wan, S.; Zhang, L.; Zhang, X. An ATP-Regulated Ion Transport Nanosystem for Homeostatic Perturbation Therapy and Sensitizing Photodynamic Therapy by Autophagy Inhibition of Tumors. *ACS Cent. Sci.* **2019**, *5*, 327–340. [CrossRef]
28. Eom, H.; Choi, J. Clathrin-Mediated Endocytosis is Involved in Uptake and Toxicity of Silica Nanoparticles in Caenohabditis Elegans. *Chem. Biol. Interact.* **2019**, *311*, 108774. [CrossRef]
29. Yu, Q.; Liu, M.; Wu, S.; Wei, X.; Xiao, H.; Yi, Y.; Cheng, H.; Wang, S.; Zhang, Q.; Qin, Q.; et al. Specific Aptamer-Based Probe for Analyzing Biomarker MCP Entry into Singapore Grouper Iridovirus-Infected Host Cells via Clathrin-Mediated Endocytosis. *Front. Microbiol.* **2020**, *11*, 1206. [CrossRef] [PubMed]
30. Han, B.; Xie, W.; Zhang, Y.; Zhou, S.; Yang, J.; Wang, R.; Sun, Y.; Wang, X.; Xu, J.; Chen, D.; et al. The Influx/Efflux Mechanisms of D-Peptide Ligand of nAChRs Across the Blood–brain Barrier and its Therapeutic Value in Treating Glioma. *J. Control. Release* **2020**, *327*, 384–396. [CrossRef] [PubMed]

31. Selo, M.A.; Delmas, A.; Springer, L.; Zoufal, V.; Sake, J.A.; Clerkin, C.G.; Huwer, H. Tobacco Smoke and Inhaled Drugs Alter Expression and Activity of Multidrug Resistance-Associated Protein-1 (MRP1) in Human Distal Lung Epithelial Cells in vitro. *Front. Bioeng. Biotechnol.* **2020**, *8*, 1030. [CrossRef] [PubMed]
32. Xie, Y.; Zhang, D.; Zhang, J.; Yuan, J. Metabolism, Transport and Drug–Drug Interactions of Silymarin. *Molecules* **2019**, *24*, 3693. [CrossRef]
33. Jaradat, A.; Macedo, M.H.; Sousa, F.; Arkill, K.; Alexander, C.; Aylott, J.; Sarmento, B. Prediction of the Enhanced Insulin Absorption Across a Triple Co-Cultured Intestinal Model using Mucus Penetrating PLGA Nanoparticles. *Int. J. Pharm.* **2020**, *585*, 119516. [CrossRef] [PubMed]
34. Maruyama, M.; Nishida, Y.; Tanaka, H.; Minami, T.; Ogawara, K.; Miyake, M.; Takamura, Y.; Kakuta, H.; Higaki, K. Analysis of Absorption-Enhancing Mechanisms for Combinatorial use of Spermine with Sodium Taurocholate in Caco-2 Cells. *Eur. J. Pharm. Biopharm.* **2022**, *180*, 332–343. [CrossRef] [PubMed]
35. Yoshida, S.; Miwa, H.; Kawachi, T.; Kume, S.; Takahashi, K. Generation of Intestinal Organoids Derived from Human Pluripotent Stem Cells for Drug Testing. *Sci. Rep.* **2020**, *10*, 5989. [CrossRef]
36. Araujo, M.; Beekman, J.K.; Mapa, M.S.T.; MacMahon, S.; Zhao, Y.; Flynn, T.J.; Flannery, B.; Mossoba, M.E.; Sprando, R.L. Assessment of Intestinal Absorption/Metabolism of 3-Chloro-1,2-Propanediol (3-MCPD) and Three 3-MCPD Monoesters by Caco-2 Cells. *Toxicol. Vitr.* **2020**, *67*, 104887. [CrossRef]
37. Tremmel, M.; Kiermaier, J.; Heilmann, J. In Vitro Metabolism of Six C-Glycosidic Flavonoids from *Passiflora incarnata* L. *Int. J. Mol. Sci.* **2021**, *22*, 6566. [CrossRef]
38. Smit, B.; Chinaka, C.C.; Scott, A.A.; Gaiduschek, K.; Hatje, E.; Kuballa, A.; Coulson, S.; Finlayson, W.; Katouli, M. Efficacy of Selected Live Biotherapeutic Candidates to Inhibit the Interaction of an Adhesive-Invasive Escherichia Coli Strain with Caco-2, HT29-MTX Cells and their Co-Culture. *Biomedicines* **2022**, *10*, 2245. [CrossRef]
39. Lv, Q.; He, Q.; Wu, Y.; Chen, X.; Ning, Y.; Chen, Y. Investigating the Bioaccessibility and Bioavailability of Cadmium in a Cooked Rice Food Matrix by using an 11-Day Rapid Caco-2/HT-29 Co-Culture Cell Model Combined with an in Vitro Digestion Model. *Biol. Trace Elem. Res.* **2019**, *190*, 336–348. [CrossRef] [PubMed]
40. Lian, P.; Henricks, P.A.J.; Wichers, H.J.; Folkerts, G.; Braber, S. Differential Effects of Oligosaccharides, Antioxidants, Amino Acids and PUFAs on Heat/Hypoxia-Induced Epithelial Injury in a Caco-2/HT-29 Co-Culture Model. *Int. J. Mol. Sci.* **2023**, *24*, 1111. [CrossRef] [PubMed]
41. Lian, P.; Braber, S.; Varasteh, S.; Wichers, H.J.; Folkerts, G. Hypoxia and Heat Stress Affect Epithelial Integrity in a Caco-2/HT-29 Co-Culture. *Sci. Rep.* **2021**, *11*, 13186. [CrossRef] [PubMed]
42. Chen, X.; Elisia, I.; Kitts, D.D. Defining Conditions for the Co-Culture of Caco-2 and HT29-MTX Cells using Taguchi Design. *J. Pharmacol. Toxicol. Methods* **2010**, *61*, 334–342. [CrossRef] [PubMed]
43. Alagawany, M.; Elnesr, S.S.; Farag, M.R.; Tiwari, R.; Yatoo, M.I.; Karthik, K.; Michalak, I.; Dhama, K. Nutritional Significance of Amino Acids, Vitamins and Minerals as Nutraceuticals in Poultry Production and Health—A Comprehensive Review. *Vet. Q.* **2021**, *41*, 1–29. [CrossRef]
44. Guo, H.; Tong, Y.; Wang, H.; Zhang, J.; Li, Z.; Abbas, Z.; Yang, T.; Liu, M.; Chen, P.; Hua, Z.; et al. Novel Hybrid Peptide Cathelicidin 2 (1-13)-Thymopentin (TP5) and its Derived Peptides with Effective Antibacterial, Antibiofilm, and Anti-Adhesion Activities. *Int. J. Mol. Sci.* **2021**, *22*, 11681. [CrossRef]
45. Mitina, N.; Riabtseva, A.; Paiuk, O.; Finiuk, N.; Slouf, M.; Pavlova, E.; Kobylinska, L.; Lesyk, R.; Hevus, O.; Garamus, V.; et al. Molecular Design, Synthesis, and Properties of Surface-Active Comb-Like PEG-Containing Polymers and Derived Supramolecular Structures for Drug Delivery. In *Biomedical Nanomaterials*; Springer International Publishing: Cham, Switzerland, 2021; pp. 17–57.
46. Ogunjobi, J.K.; McElroy, C.R.; Clark, J.H.; Thornthwaite, D.; Omoruyi, O.E.; Farmer, T.J. A Class of Surfactants via PEG Modification of the Oleate Moiety of Lactonic Sophorolipids: Synthesis, Characterisation and Application. *Green Chem.* **2021**, *23*, 9906–9915. [CrossRef]
47. Zietek, T.; Giesbertz, P.; Ewers, M.; Reichart, F.; Weinmüller, M.; Urbauer, E.; Haller, D. Organoids to Study Intestinal Nutrient Transport, Drug Uptake and Metabolism—Update to the Human Model and Expansion of Applications. *Front. Bioeng. Biotechnol.* **2020**, *8*, 577656. [CrossRef]
48. Zhang, X.; Li, N.; Zhang, S.; Sun, B.; Chen, Q.; He, Z.; Luo, C.; Sun, J. Emerging Carrier-free Nanosystems Based on Molecular Self-assembly of Pure Drugs for Cancer Therapy. *Med. Res. Rev.* **2020**, *40*, 1754–1775. [CrossRef]
49. Li, J.; Zhang, Y.; Yu, M.; Wang, A.; Qiu, Y.; Fan, W.; Hovgaard, L.; Yang, M.; Li, Y.; Wang, R.; et al. The Upregulated Intestinal Folate Transporters Direct the Uptake of Ligand-Modified Nanoparticles for Enhanced Oral Insulin Delivery. *Acta Pharm. Sin. B* **2022**, *12*, 1460–1472. [CrossRef]
50. Wright, L.; Joyce, P.; Barnes, T.J.; Lundmark, R.; Bergström, C.A.S.; Hubert, M.; Prestidge, C.A. A Comparison of Chitosan, Mesoporous Silica and Poly(Lactic-Co-Glycolic) Acid Nanocarriers for Optimising Intestinal Uptake of Oral Protein Therapeutics. *J. Pharm. Sci.* **2021**, *110*, 217–227. [CrossRef]
51. Salah, E.; Abouelfetouh, M.M.; Pan, Y.; Chen, D.; Xie, S. Solid Lipid Nanoparticles for Enhanced Oral Absorption: A Review. *Colloids Surf. B Biointerfaces* **2020**, *196*, 111305. [CrossRef]
52. Arai, M.; Komori, H.; Fujita, D.; Tamai, I. Uptake Pathway of Apple-Derived Nanoparticle by Intestinal Cells to Deliver its Cargo. *Pharm. Res.* **2021**, *38*, 523–530. [CrossRef]

53. Clausen, A.E.; Kast, C.E.; Bernkop-Schnürch, A. The Role of Glutathione in the Permeation Enhancing Effect of Thiolated Polymers. *Pharm. Res.* **2002**, *19*, 602–608. [CrossRef]
54. Wingler, K.; Müller, C.; Schmehl, K.; Florian, S.; Brigelius-Flohé, R. Gastrointestinal Glutathione Peroxidase Prevents Transport of Lipid Hydroperoxides in CaCo-2 Cells. *Gastroenterology* **2000**, *119*, 420–430. [CrossRef]
55. Chen, L.; Lin, X.; Teng, H. Emulsions Loaded with Dihydromyricetin Enhance its Transport through Caco-2 Monolayer and Improve Anti-Diabetic Effect in Insulin Resistant HepG2 Cell. *J. Funct. Foods* **2020**, *64*, 103672. [CrossRef]
56. Ma, Z.; Lim, L.-Y. Uptake of Chitosan and Associated Insulin in Caco-2 Cell Monolayers: A Comparison between Chitosan Molecules and Chitosan Nanoparticles. *Pharm. Res.* **2003**, *20*, 1812–1819. [CrossRef]
57. Chen, X.; Wang, J.; Yang, Y.; Li, J.; Chen, Z. Natural Product as Substrates of ABC Transporters: A Review. *Recent Pat. Anti-Cancer Drug Discov.* **2021**, *16*, 222–238. [CrossRef]
58. Peng, Y.; Chen, L.; Ye, S.; Kang, Y.; Liu, J.; Zeng, S.; Yu, L. Research and Development of Drug Delivery Systems Based on Drug Transporter and Nano-Formulation. *Asian J. Pharm. Sci.* **2020**, *15*, 220–236. [CrossRef] [PubMed]
59. Mayati, A.; Moreau, A.; Le Vée, M.; Stieger, B.; Denizot, C.; Parmentier, Y.; Fardel, O. Protein Kinases C-Mediated Regulations of Drug Transporter Activity, Localization and Expression. *Int. J. Mol. Sci.* **2017**, *18*, 764. [CrossRef] [PubMed]
60. Pangeni, R.; Kang, S.; Jha, S.K.; Subedi, L.; Park, J.W. Intestinal Membrane Transporter-Mediated Approaches to Improve Oral Drug Delivery. *J. Pharm. Investig.* **2021**, *51*, 137–158. [CrossRef]
61. Azman, M.; Sabri, A.H.; Anjani, Q.K.; Mustaffa, M.F.; Hamid, K.A. Intestinal Absorption Study: Challenges and Absorption Enhancement Strategies in Improving Oral Drug Delivery. *Pharmaceuticals* **2022**, *15*, 975. [CrossRef] [PubMed]
62. Macedo, M.H.; Barros, A.S.; Martínez, E.; Barrias, C.C.; Sarmento, B. All Layers Matter: Innovative Three-Dimensional Epithelium-Stroma-Endothelium Intestinal Model for Reliable Permeability Outcomes. *J. Control. Release* **2022**, *341*, 414–430. [CrossRef]
63. Husain, A.; Makadia, V.; Valicherla, G.R.; Riyazuddin, M.; Gayen, J.R. Approaches to Minimize the Effects of P-glycoprotein in Drug Transport: A Review. *Drug Dev. Res.* **2022**, *83*, 825–841. [CrossRef]
64. Chambers, I.G.; Kumar, P.; Lichtenberg, J.; Wang, P.; Yu, J.; Phillips, J.D.; Kane, M.A.; Bodine, D.; Hamza, I. MRP5 and MRP9 Play a Concerted Role in Male Reproduction and Mitochondrial Function. *Proc. Natl. Acad. Sci. USA* **2022**, *119*, e21116171. [CrossRef] [PubMed]
65. Yang, D.; Zhang, Y.; Lei, J.; Li, S.; He, L.; Tang, D.; Xu, C.; Zhang, L.; Wen, J.; Lin, H.; et al. Discovery of Fused Benzimidazole-Imidazole Autophagic Flux Inhibitors for Treatment of Triple-Negative Breast Cancer. *Eur. J. Med. Chem.* **2022**, *240*, 114565. [CrossRef] [PubMed]
66. Chu, Y.; Zhu, Y.; Zhang, Y.; Liu, X.; Guo, Y.; Chang, L.; Yun, X.; Wei, Z.; Xia, Y.; Dai, Y. Tetrandrine Attenuates Intestinal Epithelial Barrier Defects Caused by Colitis through Promoting the Expression of Occludin via the AhR-miR-429 Pathway. *FASEB J.* **2021**, *35*, e21502. [CrossRef] [PubMed]
67. Ren, Y.; Wu, W.; Zhang, X. The Feasibility of Oral Targeted Drug Delivery: Gut Immune to Particulates? *Acta Pharm. Sin. B* **2022**, *13*, 2544–2558. [CrossRef] [PubMed]
68. Rao, R.; Liu, X.; Li, Y.; Tan, X.; Zhou, H.; Bai, X.; Yang, X.; Liu, W. Bioinspired Zwitterionic Polyphosphoester Modified Porous Silicon Nanoparticles for Efficient Oral Insulin Delivery. *Biomater. Sci.* **2021**, *9*, 685–699. [CrossRef]

pharmaceutics

MDPI

Article

Enhancing Oral Delivery of Biologics: A Non-Competitive and Cross-Reactive Anti-Leptin Receptor Nanofitin Demonstrates a Gut-Crossing Capacity in an Ex Vivo Porcine Intestinal Model

Solene Masloh [1,2,3,4], Anne Chevrel [2], Maxime Culot [1], Anaëlle Perrocheau [2], Yogeshvar N. Kalia [3,4], Samuel Frehel [2], Rémi Gaussin [2], Fabien Gosselet [1], Simon Huet [2,*], Magali Zeisser Labouebe [3,4,*] and Leonardo Scapozza [3,4]

1 Blood Brain Barrier Laboratory, Faculty of Science Jean Perrin, Artois University, UR 2465, Rue Jean Souvraz, 62300 Lens, France; maxime.culot@univ-artois.fr (M.C.); fabien.gosselet@univ-artois.fr (F.G.)

2 Affilogic, 24 Rue de la Rainière, 44300 Nantes, France; anaelle@affilogic.com (A.P.); remi@affilogic.com (R.G.)

3 School of Pharmaceutical Sciences, University of Geneva, 1 Rue Michel Servet, 1201 Geneva, Switzerland; leonardo.scapozza@unige.ch (L.S.)

4 Institute of Pharmaceutical Sciences of Western Switzerland, University of Geneva, 1 Rue Michel Servet, 1201 Geneva, Switzerland

* Correspondence: simon@affilogic.com (S.H.); magali.zeisser@unige.ch (M.Z.L.)

Abstract: Biotherapeutics exhibit high efficacy in targeted therapy, but their oral delivery is impeded by the harsh conditions of the gastrointestinal (GI) tract and limited intestinal absorption. This article presents a strategy to overcome the challenges of poor intestinal permeability by using a protein shuttle that specifically binds to an intestinal target, the leptin receptor (LepR), and exploiting its capacity to perform a receptor-mediated transport. Our proof-of-concept study focuses on the characterization and transport of robust affinity proteins, known as Nanofitins, across an ex vivo porcine intestinal model. We describe the potential to deliver biologically active molecules across the mucosa by fusing them with the Nanofitin 1-F08 targeting the LepR. This particular Nanofitin was selected for its absence of competition with leptin, its cross-reactivity with LepR from human, mouse, and pig hosts, and its shuttle capability associated with its ability to induce a receptor-mediated transport. This study paves the way for future in vivo demonstration of a safe and efficient oral-to-systemic delivery of targeted therapies.

Keywords: biotherapeutics; permeability; shuttle; leptin receptor; Nanofitins; ex vivo; porcine intestinal model; receptor-mediated transport; oral-to-systemic delivery

1. Introduction

Recombinant biological molecules, the powerful pioneers of modern medicine, referred to as biologics—encompassing entities such as antibodies, proteins, and peptides—constitute the very backbone of contemporary medical treatments [1–3]. However, unlike conventional small-molecule drugs commonly administered orally [4], they are mostly limited to parenteral injections mainly due to their sensitivity to protease degradation and their limited passive diffusion through the intestinal barrier [1]. Specifically, the poor permeability of biologics across the intestinal barrier is attributed to the presence of tight junctions at the border of intestinal epithelial cells which hinder their paracellular transport [5], as well as to the enzymes and transporters expressed by these cells which limit their transcellular passage to specific active mechanisms [6–9]. While the stability in the GI tract of biologics can be solved by gastro-resistant formulation, enabling the permeability of biologics through the intestinal barrier remains a critical factor in achieving successful oral-to-systemic delivery of targeted biologics-based therapies.

Harnessing the active translocation mechanisms employed by receptors for biomolecule passage through biological barriers has shown promise for drug transport in preclinical studies, particularly across the blood–brain barrier (BBB) that isolates the brain from the bloodstream [10–12]. This strategy, known as molecular trojan horse or receptor-mediated transcytosis (RMT), involves targeting various receptors of natural ligands, including the transferrin receptor [13,14], the low-density lipoprotein receptor [14,15], and the insulin receptor [12,16], which can trigger the internalization and transport of their natural ligand across biological barriers. Adopting a similar strategy to facilitate the translocation of biologics across the intestinal barrier could enable their systemic delivery after oral administration.

Several receptors, including the neonatal Fc receptor [17,18] and LepR [19,20], have been partially characterized for their involvement in the active transport of protein-based ligands across the intestinal epithelium, despite the scarcity of information available in this field. The LepR, a member of the class I cytokine receptor family, exists in various isoforms resulting from alternative splicing [21,22] (long, short, or secretory). The membrane-bound isoforms share common extracellular and transmembrane domains, whereas their intracellular regions differ in size and amino-acid sequence. They have an identical affinity for the leptin since the ligand-binding region is located on the shared extracellular segment [23]. Evidence suggests that LepR facilitates a specific, saturable, and energy-dependent process for the transcytosis of leptin across the intestinal barrier [19,24]. Leptin interacts with the extracellular domain of the receptor present on the apical membrane of enterocytes and is internalized by the cells through their endosomal compartments. The leptin-LepR complex is then packaged and discharged on the basolateral membrane to reach the blood circulation across the capillary endothelial cells [24]. Given its biological significance, LepR presents itself as a compelling receptor for RMT.

Our present strategy to enhance the transport of biologics across the intestinal barrier relies on Nanofitins targeting the LepR (anti-LepR Nanofitins), which offer a combination of protein robustness, modularity, and tunable specificity. These small single-chain binding proteins of 7 kDa, devoid of cysteine residues, are derived from the naturally hyper thermostable protein Sac7d [25,26], or more generally from the Sul7d family [27]. They can be custom-engineered for high specificity and affinity toward a target, as already demonstrated against a variety of biological targets [28–31]. Importantly, they maintain the stability of their parental protein, including resistance to extreme pH levels (pH 1–13) and the harsh intestinal environment [28]. With their N- and C-termini located on opposite faces of their binding site, they can be easily assembled to a cargo molecule, either via chemical conjugation or genetic fusion, while preserving their individual properties [32].

In this proof-of-concept study, we investigate the potential of employing a delivery strategy based on anti-LepR Nanofitins as molecular shuttles to enhance the transport of biologics through the intestine. In vitro, our approach involved developing Nanofitins targeting the LepR. The target product profile included non-competition with the leptin binding to its receptor, aimed at improving safety by minimizing competition with endogenous ligands, and cross-reactivity with receptors from human, mouse, and pig hosts to suit relevant ex vivo and in vivo preclinical models. Ex vivo, we successfully demonstrated the potential of an anti-LepR Nanofitin candidate as an efficient carrier for transporting functional cargo proteins across the intestinal barrier, suggesting the potential of the NF scaffold for application in oral biologics delivery strategies.

2. Materials and Methods

2.1. Reagents

Horseradish peroxidase(HRP)-conjugated RGS-His antibody used for detection of Nanofitins was part of a detection kit from Qiagen (Hilden, Germany, cat. no. 34460). Rabbit monoclonal antibody against the LepR (cat. no. MA5-35247) and goat anti-rabbit secondary antibody (cat. no. 35565) used for Western blot were purchased from Thermo Fischer Scientific (Waltham, MA, USA). Pierce™ protein-free blocking buffer (cat. no. 37585), 3,3′,5,5′-tétraméthylbenzidine (TMB) for ELISA revelation (cat. no. 34022), Pierce Bicinchoninic acid (BCA) protein assay kit used to determine concentrations of lysates or fluorescently labeled Nanofitins (cat. no. 23225),

DMEM with GlutaMAX™ Supplement (cat. no. 10566016), fetal calf serum (cat. no. 16010167), penicillin–streptomycin (cat. no. 15140122), and finally, the lipofectamine™ 2000 used for transfections (cat. no. 11668019) were also from Thermo Fischer Scientific. Recombinant human leptin (cat. no. 398-LP), recombinant human LepR (rhLepR), and recombinant mouse LepR (rmLepR) (cat. no. 389-LR-100/CF and cat.no. 497-LR-100/CF), the last two being expressed as a Fc fusion, were from R&D systems (Minneapolis, MN, USA), as well as the Alexa-Fluor 647-conjugated anti-LepR antibody (cat. no. FAB867P) and the Alexa-fluor 647-conjugated anti-His-tag antibody (cat. no. IC0501R) used for cellular assays. N-(5-Fluoresceinyl)-maleimide, human serum albumin (HSA, cat. no. SRP6182), phosphatase (cat. no P2850 and cat. no P5726)/protease (cat. no P8340) inhibitor cocktails, and Sera-mag SpeedBeads Protein A/G (cat. no. GE17152104010150) were obtained from Sigma-Aldrich (St.-Louis, MO, USA). HepG2 (cat. no. ab166833), HEK293 (cat. no. ab7902)m and HeLa (cat. no. ab150035) cell lysates were from Abcam (Cambridge, United Kingdom). Finally, the accutase solution (cat. no. SCR005) for cellular assays and the BugBuster® Protein Extraction Reagent (cat. no. 70584) were obtained from Merck (Kenilworth, NJ, USA).

2.2. In Vitro Selection by Ribosome Display and Preliminary Screening

2.2.1. In Vitro Selection by Ribosome Display

A combinatorial library of Nanofitins was generated following the protocol described in the literature with minor modifications [25,33]. In brief, the library was prepared with two successive overlapping PCRs using degenerated oligonucleotides at randomized positions encoded by trimer codons of naturally occurring amino acids (except cysteine). The 5′- and 3′-flanking regions necessary for the in vitro technique were then supplemented with a final PCR [34]. After the amplification of the library, a transcription was realized to start the in vitro selection process.

The ribosome display procedure was performed at 4 °C, following the protocol described by Mouratou et al. [25,33], with the rhLepR chimera (recombinant extracellular domain of the hLepR fused to the Fc portion of human IgG1) as the target of interest. The target was not biotinylated as described in the initial protocol since we took advantage of the Fc fusion to perform an immobilization on protein A beads. Four rounds of selection have been performed to isolate high affinity binders. The intensive washing was gradually increased to apply a higher selection pressure (round 1: eight washes of 20 s; round 2: eight washes of 3 min; round 3: eight washes of 15 min; and round 4: four washes of 15 min followed by four washes of 30 min).

2.2.2. Isolation of Clones

The amplified DNA sequences recovered from the last round of selection were cloned between BamHI and HindIII restriction sites in a modified pQE-30 expression vector (Qiagen, Hilden, Germany) called pAFG12. The cloning of the DNA material inside this plasmid enabled the expression of Nanofitins with *Aequorea coerulescens* green fluorescent protein (acGFP) fused at their C-terminus using the linker sequence GSAGSAAGSGEF. *Escherichia coli* DH5α LacIq strain (Invitrogen, Waltham, MA, USA) was then transformed with the ligation mixtures using the manufacturer's protocol. Following bacteria transformation, 95 fluorescent clones selected on yeast extract tryptone (2YT)-agar plates with ampicillin (100 μg/mL) and kanamycin (25 μg/mL) were picked and seeded into a 96-deep-well plate filled with 0.75 mL of 2YT medium complemented with antibiotics and 1% glucose in each well. After an overnight culture at 37 °C under shaking (600 rpm), 200 μL of each culture were used to inoculate in mirror another 96-deep-well plate containing 1.25 mL of 2YT medium supplemented with ampicillin (100 μg/mL), kanamycin (25 μg/mL), and 0.1% glucose. Also, 10 μL of the same precultures were deposed on a 96-well agar plate with ampicillin at 100 μg/mL for sequencing using the oligo Qe30_for CTTTCGTCTTCACCTCGA (Plateseq Service, Eurofins). The deep-well plate was incubated during 3 h at 37 °C and 600 rpm before the addition of 50 μL of IPTG to reach a concentration of 0.5 mM (isopropyl β-D-1-thiogalactopyranoside, Sigma-Aldrich, cat. no. I5502) used to induce the expression of Nanofitins. This step was followed by another incubation under shaking (600 rpm) at 30 °C for 4 h. After induction, cells were pelleted via a centrifugation of 20 min at 2000× *g* and the supernatants were discarded. Then, Nanofitins were extracted via cell lysis with 100 µL/well of BugBuster protein extraction reagent (Novagen, Madison, WI, USA, cat. no. 70584) for 1 h at room temperature (RT). Finally, 350 µL of tris-buffered saline (TBS, 20 mM Tris-HCl, 150 mM NaCl, pH 7.4) were added and cell debris were pelleted by 20 min of centrifugation at 2000× *g*. The supernatants were used to perform a first screening of Nanofitins generated against the rhLepR.

2.2.3. Preliminary Screening by ELISA

Enzyme-linked immunosorbent assays (ELISA) were performed according to standard protocols. Briefly, rhLepR diluted at 5 µg/mL in TBS (100 µL/well) was immobilized on 96-well flat-bottomed Nunc MaxiSorp plates (Thermo Fischer Scientific) incubated at 4 °C overnight or 1 h at RT. Plates were then washed 3 times with TBS (300 µL/well) and blocked for 1 h at RT under shaking (600 rpm) with 300 µL/well of TBS-bovine serum albumin 0.5% (*w*/*v*) (BSA, Sigma-Aldrich). Each of the following steps (except revelation) was followed by an incubation of 1 h at RT and 4 washes with TBS-Tween 20 0.1% (TBST). After the blocking, 100 µL of crude *E. coli* extracts were added to the wells with or without the immobilized target. In order to detect specific binding of Nanofitins, an HRP-conjugated RGS-His antibody diluted 4000 times in TBST was used. The revelation was performed 1 h later with TMB (3,3′,5,5′-tetramethylbenzidine) and stopped after 5 min with the addition of H_2SO_4 solution (2 N, 50 µL/well). Finally, absorbance was measured at 450 nm on a Varioskan ELISA plate reader (Thermo Fischer Scientific).

2.3. *Production of Nanofitins*

Following four rounds of ribosome display, the most relevant anti-LepR Nanofitins were selected for subsequent investigations. This selection was based on an analysis of the sequences of the isolated clones and a preliminary screening of their affinity for the rhLepR. Plasmids coding for the most interesting candidates were ordered from Genscript (Piscataway, NJ, USA), performing gene synthesis and subcloning into a pet21a(+) vector between the NdeI/BlpI cloning site. The same approach for the Nanofitin fusions was undertaken with Genscript: gene synthesis of Nanofitin (NF1) and Nanofitin (NF2) linked by a nucleotide sequence coding for a $(G_4S)_2$ linker between NF1 and NF2 and subsequent subcloning. All protein constructs carry an RGS-His_6 tag at the C-termini of the construct. Also, the most interesting candidates chosen to perform the ex vivo study following the characterization, as well as the Nanofitin fusions, carry a unique cysteine at the N-termini of the construct to be able to perform a regioselective conjugation to a fluorescent marker. Nanofitins were expressed in BL21 Gold (DE3) strain of *E. coli* (Agilent technologies, Santa Clara, CA, USA) following a bacterial transformation. Their precultures, grown at 37 °C overnight in 2YT medium with ampicillin (100 µg/mL), tetracyclin (5 µg/mL), and 1% of glucose (*w*/*v*), were diluted 20 times in a similar medium with glucose at 0.1% (*w*/*v*). Cultures were then incubated at 37 °C until the mid-log phase. Once optical density at 600 nm reached 0.8 to 1, Nanofitins expression was triggered by addition of IPTG at 0.5 mM for 4 h at 30 °C. After 45 min of centrifugation at 3220× *g*, pelleted cells were resuspended in a lysis buffer (1× BugBuster Protein Extraction Reagent, 5 µg/mL DNaseI, 20 mM Tris, 500 mM NaCl, 25 mM imidazole, pH 7.4) at RT during 15 min under stirring. Following this lysis, another centrifugation of 45 min was carried out to eliminate cell debris. The His-tagged Nanofitins from the supernatants were then filtered (0.45 µm) and purified on an immobilized metal ion affinity chromatography using HisTrap HP column (Cytiva, Marlborough, MA, USA) or bulk Ni-NTA resin (Ozyme, 635660). Finally, Nanofitins were eluted with a buffer composed of 20 mM Tris, 500 mM NaCl, and 500 mM of imidazole, pH 7.4. Concentrations of the Nanofitins were determined from absorbance at 280 nm with a Biospectrometer (Eppendorf, Hamburg, Germany).

2.4. Biochemical Characterization of Nanofitins

2.4.1. Binding Assays: Determination of the Affinity, Kinetics of Interaction, and the Competition Profile with Leptin

ELISA

ELISAs were performed according to the protocol described in Section 2.3. Either rhLepR (5 µg/mL), rmLepR (5 µg/mL), or HSA (2.5 µg/mL), diluted in TBS, were immobilized on 96-well flat-bottom Nunc MaxiSorp plates (Thermo Fischer Scientific). The blocking step was performed with Pierce™ Protein-Free (TBS) Blocking Buffer when the plates were coated with HSA. EC_{50} were determined by adding 100 µL/well of purified Nanofitins from 10^{-12} to 10^{-5} M after the blocking step, with 10-fold dilutions, with or without the immobilized target. Binding curves were fitted following the measurement of the absorbance at 450 nm on a Varioskan plate reader, and EC_{50} were calculated using GraphPad Prism 7.0 software (GraphPad Software, Inc., San Diego, CA, USA).

Competition experiments with the natural ligand were performed with purified Nanofitins at their maximum concentration, providing a linear ELISA signal (from 2 nM for the best affinities, to 5 µM for weaker binders) with leptin at 100 nM.

This methodology has also been used to evaluate the binding activity of Nanofitins after ex vivo transport experiments. Samples recovered from these assays were applied instead of the purified Nanofitins. The Nanofitin solutions of the initial donors (solutions in the donor chambers at the beginning of the experiments) were diluted at the same concentrations than the Nanofitins solutions recovered from the serosal chambers (receivers) after 120 min: 1000 and 660 times, respectively, for 1-F08 and 1-F08-NF2. For the dimeric construct, samples were tested separately against immobilized rhLepR and HSA.

Binding Kinetics Assays by Bio-Layer Interferometry

Additional characterization of Nanofitins interactions with the rhLepR was performed by bio-layer interferometry (BLI) on Octet RED96 system (ForteBio, Fremont, CA, USA). Prior to the experiments, protein A biosensors (ForteBio, cat. no. 18-5010) were rehydrated for 10 min in a 96-well plate filled with 200 µL of TBS and equilibrated in TBS-BSA 0.01%-Tween 20 0.002%. Unless specified, all steps were performed in this latter buffer. Biosensors were then functionalized with rhLepR diluted at 5 µg/mL until the threshold of 1 nm was reached. After an equilibration of 60 s in the buffer, associations were measured by exposing the sensors to a concentration range of Nanofitins (333, 111, 37, 12.3, 4.1, and 1.4 nM) alongside a condition without Nanofitin used as reference. For each protein, the sequence of association and dissociation steps (180 s each) was followed by a regeneration of the sensors with 3 cycles alternating 10 s in glycine (10 mM, pH 2) and 10 s in TBS. All steps were performed under continuous 1000 rpm shaking at 30 °C. Sensorgrams were analyzed with the Octet Data Analysis software 11.1 (ForteBio) and fitted with a 1:1 binding model providing K_D, the equilibrium binding constant in M; k_{on}, the association rate constant in $M^{-1}s^{-1}$; and k_{off}, the dissociation rate constant in s^{-1}.

2.4.2. Cross-Reactivity: Cell Transfection and Flow Cytometry

HEK293 (human embryonic kidney 293, CRL-1573) cells, obtained from ATCC (Rockville, MD, USA), were grown at 37 °C in a humidified atmosphere (95% O_2 and 5% CO_2) and in DMEM with GlutaMAX™ supplemented with 10% of fetal calf serum and 1% of penicillin/streptomycin. Once cells reached 70–90% confluence, they were washed with PBS and collected with an accutase solution. HEK293 cells were then seeded at 2.1×10^6 cells into 10 cm petri dishes. After 24 h, cells were transfected using the manufacturer's protocol (Thermo Fischer Scientific) with 15 µg of plasmid containing the long isoform nucleic sequence of human, pig, or mouse LepR (fused at their C-terminal to the GFP), and 30 µL of lipofectamine 2000 reagent. The growth media was replaced 5 h after the transfection. Two days later, cells were collected with accutase and blocked in cold PBS-BSA 1% (*w*/*v*) at 2×10^6 cells/mL for at least 30 min. Dilutions and washes were performed in the same buffer. Cells were then split into a 96-well conical bottom plate, pelleted by centrifugation (1 min at 750× *g*), and incubated for 30 min on ice with either an anti-LepR Nanofitin (1 μM, 100 μL/well) or an irrelevant Nanofitin (Irr-NF; 1 μM, 100 μL/well) or PBS-BSA 1% (*w*/*v*). Following that step, HEK293 cells were washed 3 times with 200 μL of PBS by centrifugation (1 min at 750× *g*), and cells previously incubated with Nanofitins were resuspended with the anti-His-tag antibody for 45 min on ice, whereas cells that were incubated with PBS-BSA 1% (*w*/*v*) were resuspended either with the anti-His-tag antibody (0.25 μg/mL, 100 μL/well) used as negative controls, or the anti-LepR antibody (0.3 μg/mL, 100 μL/well) used as a positive control. Both control antibodies are conjugated with Alexa-Fluor 647 for detection. Then, 3 washes were performed for all conditions and cells were resuspended into 200 μL of cold PBS-BSA 1% at a final concentration of 10^5 cells/mL until analysis. The binding was recorded on viable single cells and on the allophycocyanine (APC) channel using a CytoFLex Flow Cytometer (Beckman Coulter, Brea, CA, USA), and data were analyzed with the CytExpert Sofware (Beckman Coulter).

2.5. *Preparation for Ex Vivo Experiments*

2.5.1. Recovery and Transport of Porcine Intestinal Tissue

Directly after the animal slaughter, fresh porcine mid-jejunum was recovered from a 6-month-old Swiss noble pig (slaughter house of Loëx, Bernex, Switzerland) [35]. Tissue was rinsed with ultrapure water and immersed into oxygenated (95% O_2 and 5% CO_2, PanGas AG, Dagmersellen, Switzerland) cold krebs-bicarbonate ringer buffer (KBR, 120 mM NaCl, 20 mM $NaHCO_3$, 11 mM glucose, 5.5 mM KCl, 2.5 mM $CaCl_2$, 1.2 mM $MgCl_2$, 1.2 mM NaH_2PO_4, at pH 7.4). The tissue was kept under oxygenation until the beginning of the experiment.

2.5.2. Validation of the LepR Expression on Porcine Intestinal Tissue by Western Blot

To generate porcine intestinal tissue lysate for the evaluation of the LepR expression by Western blot, a small part of the porcine jejunum segment was crushed with liquid nitrogen, recovered in Radioimmunoprecipitation assay buffer (RIPA, 1 mM EDTA, 0.5 mM EGTA, 1% Triton X-100, 0.1% sodium deoxycholate, 0.1% SDS, 140 mM NaCl) supplemented with 1% of protease and phosphatase inhibitor cocktails then sonicated (3 times: 10 s, 5 cycles, 10%). Supernatant was recovered after 10 min of centrifugation (10,000 rpm, 4 °C) and proteins concentration was determined using a BCA protein assay kit. Then, 15 μg of porcine jejunum lysate, HepG2 cell lysate used as a positive control, HEK293 cell lysate used as negative controls, and a prestained protein ladder were separated on a 12% SDS-PAGE gel and transferred overnight at 4 °C to a nitrocellulose membrane (Cytiva). Blocking of the membrane during 4 h at RT was realized in TBST-BSA 3% (*w*/*v*) and followed by an incubation of 2 h at RT with a rabbit monoclonal antibody diluted 500 times, recognizing the long isoform of the LepR. After 3 washes of 10 min in TBST, an incubation of 2 h was carried out with a secondary anti-rabbit antibody diluted 10,000 times. The membrane was then washed 4 times and immunoreactivity was detected using chemiluminescence on the Odyssey imaging system (LiCor Biotechnology, Lincoln, NE, USA).

2.5.3. Labeling of Nanofitins for Ex Vivo Transport Experiments

Anti-LepR Nanofitin and the irrelevant Nanofitin quantification for the ex vivo assays was performed via direct measurement of the fluorescence coming from the fluorescein conjugated Nanofitins. A regioselective conjugation of maleimide–fluorescein was performed on a unique engineered cysteine at the N-terminus of the Nanofitins. The modified Nanofitins were expressed from plasmid constructs, as described in Section 2.3, and dialyzed in Hepes-NaCl buffer (20 mM Hepes, 150 mM NaCl, pH 7.4) with SnakeSkin™ Dialysis Tubing 3.5K MWCO (Thermo Fischer Scientific). For the dimers, the single cysteine was added at the N-terminus of the constructs, i.e., at the N-terminus of the of the anti-LepR 1-F08 or the irrelevant Nanofitin domain.

Nanofitins were diluted at 5 mg/mL in Hepes-NaCl and reduced overnight at 4 °C with TCEP-HCl (Thermo Fischer Scientific) at a final concentration of 1 mM. The following day, N-(5-Fluoresceinyl)-maleimide was solubilized in dimethylsulfoxyde (DMSO) and added 10 times in excess to the reduced proteins. Solutions were left 2 h under stirring and argon at RT. Then, free dye was removed using a PD10 desalting column (GE Healthcare, Chicago, IL, USA), equilibrated with Hepes-NaCl, and the fluorescently labeled Nanofitins were concentrated until at least 10 mg/mL with 3 kDa protein concentrators (Thermo Fischer Scientific). Finally, protein concentrations were determined with a BCA Protein Assay Kit and their binding activity was validated by ELISA.

2.5.4. Calibration of the Ussing Chambers and Porcine Intestinal Tissue Preparation

Anti-LepR Nanofitinstransport across porcine intestinal tissue was evaluated ex vivo in the Ussing chambers system [35]. To calibrate the system, two pairs of Ag/AgCl-electrodes were first inserted into tips filled with a mixture of 3% agar in KCl 3 M and connected to each chamber. Then, mucosal (donor) and serosal (receiver) compartments of the Ussing chambers were filled with 7 mL of preheated KBR (38 °C), and differences of voltage between the two pairs of electrodes, as well as the electrical resistance of the buffer, were removed. During this step, a circulating water bath ED-5 (Julabo GmbH, Seelbach, Germany) was used to regulate the temperature of the chambers (porcine body temperature: 38 °C). The system was also under constant oxygenation with a mixture of 95% O_2 and 5% CO_2 to keep the tissue viable and avoid unstirred layer formation.

At this stage, the tissues were mounted into the sliders. The intestine was first opened along the mesenteric border to remove the serosa and tunica muscularis via blunt dissection with fine scissors and tweezers. Then, segments of approximatively 1.5 cm^2 were cut off, while being careful to avoid areas with Peyer's Patches, and each of them was mounted on a slider (Physiologic instruments, San Diego, CA, USA) with an exposed surface area of 1.26 cm^2. Then, the KBR buffer was removed, and the sliders were inserted between the donor and receiver compartments. After 30 min of equilibration of the tissues with preheated KBR, chambers were emptied again, and the buffer of the receiver compartments was replaced with fresh KBR to prevent a possible impact of endogenous material released during the equilibration. All segments were set within 60 min following the animal death into the Ussing chambers system. It was later coupled to a VCC MC6 Multichannel Voltage–Current Clamp (Physiologic Instruments) to monitor the setup integrity by continuous measurements of the transepithelial electrical resistance (TEER, in $\Omega\cdot cm^2$).

2.6. *Ex Vivo Transport Evaluation of Nanofitins Targeting the LepR*

To evaluate the anti-LepR Nanofitins transport across porcine intestinal tissue, they were diluted in KBR at 90 µM. The irrelevant Nanofitin was diluted at the same concentration. With the limit of quantification by fluorescence in KBR being 18 ng/mL, the used concentration allowed for a quantification of the fluorescent proteins added into the mucosal compartments as low as 0.0019%. Then, each donor compartment was filled with 7 mL of the Nanofitin solutions. For competition assays, a 9-fold excess of unlabeled anti-LepR Nanofitin 1-F08 (800 µM) was also added to the mucosal compartments. After 120 min of experiment (maximal viability duration of the intestinal tissue in Ussing chambers [6]), tissues exhibiting a TEER value below 15 $\Omega\cdot cm^2$ were omitted from the dataset as this threshold reliably indicates a loss of integrity [36]. Final donor and receiver samples were recovered from the compartments of the other chambers.

Although the common analytical method employed to quantify small molecules following transport experiments lean on UHPLC-MS/MS [35], we chose fluorescence to measure the transported Nanofitins given the higher sensitivity of this method for these proteins. To that end, the Nanofitins in the donor compartment at the beginning of the experiment (initial) and after 120 min (final) were diluted 500 times in KBR to fit into the detection range fixed by a calibration curve performed in KBR with solutions ranging from 0.8 to 900 nM (each dilution was performed in triplicate). The buffer was used as a blank. In contrast to the Nanofitins in the donor solution, the Nanofitins in the receiver compartment were used undiluted (each solution was tested in triplicate). A total of 200 µL of all the samples were then added into a black Nunc MicroWell 96-Well Optical-Bottom plate (Thermo Fischer Scientific). Fluorescence (λex: 490 nm; λem: 525 nm) was measured by a CLARIOstar Plus plate reader (BMG Labtech, Ortenberg, Germany).

In order to determine the percentages of transported Nanofitins (anti-LepR Nanofitins or irrelevant Nanofitin) in the receiver compartments at the end of the experiments, the following equations were used with the masses determined by the fluorescence calibration curve and considering the used dilutions:

$$\text{Transported Nanofitin (\% initial donor)} = \frac{\text{mass transported in the receiver after 120 min}}{\text{mass in the donor compartment at the onset}} \times 100, \quad (1)$$

$$\text{Final donor (\% initial donor)} = \frac{\text{mass in the donor compartment after 120 min}}{\text{mass in the donor compartment at the onset}} \times 100 \quad (2)$$

2.7. Statistical Analysis

All statistical analyses were performed using the GraphPad Prism 7.0 software. Data are presented as the mean ± standard deviation (SD). The results obtained were evaluated with the Student's *t*-test. The significance level was fixed at $\alpha = 0.05$.

3. Results

3.1. Characterization of Nanofitins Targeting the LepR

3.1.1. Selection of Nanofitins Targeting the LepR for Ex Vivo Transport Experiments

To identify Nanofitins binding to the extracellular domain of the hLepR, a combinatorial library of variants was challenged through four rounds of ribosome display using the rhLepR as the target. Following the final selection round, the enriched library was subcloned and transformed in *E. coli*, and 95 single clones were isolated for a preliminary screening fused with acGFP against the rhLepR by ELISA. Clones were ranked based on their binding signal ratio on the rhLepR versus non-specific binding signal in the absence of the target (Figure S1A). The enrichment of specific hits led to the isolation of 53 unique validated clones exhibiting a specific signal on rhLepR at least twice superior to the non-specific signal (Figure S1B). These clones were categorized into four families based on similarities in amino acid patterns within their binding site.

Subsequently, a representative panel of 20 hits, selected based on their binding signal-to-noise ratio and sequence diversity within and between families, was produced in the same format for further characterization. Various binding profiles were identified among these clones. A competition assay with the natural ligand, the leptin, also revealed that all clones from family 1 displayed a binding ratio close to 1, demonstrating a specific interaction with rhLepR on an epitope distinct from that of leptin. Conversely, families 2, 3, and 4 exhibited binding ratios of 2 or higher, suggesting binding to an epitope that overlapped, at least partially, with the leptin binding site (Figure 1A). Finally, cross-reactivity experiments performed with rmLepR showed that clones from family 1 present a similar binding signal to the mouse and human targets, whereas the others have a higher binding signal than the mouse receptor (Figure 1B). These results demonstrate that the identified Nanofitins target at least two distinct epitopes on the LepR.

We focused the next stages of the study on anti-LepR Nanofitins 1-F08 and 1-D07 from family 1. This family comprised Nanofitin candidates displaying two essential features from the target product profile: non-competition with the binding of the natural ligand to prevent any interference with natural physiological processes [37,38]; and binding both the murine and human forms of the receptor to facilitate translatability during preclinical evaluations. Within family 1, 1-F08 and 1-D07 were chosen due to their differing ELISA response levels, suggesting distinct affinities.

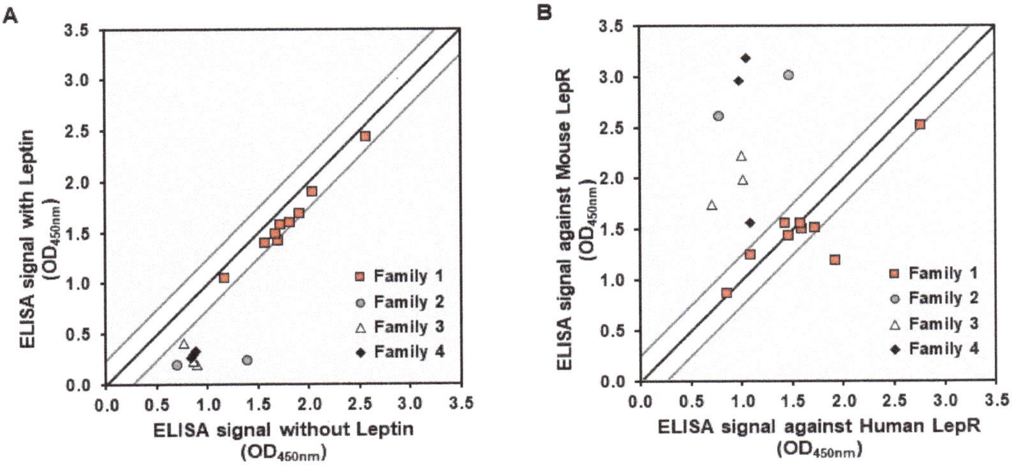

Figure 1. Characterization of Nanofitins targeting the LepR. (**A**) Signals obtained in a competition ELISA with Nanofitins tested on immobilized rhLepR in the presence or absence of leptin. (**B**) Signals obtained with a cross-reactivity ELISA with Nanofitins tested on immobilized rhLepR or rmLepR. Signal ratio of 1:1 is indicated by a black line, with a delimitation of ±0.25 absorbance units.

3.1.2. Binding Characterization of Selected Nanofitins

Recognizing the significance of affinity in BBB studies for modulating active transport across cellular barriers [39], we conducted a more in-depth characterization of the binding affinity of both 1-F08 and 1-D07 in a format without acGFP (Figure 2).

A

Nanofitin	EC_{50} (M)	K_D (M)	k_{on} ($M^{-1}s^{-1}$)	k_{off} (s^{-1})
1-F08	2.94×10^{-10}	9.56×10^{-9}	1.63×10^{6}	1.56×10^{-2}
1-D07	3.57×10^{-8}	8.30×10^{-7}	4.21×10^{5}	3.49×10^{-1}

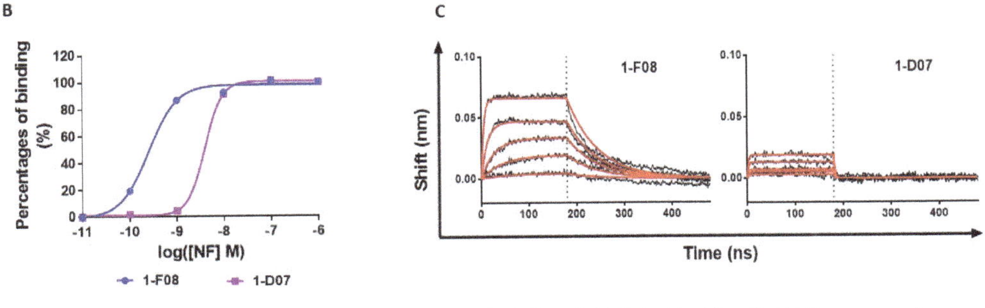

Figure 2. Characterization of the interaction of 1-F08 and 1-D07 with rhLepR. (**A**) Summary of binding parameters (EC_{50}, K_D, k_{on}, and k_{off}) of 1-F08 and 1-D07 (n = 1). (**B**) ELISA binding curves of 1-F08 and 1-D07 on the immobilized rhLepR (n = 1). Signal normalization was achieved by setting the highest binding signal obtained for each protein as 100%. (**C**) BLI binding profiles (association for 180 s followed by dissociation for 300 s) of 1-F08 and 1-D07 (n = 1). The concentrations represented start from 111 nM for 1-F08 and 333 nM for 1-D07 (followed by successive one-third dilutions). Raw data are represented in black sensorgrams, whereas fitted sensorgrams are in red.

The EC_{50} values obtained in ELISA indicated a higher relative affinity for 1-F08 (0.29 nM) compared to 1-D07 (35.70 nM) (Figure 2A,B). Moreover, we investigated the binding kinetic parameters of these two anti-LepR Nanofitins by BLI. The sensorgrams confirmed the high affinity of 1-F08 for the target (K_D = 9.56 nM) and emphasized the strong contribution of the on-rate to its affinity with rapid association kinetics ($k_{on} = 1.63 \times 10^6\ M^{-1}s^{-1}$) (Figure 2A,C). Conversely, 1-D07 exhibited a lower affinity for the target (K_D = 830 nM) compared to 1-F08. Notably, 1-D07 demonstrated a slower association rate ($k_{on} = 4.21 \times 10^5\ M^{-1}s^{-1}$) than 1-F08, as well as a faster dissociation from the target ($k_{off} = 3.49 \times 10^{-1}\ s^{-1}$ for 1-D07 and $k_{off} = 1.56 \times 10^{-2}\ s^{-1}$ for 1-F08), leading to a distinctive square waveform profile.

3.1.3. In Vitro Evaluation of Nanofitins Cross-Reactivity on Transfected HEK293 Cells

As shown in Figure 1B, cross-reactivity was detected on human and murine isolated receptors. This was further supported by assessing the specific binding of Nanofitins on cell models expressing the LepR from different species. To that end, HEK293 cells were transiently transfected with plasmids encoding for the long isoform of the LepR from human, mouse, and swine. This approach aimed to encompass all relevant models likely to be used for the preclinical evaluation of the transport abilities of the anti-LepR Nanofitin-based shuttle. Transfection efficiency was monitored by measuring cells fluorescence since each LepR was fused with GFP to facilitate cell selection. The expression of receptors at the cell membranes was confirmed by the specific binding of a labeled anti-LepR antibody on transfected cells compared to non-transfected cells (Figure S2).

The binding of 1-F08 and 1-D07 was tested at 1 μM by flow cytometry and was normalized with the anti-LepR antibody binding signal on cells (Figure 3). The anti-His antibody alone and an irrelevant Nanofitin were also tested to establish the correlation between signal positivity and the presence of specific anti-LepR Nanofitins (Table S1). Furthermore, the absence of Nanofitin binding on non-transfected HEK293 cells was confirmed in each assay.

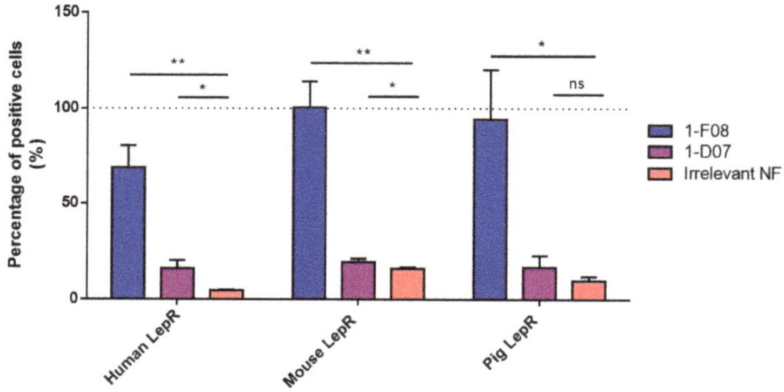

Figure 3. Binding of 1-F08 (n = 4) and 1-D07 (n = 4) on HEK293 cells transfected with the human, mouse, and pig LepR, analyzed by flow cytometry. The binding signals were normalized with the anti-LepR antibody binding signal (100%, represented by the dashed line) and expressed as a percentage of positive cells. An irrelevant Nanofitin (n = 2) was used as a negative control. Results are expressed as mean values ± SD (unpaired Student's *t*-test; ns, non-significant ($p > 0.05$); * $p < 0.05$, ** $p < 0.01$).

The data presented in Figure 3 revealed that both anti-LepR Nanofitins bind to the hLepR, as demonstrated by their significantly higher signal on cells compared to the negative control. Their level of positivity aligns with their respective affinities determined in Figure 2. Additionally, 1-F08 recognizes the membrane-bound porcine LepR and the mouse LepR, confirming its cross-reactivity with these targets. We observed minimal to no cross-reactivity with the anti-LepR Nanofitin 1-D07, attributed to its lower affinity in conjunction with higher background signals on these cell models.

3.2. Experimental Setup Validation for Ex Vivo Studies

3.2.1. LepR Expression in Porcine Jejunum Lysate

Since the jejunum exhibits the most active carrier-mediated transport in the intestine [40], our focus for the ex vivo studies was directed toward this particular segment of the GI tract. To investigate the expression of LepR in this tissue, we conducted an immunoblot analysis. The immunoblot revealed a band at the expected molecular weight (130 kDa) in the porcine jejunum lysate, which was absent in the negative control (HEK293 cell lysate). The same band, representing the long isoform of the receptor, was identified in the positive control (HepG2 lysate, Figure S3). These results validate the expression of LepR in the porcine jejunum and underscore the relevance of using an ex vivo model of porcine origin to evaluate the intestinal transport of Nanofitins targeting this receptor.

3.2.2. Nanofitins Fluorescently Labeled

The anti-LepR Nanofitins and the irrelevant Nanofitin were fluorescently labeled using N-(5-Fluoresceinyl)-maleimide. We determined the EC_{50} of the labeled constructs by ELISA on immobilized rhLepR. No discernible impact of the labeling was observed on the binding activities of the anti-LepR Nanofitins. The EC_{50} values obtained (4.23×10^{-10} M and 2.89×10^{-8} M for fluorescent 1-F08 and 1-D07, respectively, Table S2) fell within a similar range to those determined for the unlabeled proteins (2.94×10^{-10} and 3.57×10^{-8} M for 1-F08 and 1-D07, respectively, Figure 2).

3.3. Investigation of Receptor-Mediated Transport across the Intestinal Barrier

3.3.1. Specific Transintestinal Shuttle Activity of Non-Competitive Anti-LepR Nanofitins

The ability of fluorescein-labeled 1-F08 and 1-D07 to cross the intestinal barrier was assessed in comparison to an irrelevant Nanofitin used as a negative control (Figure 4).

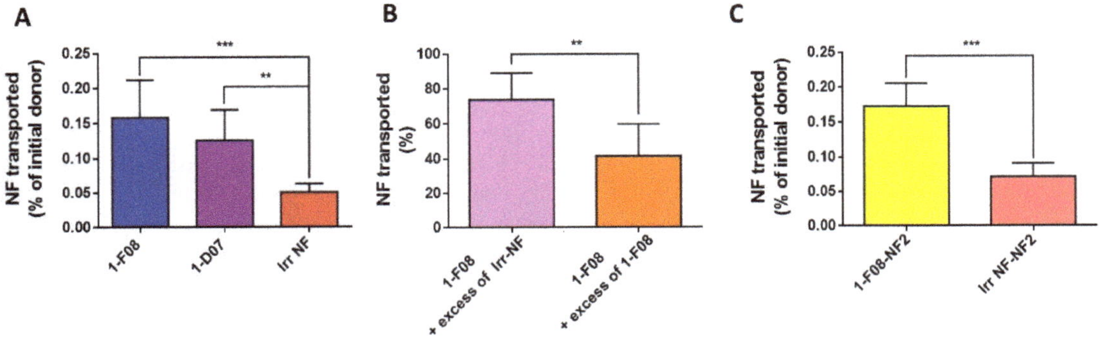

Figure 4. Ex vivo transport experiments across porcine intestinal tissue performed with (**A**) labeled anti-LepR Nanofitins 1-F08 (n = 10), 1-D07 (n = 4), and an irrelevant Nanofitin (n = 6) at 90 µM; (**B**) labeled 1-F08 at 90 µM in the presence of a 9-fold excess of unlabeled 1-F08 (1-F08 + excess of 1-F08, n = 6) or unlabeled irrelevant Nanofitin (1-F08 + excess of Irr-NF, n = 8); or (**C**) labeled 1-F08-NF2 (n = 4) and labeled irrelevant NF-NF2 (Irr NF-NF2, n = 5) tested at 90 µM. The masses used to calculate the percentages of initial donor transported were determined by fluorescence. The percentages of Nanofitin transported (**B**) were normalized with the percentage of labeled 1-F08 transported in the absence of an excess of unlabeled Nanofitin. Results are expressed as mean values ± SD (unpaired Student's *t*-test; ** $p < 0.01$, *** $p < 0.001$).

Continuous monitoring by TEER measurements yielded a mean TEER of $45 \pm 16\ \Omega\cdot cm^2$ (n = 53) at the conclusion of the incubation period of labeled Nanofitins in the donor (mucosal) compartments of the Ussing chambers. This value closely resembles the reported ex vivo measurements for porcine ($42 \pm 14\ \Omega\cdot cm^2$) [35] and human intestines ($34 \pm 12\ \Omega\cdot cm^2$) [41], confirming the integrity of each considered intestinal segment. The percentages of labeled Nanofitins found in the receiver compartments were calculated relative to the quantity of material applied in the donor compartments, determined using the calibration curve equation (an example of such a calibration curve is provided in Figure S4).

The anti-LepR Nanofitin displaying the highest passage across the intestinal barrier is 1-F08 (0.16% of the initial donor or 11.59 ± 4.40 μg) demonstrated a 3.2-fold increase compared to the calculated passage for the irrelevant NF (0.05% of the initial donor or 4.02 ± 0.98 μg) (Figure 4A). Similarly, the passage percentage of 1-D07 is significantly higher than the negative control, presenting a 2.6-fold difference (0.13% of the initial donor, or 10.51 ± 3.66 μg). These data demonstrate that LepR-binding Nanofitins exhibit a greater capability to cross the intestinal barrier compared to the irrelevant Nanofitin, suggesting a potential role of LepR in their transport. Notably, due to its superior ex vivo transport efficacy and higher in vitro affinity for the LepR, 1-F08—belonging to the same family as 1-D07—was chosen for further investigation of the receptor-mediated transport across the intestinal barrier.

To further validate the potential specific interaction driving the transportation of 1-F08 across the intestinal barrier, we conducted a competitive assay. This involved employing labeled 1-F08 along with an excess of either unlabeled 1-F08 or an irrelevant Nanofitin in the donor compartment, in comparison to labeled 1-F08 used solely (for normalization). When an excess of unlabeled irrelevant Nanofitin was introduced, it resulted in a modest 28% reduction in the transported amount of labeled 1-F08 in the receiver compartments. However, the addition of unlabeled 1-F08 led to a notably higher reduction, showing a 58% decrease (Figure 4B). These results suggest a specific passage mechanism for 1-F08, likely triggered by its binding to the LepR.

The ability of 1-F08 to transport a cargo protein was also evaluated by fusing the anti-LepR Nanofitin with a second Nanofitin (NF2) specific to HSA [28], serving as a model protein for potential carriage by the shuttle. We assessed the binding activity of 1-F08-NF2 on the rhLepR and HSA by ELISA. Similar EC_{50} values were obtained on the rhLepR for 1-F08, whether tested as a monomer or as a dimeric construct (Table S3), indicating consistent binding activity on the rhLepR. Furthermore, the low EC_{50} obtained for HSA aligns with the reported high affinity of this Nanofitin for HSA [28]. Thus, both Nanofitins conserved their respective binding activities in genetic fusion. Following this validation, the dimeric construct was labeled with fluorescein, and its binding conservation was confirmed by ELISA.

The transport of 1-F08-NF2 was evaluated ex vivo against a labeled dimeric construct, wherein 1-F08 is substituted by an irrelevant Nanofitin (Irr NF-NF2). The results reveal that the passage percentage of 1-F08-NF2 (0.17% of the initial donor, or 26.24 ± 4.91 μg) is significantly higher compared to the negative control Irr NF-NF2 (0.06% of the initial donor, 11.33 ± 3.01 μg), showing a 2.7-fold difference. Moreover, similar crossing efficiency was observed for 1-F08 alone and 1-F08-NF2 (0.16% and 0.17% of the initial donors, respectively) (Figure 4C). These data demonstrate that the molecular shuttle 1-F08 can promote the transport of a cargo (NF2) across the intestinal barrier as efficiently as in the absence of a cargo.

3.3.2. Nanofitin Activity Conservation after Mucosal Transport

In order to assess the binding activity of the monomeric and dimeric constructs subsequent to their transit through porcine jejunum, ex vivo samples of 1-F08 and 1-F08-NF2, retrieved from receiver compartments after 120 min, were tested by ELISA (Figure 5). These samples were compared to those obtained from their respective initial donors, which were diluted in KBR at the same concentration. The specificity of the signals was validated by the low absorbance observed in wells without target for all samples.

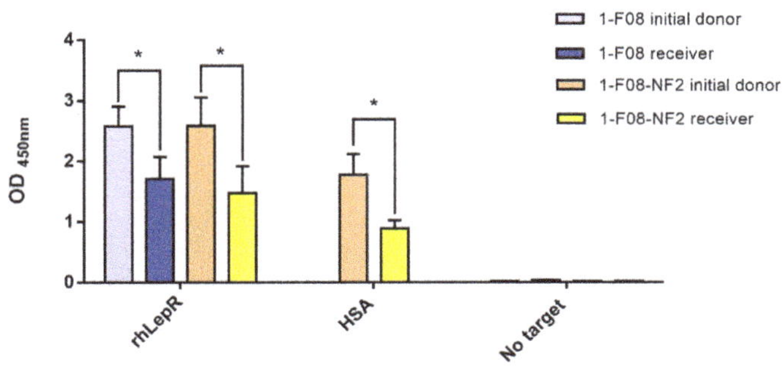

Figure 5. Binding activity of ex vivo samples evaluated on immobilized rhLepR or HSA. The initial donor samples of 1-F08 (n = 4) and 1-F08-NF2 (n = 3) were diluted at the same concentrations as their respective receiver samples. Specificity of Nanofitins binding was validated on wells without target. Results are expressed as mean values ± SD (unpaired Student's t-test; * $p < 0.05$).

The results demonstrate that both 1-F08 and the dimeric construct maintained their capability to bind the rhLepR target after crossing the intestinal epithelium. Additionally, this validates the structural integrity of a substantial portion of the protein fusion 1-F08-NF2, as the RGS-His detection tag was genetically appended to the C-terminus of NF2. Furthermore, the Nanofitin cargo (NF2) within the dimeric construct exhibits binding to its target, HSA, suggesting the shuttle's capacity to transport an active protein. Nevertheless, the binding signals of 1-F08 and 1-F08-NF2 receiver samples on rhLepR exhibit reductions of 33% and 42%, respectively, in comparison to the binding signals obtained with their initial donors at equivalent concentrations. Similarly, the binding signals of the dimeric construct from receiver samples, assessed on immobilized HSA, exhibit a reduction by half compared to those obtained from the initial donor. Hence, further investigations are warranted to elucidate the underlying factors contributing to the observed differences in binding signals. These variations might arise from protein derivatization, potential partial denaturation, or artifacts associated with the in vitro and ex vivo methods.

4. Discussion

The oral administration of systemically bioavailable biologics presents considerable challenges due to their vulnerability to the harsh conditions of the GI tract and their limited absorption through the intestinal barrier [1,42,43]. Overcoming these obstacles requires a strategy that facilitates active and specific mucosal transport while withstanding chemical and proteolytic stresses from the buccal cavity to the intestine. Additionally, it is crucial for the carrier to exhibit controlled conjugation or fusion compatibility [30,31,44], enabling therapeutic activity and precise modulation of clearance once in the bloodstream [28]. In this study, we demonstrate the potential of Nanofitins, engineered from a 7 kDa hyperstable protein scaffold [25,26,45], to selectively target the LepR [19] and trigger the receptor-mediated transport of protein payloads from the gut lumen to the bloodstream, as demonstrated using an ex vivo model.

The anti-LepR Nanofitin target product profile was meticulously designed during the early stages of the project, considering its pivotal role in transitioning from wet lab experiments to preclinical studies and subsequent human use. Key criteria were given priority as follows: selecting Nanofitins that recognize the human LepR with non-overlapping epitopes compared to the natural ligand emerged as a primary focus. This strategy aimed to bolster efficiency and safety by mitigating risks associated with competition with endogenous ligands present at physiological concentrations, thereby reducing potential interference with normal biological functions [24,46,47]. Secondly, substantial emphasis was placed on identifying a Nanofitin capable of cross-reaction with mouse and pig species. This cross-reactivity facilitates the use of ex vivo and in vivo models during preclinical stages while upholding a high level of translatability. Furthermore, although preclinical efficacy studies may occasionally use humanized animals [48,49], they are commonly based on murine pathological models. Thus, the inclusion of Nanofitins exhibiting inter-species cross-reactivity obviates the necessity for numerous animal models specific to each active pharmaceutical ingredient, streamlining effective transport across the intestinal barrier.

To assess the transport capability of anti-LepR Nanofitins, we established a setup using porcine intestinal sections within Ussing chambers [35]. This approach provided a controlled experimental environment, enabling us to focus specifically on studying the transport process without the influence of systemic factors encountered in vivo. Beyond exploring the transport mechanism, this ex vivo model offered an opportunity to refine experimental techniques, optimize protocols, and gather valuable insights before transitioning to in vivo studies. Consequently, this strategy empowered informed decision-making, elevating the likelihood of success while reducing dependence on animal subjects [50,51]. In addition to ethical considerations, prior studies have highlighted a strong resemblance between porcine and human intestinal tissues in macroscopic and microscopic characteristics, establishing the porcine model as a reliable predictor of drug absorption in humans [52,53]. While acknowledging that reducing an entire digestive organ to a tissue section in a laboratory setting only partially mirrors the physiological diversity along the intestinal tract, we focused on the jejunal region due to its relevance to this study. Notably, the jejunum exhibits the highest degree of carrier-mediated transport in the gut, making it particularly suitable for our investigations [40,54]. Moreover, our validation of the presence of the long isoform of the LepR—responsible for leptin's intestinal transcytosis [19]—in porcine jejunal tissue (Figure S3) reinforced the suitability of our ex vivo model. Thus, this ex vivo system emerges as a reliable mimic of the human intestine, pivotal for preclinical investigations and for evaluating the efficacy of the anti-LepR Nanofitins. This study marks a significant advancement by utilizing the porcine intestinal model within Ussing chambers to assess the transport of biologics, expanding from its conventional usage restricted to small compounds [35]. It represents a noteworthy progression in comprehending gastrointestinal transport mechanisms through an ex vivo model and underscores the pioneering nature of this research, potentially opening new avenues in the field of oral drug delivery and therapeutic applications.

To initiate our study, we conducted a successful screening of the Nanofitins library, leading to the identification of four major families. Notably, Nanofitins from family 1 exhibited binding to the LepR that remained unaffected by the presence of human leptin, distinguishing them from Nanofitins from the other families (Figure 1A). This competitive behavior coincided with the results of cross-reactivity screening, wherein family 1 Nanofitins displayed ELISA signals independent of the target host (Figure 1B). As an outcome, we selected 1-F08 as the primary candidate for the proof-of-concept study. Acknowledging the limited understanding of the optimal parameters required to trigger active passage and enhance intestinal permeability of biologics [12,39], we included its homologue 1-D07, possessing lower affinity (a two-log difference in EC_{50} and K_D values (Figure 2)) for characterization alongside 1-F08.

We hypothesized that this affinity disparity significantly impacts the binding to cell surface receptors, as evidenced by flow cytometry analysis following transient transfection of human, mouse, and pig LepR in HEK293 cells (Figure 3). While 1-F08 exhibited robust labeling of LepR-positive cells in all conditions, 1-D07 yielded modest signals with the human target, and the cross-reactivity could not be confirmed in a cellular context. However, both candidates showed promise in assessing our strategy regarding the ability of Nanofitins targeting LepR to cross the intestinal barrier using the ex vivo porcine model.

Transport experiments conducted using the Ussing chamber system revealed that 1-F08 and 1-D07 exhibited a 3.6-fold- and 2.5-fold-higher crossing ability, respectively, from the mucosal to the serosal compartment compared to the irrelevant Nanofitin (Figure 4A). Consistent with recent studies on FcRn-mediated transcytosis [39], we observed a correlation between increased affinity for the target receptor and enhanced transport across the intestinal barrier. Additionally, competition experiments demonstrated a significant hindrance, with a 58% decrease in the intestinal transport of labeled 1-F08 in the presence of an excess of unlabeled 1-F08, while only a 26% decrease was observed with the unlabeled irrelevant Nanofitin (Figure 4B). These findings suggest the saturation of the LepR epitope targeted by unlabeled 1-F08, impeding the interaction between the fluorescent protein and the receptor. Then, we tested a construction composed of 1-F08 with NF2, an anti-HSA Nanofitin [28], to illustrate the transportation of other biological molecules, in that case another protein fused genetically to 1-F08 (Figure 4C). The results strongly support the notion that anti-LepR Nanofitins from family 1 can serve as a shuttle for the transportation of other biologics, as demonstrated by the specific transport of the anti-HSA Nanofitin, NF2. These results further validate the concept that 1-F08 uses a cargo-size-independent mechanism [55], addressing the challenge of transporting diverse biological molecules, such as a protein, across the intestinal mucosa.

Using the ex vivo model samples, we demonstrated the effective transport of both monomers and dimers of Nanofitins including the 1-F08 moiety, while retaining their specific binding activity. This was exemplified by the successful transport of the anti-LepR 1-F08 and anti-LepR/anti-HSA 1-F08-NF2 constructs (Figure 5). Despite acknowledging a partial reduction in the binding signals of the constructs in the serosal compartments, these results affirm the integrity of the multimeric assembly detected by ELISA on the rhLepR. Notably, the anti-LepR activity was elicited by the N-terminus moiety, while the detection tag was located at the C-terminus of the NF2. These data show the preserved binding activity of the constructs and highlight the significant potential of 1-F08 as a gut-to-blood shuttle for delivering active molecules with therapeutic purposes. However, it is important to consider the challenges posed by gastric and intestinal fluids [42], as well as the consecutive requirements for stability in future constructs. These considerations become particularly crucial for successful oral delivery of therapeutic molecules with maintained efficacy. Robust moieties, such as small molecules, peptides, or Nanofitin-based compounds, may offer improved resistance to the demanding conditions of the GI tract. Various strategies [4,6] can be explored to address the challenging conditions of the GI tract, warranting consideration for the forthcoming preclinical experiments subsequent to this proof-of-concept study.

Translating the findings of our study into in vivo drug bioavailability and subsequent therapeutic effect necessitates further investigation. Our initial results demonstrate the transport capabilities of anti-LepR 1-F08, capable of transporting itself and another Nanofitin domain at similar rates (NF2). This is exemplified by the observation that the dimeric construct, with a molecular weight twice that of the monomer, appeared in double the mass of the monomer in the receiver compartment. We envision the potential addition of more moieties, especially at the C-terminus of 1-F08, in future biotherapeutics. Additionally, the 1.26 cm^2 of jejunal surface exposed in an Ussing chamber represents only a fraction of the available surface in the human jejunum, estimated at approximately one 1000th to one 10,000th depending on diameter and length [56]. Assuming linear rate conversion, the 26.24 µg of 1-F08-NF2 available in the serosal compartment after 2 h could translate to a dosage range from hundreds of µg/kg to single-digit mg/kg after each administration. These expected blood titers underscore the potential of the anti-LepR shuttle for real therapeutic applications, enhanced by the ability to fine-tune blood accumulation through the use of an anti-HSA moiety [28] in the final product. Furthermore, Nanofitin-based molecules are notably smaller than monoclonal antibodies. As a consequence, an equivalent molar dose of the pharmaceutical ingredient falls within the standard range of circulating monoclonal antibodies, starting from 1 mg/kg [57,58]. These prospects will undergo further assessment, considering numerous factors influencing final serum bioavailability, including: (i) actual exposure to the intestine, accounting for a transit time through the human intestine of up to 6 h [56]; (ii) expression levels of LepR across the human gut tract, evidenced at the RNA level from the stomach to the rectum, not limited to the jejunum [59–61]; (iii) receptor turnover rate, crucial for optimizing dosing regimens and determining the administration frequency [62]. These considerations are paramount in ensuring the successful and effective utilization of biologics in therapeutic applications.

5. Conclusions

In summary, this ex vivo proof-of-concept study has yielded compelling insights supporting several critical observations. First, it demonstrates the efficacy of LepR as a target capable of initiating a specific transport mechanism, showcasing the potential for leveraging this receptor in designing innovative oral-to-systemic delivery strategies. Second, the study conclusively demonstrates that a Nanofitin targeting a distinct epitope from the natural ligand of the LepR can efficiently traverse the intestinal barrier via a translocation mechanism, highlighting the promise of anti-LepR Nanofitins as carriers for overcoming biological barriers. Moreover, this study has established the potential of 1-F08 as a shuttle by enhancing the permeability of other biologically active molecules, aligning with the growing demand for efficient drug delivery systems in the field of biologics.

With these impactful findings, our research can embark on the next phase of advancement. This forthcoming stage will involve a comprehensive evaluation of the in vivo transport dynamics of 1-F08, engineered to incorporate a stable, biologically active cargo in rodent models. This crucial step bridges the gap between ex vivo insights and real-world applications, offering valuable insights into the construct's behavior within the complexities of living organisms. It marks a critical steppingstone toward translating our innovative approach into potential clinical applications.

6. Patents

The innovative findings presented in this manuscript have led to the development of a patent entitled "Polypeptides as Carrier for Intestinal Barrier Crossing" (application number: EP21306709.3; file date: 5 December 2021). The patent, filed based on the novel discoveries reported herein, covers the unique application of Nanofitins as carriers facilitating the transport of therapeutic compounds across the intestinal barrier. The inventive approach outlined in this manuscript forms the basis for the claims made in the patent application, highlighting the potential for significant advancements in drug delivery systems.

Supplementary Materials: The following supporting information can be downloaded at https://www.mdpi.com/article/10.3390/pharmaceutics16010116/s1: Figure S1: Ratio of binding signals of Nanofitins on the rhLepR and non-specific binding signals in absence of target obtained by ELISA. (A) Binding signal-to-noise ratio of the 95 clones isolated for a pre-liminary screening. (B) Binding signal-to-noise ratio of 53 unique clones selected for their ratio superior to 2 and divided into four families based on similarities of amino acid patterns in their binding site; Figure S2: Binding of the anti-LepR antibody on non-transfected HEK293 cells (n = 3) or cells transfected with human (n = 3), mouse (n = 3), and pig (n = 3) LepR, analyzed by flow cytometry. Signal intensities correlate with receptor presence and the percentage of homology with human LepR. The binding signals were expressed as a percentage of positive cells. Results are expressed as mean values ± SD (unpaired Student's *t*-test; * $p < 0.05$, ** $p < 0.01$, *** $p < 0.001$); Figure S3: Identification of the LepR on porcine jejunum lysate. The immunoblot was performed on the lysates using an antibody generated against an intracellular epitope of the long isoform of the LepR. HEK293 cell lysate was used as a negative control, whereas the HepG2 cell lysate was used as a positive control; Figure S4: Example of a calibration curve of the concentration of Nanofitin (nM) in function of the fluorescence (RFU); Table S1: Binding of 1-F08 (n = 4) and 1-D07 (n = 4)) on HEK293 cells transfected with the human, mouse, and pig LepR, analyzed by flow cytometry. The binding signals were normalized with the anti-LepR antibody binding signal expressed as percentage of positive cells. Anti-His antibody (n = 4) and an irrelevant NF (Irr-NF; n = 4) were used as negative controls. Results are expressed as mean values ± SD; Table S2: EC_{50} of labeled 1-F08 and 1-D07 determined by ELISA on the immobilized rhLepR; Table S3: EC_{50} of 1-F08 and the dimeric construct (1-F08-NF2) determined by ELISA on immobilized rhLepR or HSA.

Author Contributions: Conceptualization, S.M., A.C., S.H., M.C. and M.Z.L.; methodology, S.M., A.C., S.H., A.P., M.C. and M.Z.L.; validation, S.M., A.C., S.H., M.C. and M.Z.L.; formal analysis, S.M., A.C., S.H., M.C. and M.Z.L.; investigation, S.M., A.C., S.H., A.P., R.G., S.F. and M.Z.L.; resources, S.M., A.P., R.G., S.F., Y.N.K., L.S. and M.Z.L.; writing—original draft preparation, S.M., A.C., S.H., M.C. and M.Z.L.; writing—reviw and editing, S.M., A.C., S.H., M.C., F.G., M.Z.L. and L.S.; visualization, S.M., A.C., A.P., S.H., M.C. and M.Z.L.; supervision, A.C., S.H., M.C., M.Z.L. and L.S.; project administration, A.C., S.H., M.C., M.Z.L. and L.S.; funding acquisition, A.C., M.C., M.Z.L. and L.S. All authors have read and agreed to the published version of the manuscript.

Funding: This project was sponsored by a grant from Eurostars/the European Commission via Banque Publique d'Investissement for France and Innosuisse for Switzerland—grant number: E! 114171.

Institutional Review Board Statement: Not applicable.

Informed Consent Statement: Not applicable.

Data Availability Statement: Data are contained within the article.

Acknowledgments: We express our deep gratitude to the dedicated staff at the slaughterhouse; their unwavering assistance made this study possible.

Conflicts of Interest: A.C., A.P., R.G., S.F., and S.H. hold employment in Affilogic. The Nanofitin technology described in this study, commercialized by Affilogic, uses the patent application owned by Institut Pasteur and Centre National de la Recherche Scientifique (CNRS): "OB-fold used as scaffold for engineering new specific binders"; PCT/IB2007/004388. Affilogic SAS, Nantes, France, provided support for the study and participated in study design, conducted the study, and provided data collection, management, and interpretation. This does not alter the authors' adherence to all the journal policies on sharing data and materials.

References

1. Zhu, Q.; Chen, Z.; Paul, P.K.; Lu, Y.; Wu, W.; Qi, J. Oral delivery of proteins and peptides: Challenges, status quo and future perspectives. *Acta Pharm. Sin. B* **2021**, *11*, 2416–2448. [CrossRef] [PubMed]
2. Lagassé, H.D.; Alexaki, A.; Simhadri, V.L.; Katagiri, N.H.; Jankowski, W.; Sauna, Z.E.; Kimchi-Sarfaty, C. Recent advances in (therapeutic protein) drug development. *F1000Research* **2017**, *6*, 113. [CrossRef]
3. Dimitrov, D.S. Therapeutic Proteins. *Methods Mol. Biol.* **2012**, *899*, 1–26.
4. Alqahtani, M.S.; Kazi, M.; Alsenaidy, M.A.; Ahmad, M.Z. Advances in Oral Drug Delivery. *Front. Pharmacol.* **2021**, *12*, 618411. [CrossRef] [PubMed]
5. Anderson, J.M.; Van Itallie, C.M. Tight junctions and the molecular basis for regulation of paracellular permeability. *Am. J. Physiol. Liver Physiol.* **1995**, *269*, G467–G475. [CrossRef] [PubMed]
6. Masloh, S.; Culot, M.; Gosselet, F.; Chevrel, A.; Scapozza, L.; Labouebe, M.Z. Challenges and Opportunities in the Oral Delivery of Recombinant Biologics. *Pharmaceutics* **2023**, *15*, 1415. [CrossRef] [PubMed]
7. Thuenauer, R.; Müller, S.K.; Römer, W. Pathways of protein and lipid receptor-mediated transcytosis in drug delivery. *Expert Opin. Drug Deliv.* **2017**, *14*, 341–351. [CrossRef]
8. Doherty, G.J.; McMahon, H.T. Mechanisms of Endocytosis. *Annu. Rev. Biochem.* **2009**, *78*, 857–902. [CrossRef]
9. Kruth, H.S. Receptor-independent fluid-phase pinocytosis mechanisms for induction of foam cell formation with native LDL particles. *Curr. Opin. Lipidol.* **2011**, *22*, 386–393. [CrossRef]
10. Willson, J. Transferrin' across the blood–brain barrier. *Nat. Rev. Drug Discov.* **2020**, *19*, 444. [CrossRef]
11. Neves, A.; van der Putten, L.; Queiroz, J.; Pinheiro, M.; Reis, S. Transferrin-functionalized lipid nanoparticles for curcumin brain delivery. *J. Biotechnol.* **2021**, *331*, 108–117. [CrossRef] [PubMed]
12. Pulgar, V.M. Transcytosis to Cross the Blood Brain Barrier, New Advancements and Challenges. *Front. Neurosci.* **2019**, *12*, 1019. [CrossRef] [PubMed]
13. Bien-Ly, N.; Yu, Y.J.; Bumbaca, D.; Elstrott, J.; Boswell, C.A.; Zhang, Y.; Luk, W.; Lu, Y.; Dennis, M.S.; Weimer, R.M.; et al. Transferrin receptor (TfR) trafficking determines brain uptake of TfR antibody affinity variants. *J. Exp. Med.* **2014**, *211*, 233–244. [CrossRef] [PubMed]
14. Guo, Q.; Zhu, Q.; Miao, T.; Tao, J.; Ju, X.; Sun, Z.; Li, H.; Xu, G.; Chen, H.; Han, L. LRP1-upregulated nanoparticles for efficiently conquering the blood-brain barrier and targetedly suppressing multifocal and infiltrative brain metastases. *J. Control. Release* **2019**, *303*, 117–129. [CrossRef] [PubMed]
15. Tian, X.; Nyberg, S.; Sharp, P.S.; Madsen, J.; Daneshpour, N.; Armes, S.P.; Berwick, J.; Azzouz, M.; Shaw, P.; Abbott, N.J.; et al. LRP-1-mediated intracellular antibody delivery to the Central Nervous System. *Sci. Rep.* **2015**, *5*, srep11990. [CrossRef] [PubMed]
16. Boado, R.J.; Zhang, Y.; Zhang, Y.; Xia, C.; Wang, Y.; Pardridge, W.M. Genetic engineering of a lysosomal enzyme fusion protein for targeted delivery across the human blood-brain barrier. *Biotechnol. Bioeng.* **2008**, *99*, 475–484. [CrossRef]

17. Hornby, P.J.; Cooper, P.R.; Kliwinski, C.; Ragwan, E.; Mabus, J.R.; Harman, B.; Dorai, H.; Giles-Komar, J. FcRn Expression and Antibody Transcytosis in Adult Human and Non-Human Primate Intestine. *FASEB J.* **2013**, *27*, 1093.3. [CrossRef]
18. Azevedo, C.; Nilsen, J.; Grevys, A.; Nunes, R.; Andersen, J.T.; Sarmento, B. Engineered albumin-functionalized nanoparticles for improved FcRn binding enhance oral delivery of insulin. *J. Control. Release* **2020**, *327*, 161–173. [CrossRef]
19. Cammisotto, P.G.; Bendayan, M.; Sané, A.; Dominguez, M.; Garofalo, C.; Levy, E. Receptor-Mediated Transcytosis of Leptin through Human Intestinal Cells In Vitro. *Int. J. Cell Biol.* **2010**, *2010*, e928169. [CrossRef]
20. Cammisotto, P.G.; Gingras, D.; Bendayan, M. Transcytosis of gastric leptin through the rat duodenal mucosa. *Am. J. Physiol. Liver Physiol.* **2007**, *293*, G773–G779. [CrossRef]
21. Gorska, E.; Popko, K.; Stelmaszczyk-Emmel, A.; Ciepiela, O.; Kucharska, A.; Wasik, M. Leptin receptors. *Eur. J. Med. Res.* **2010**, *15* (Suppl. S2), 50–54. [CrossRef] [PubMed]
22. Obradovic, M.; Sudar-Milovanovic, E.; Soskic, S.; Essack, M.; Arya, S.; Stewart, A.J.; Gojobori, T.; Isenovic, E.R. Leptin and obesity: Role and clinical implication. *Front. Endocrinol.* **2021**, *12*, 585887. [CrossRef] [PubMed]
23. Fong, T.M.; Huang, R.-R.C.; Tota, M.R.; Mao, C.; Smith, T.; Varnerin, J.; Karpitskiy, V.V.; Krause, J.E.; Van der Ploeg, L.H.T. Localization of Leptin Binding Domain in the Leptin Receptor. *Mol. Pharmacol.* **1998**, *53*, 234–240. [CrossRef]
24. Cammisotto, P.; Bendayan, M. A review on gastric leptin: The exocrine secretion of a gastric hormone. *Anat. Cell Biol.* **2012**, *45*, 1–16. [CrossRef] [PubMed]
25. Mouratou, B.; Schaeffer, F.; Guilvout, I.; Tello-Manigne, D.; Pugsley, A.P.; Alzari, P.M.; Pecorari, F. Remodeling a DNA-binding protein as a specific in vivo inhibitor of bacterial secretin PulD. *Proc. Natl. Acad. Sci. USA* **2007**, *104*, 17983–17988. [CrossRef]
26. McAfee, J.G.; Edmondson, S.P.; Datta, P.K.; Shriver, J.W.; Gupta, R. Gene Cloning, Expression, and characterization of the Sac7 proteins from the hyperthermophile *Sulfolobus acidocaldarius*. *Biochemistry* **1995**, *34*, 10063–10077. [CrossRef] [PubMed]
27. Kalichuk, V.; Kambarev, S.; Béhar, G.; Chalopin, B.; Renodon-Cornière, A.; Mouratou, B.; Pecorari, F. Affitins: Ribosome Display for Selection of Aho7c-Based Affinity Proteins. *Methods Mol. Biol.* **2020**, *2070*, 19–41. [PubMed]
28. Michot, N.; Guyochin, A.; Cinier, M.; Savignard, C.; Kitten, O.; Pascual, M.H.; Pouzieux, S.; Ozoux, M.-L.; Verdier, P.; Vicat, P.; et al. Albumin Binding Nanofitins, a new scaffold to extend half-life of Biologics—A case study with exenatide peptide. *Peptides* **2022**, *152*, 170760. [CrossRef]
29. Huet, S.; Gorre, H.; Perrocheau, A.; Picot, J.; Cinier, M. Use of the Nanofitin Alternative Scaffold as a GFP-Ready Fusion Tag. *PLoS ONE* **2015**, *10*, e0142304. [CrossRef]
30. Goux, M.; Becker, G.; Gorré, H.; Dammicco, S.; Desselle, A.; Egrise, D.; Leroi, N.; Lallemand, F.; Bahri, M.A.; Doumont, G.; et al. Nanofitin as a New Molecular-Imaging Agent for the Diagnosis of Epidermal Growth Factor Receptor Over-Expressing Tumors. *Bioconjugate Chem.* **2017**, *28*, 2361–2371. [CrossRef]
31. Mouratou, B.; Béhar, G.; Pecorari, F. Artificial Affinity Proteins as Ligands of Immunoglobulins. *Biomolecules* **2015**, *5*, 60–75. [CrossRef]
32. Huet, S.; Zeisser Labouebe, M.; Castro, R.; Jacquot, P.; Pedrault, J.; Viollet, S.; Van Simaeys, G.; Doumont, G.; Larbanoix, L.; Zindy, E.; et al. Targeted Nanofitin-drug conjugates achieve efficient tumor delivery and therapeutic effect in an EGFR-positive mouse xenograft model. *Mol. Cancer Ther.* **2023**, *22*, 1343–1351. [CrossRef] [PubMed]
33. Mouratou, B.; Béhar, G.; Paillard-Laurance, L.; Colinet, S.; Pecorari, F. Ribosome display for the selection of Sac7d scaffolds. *Methods Mol. Biol.* **2012**, *805*, 315–331.
34. Hanes, J.; Plückthun, A. In vitro selection and evolution of functional proteins by using ribosome display. *Proc. Natl. Acad. Sci. USA* **1997**, *94*, 4937–4942. [CrossRef]
35. Arnold, Y.E.; Thorens, J.; Bernard, S.; Kalia, Y.N. Drug Transport across Porcine Intestine Using an Ussing Chamber System: Regional Differences and the Effect of P-Glycoprotein and CYP3A4 Activity on Drug Absorption. *Pharmaceutics* **2019**, *11*, 139. [CrossRef]
36. Arnold, Y.E.; Kalia, Y.N. Using Ex Vivo Porcine Jejunum to Identify Membrane Transporter Substrates: A Screening Tool for Early—Stage Drug Development. *Biomedicines* **2020**, *8*, 340. [CrossRef]
37. Yarandi, S.S.; Hebbar, G.; Sauer, C.G.; Cole, C.R.; Ziegler, T.R. Diverse roles of leptin in the gastrointestinal tract: Modulation of motility, absorption, growth, and inflammation. *Nutrition* **2011**, *27*, 269–275. [CrossRef]
38. Park, H.K.; Ahima, R.S. Leptin signaling. *F1000Prime Rep.* **2014**, *6*, 73. [CrossRef] [PubMed]
39. Lawrence, S.A.; Blankenship, R.; Brown, R.; Estwick, S.; Ellis, B.; Thangaraju, A.; Datta-Mannan, A. Influence of FcRn binding properties on the gastrointestinal absorption and exposure profile of Fc molecules. *Bioorganic Med. Chem.* **2021**, *32*, 115942. [CrossRef] [PubMed]
40. Lennernäs, H. Intestinal permeability and its relevance for absorption and elimination. *Xenobiotica* **2007**, *37*, 1015–1051. [CrossRef]
41. Sjöberg, Å.; Lutz, M.; Tannergren, C.; Wingolf, C.; Borde, A.; Ungell, A.-L. Comprehensive study on regional human intestinal permeability and prediction of fraction absorbed of drugs using the Ussing chamber technique. *Eur. J. Pharm. Sci.* **2013**, *48*, 166–180. [CrossRef]
42. Homayun, B.; Lin, X.; Choi, H.-J. Challenges and Recent Progress in Oral Drug Delivery Systems for Biopharmaceuticals. *Pharmaceutics* **2019**, *11*, 129. [CrossRef]
43. Vllasaliu, D.; Thanou, M.; Stolnik, S.; Fowler, R. Recent advances in oral delivery of biologics: Nanomedicine and physical modes of delivery. *Expert Opin. Drug Deliv.* **2018**, *15*, 759–770. [CrossRef]

44. Marcion, G.; Hermetet, F.; Neiers, F.; Uyanik, B.; Dondaine, L.; Dias, A.M.M.; Da Costa, L.; Moreau, M.; Bellaye, P.; Collin, B.; et al. Nanofitins targeting heat shock protein 110: An innovative immunotherapeutic modality in cancer. *Int. J. Cancer* **2021**, *148*, 3019–3031. [CrossRef] [PubMed]
45. Krehenbrink, M.; Chami, M.; Guilvout, I.; Alzari, P.M.; Pécorari, F.; Pugsley, A.P. Artificial binding proteins (Affitins) as probes for conformational changes in secretin PulD. *J. Mol. Biol.* **2008**, *383*, 1058–1068. [CrossRef]
46. Morton, N.M.; Emilsson, V.; Liu, Y.-L.; Cawthorne, M.A. Leptin action in intestinal cells. *J. Biol. Chem.* **1998**, *273*, 26194–26201. [CrossRef]
47. Sweeney, G. Leptin signalling. *Cell. Signal.* **2002**, *14*, 655–663. [CrossRef] [PubMed]
48. Cogels, M.M.; Rouas, R.; Ghanem, G.E.; Martinive, P.; Awada, A.; Van Gestel, D.; Krayem, M. Humanized Mice as a Valuable Pre-Clinical Model for Cancer Immunotherapy Research. *Front. Oncol.* **2021**, *11*, 784947. [CrossRef]
49. Denayer, T.; Stöhr, T.; Van Roy, M. Animal models in translational medicine: Validation and prediction. *Eur. J. Mol. Clin. Med.* **2014**, *2*, 5. [CrossRef]
50. Xu, Y.; Shrestha, N.; Préat, V.; Beloqui, A. An overview of in vitro, ex vivo and in vivo models for studying the transport of drugs across intestinal barriers. *Adv. Drug Deliv. Rev.* **2021**, *175*, 113795. [CrossRef]
51. Kiani, A.K.; Pheby, D.; Henehan, G.; Brown, R.; Sieving, P.; Sykora, P.; Marks, R.; Falsini, B.; Capodicasa, N.; Miertus, S.; et al. Ethical considerations regarding animal experimentation. *J. Prev. Med. Hyg.* **2022**, *63* (Suppl. S3), E255–E266. [CrossRef]
52. Ripken, D.; Hendriks, H.F.J. Porcine Ex Vivo Intestinal Segment Model. In *The Impact of Food Bioactives on Health: In Vitro and Ex Vivo Models*; Verhoeckx, K., Cotter, P., López-Expósito, I., Kleiveland, C., Lea, T., Mackie, A., Requena, T., Swiatecka, D., Wichers, H., Eds.; Springer International Publishing: Cham, Switzerland, 2015; pp. 255–262. [CrossRef]
53. Westerhout, J.; van de Steeg, E.; Grossouw, D.; Zeijdner, E.E.; Krul, C.A.; Verwei, M.; Wortelboer, H.M. A new approach to predict human intestinal absorption using porcine intestinal tissue and biorelevant matrices. *Eur. J. Pharm. Sci.* **2014**, *63*, 167–177. [CrossRef]
54. Billat, P.A.; Roger, E.; Faure, S.; Lagarce, F. Models for drug absorption from the small intestine: Where are we and where are we going? *Drug Discov. Today* **2017**, *22*, 761–775. [CrossRef] [PubMed]
55. Pardridge, W.M.; Boado, R.J.; Patrick, D.J.; Hui, E.K.-W.; Lu, J.Z. Blood-Brain Barrier Transport, Plasma Pharmacokinetics, and Neuropathology Following Chronic Treatment of the Rhesus Monkey with a Brain Penetrating Humanized Monoclonal Antibody Against the Human Transferrin Receptor. *Mol. Pharm.* **2018**, *15*, 5207–5216. [CrossRef] [PubMed]
56. Collins, J.T.; Nguyen, A.; Badireddy, M. Anatomy, Abdomen and Pelvis, Small Intestine. In *StatPearls*; StatPearls Publishing: Treasure Island, FL, USA, 2023. Available online: http://www.ncbi.nlm.nih.gov/books/NBK459366/ (accessed on 3 August 2023).
57. Singh, S.; Kumar, N.K.; Dwiwedi, P.; Charan, J.; Kaur, R.; Sidhu, P.; Chugh, V.K. Monoclonal Antibodies: A Review. *Curr. Clin. Pharmacol.* **2018**, *13*, 85–99. [CrossRef]
58. Strik, A.S.; Wang, Y.M.C.; Ruff, L.E.; Yashar, W.; Messmer, B.T.; Mould, D.R. Individualized Dosing of Therapeutic Monoclonal Antibodies—A Changing Treatment Paradigm? *AAPS J.* **2018**, *20*, 99. [CrossRef]
59. Tissue Expression of LEPR-Summary—The Human Protein Atlas. Available online: https://www.proteinatlas.org/ENSG00000116678-LEPR/tissue (accessed on 13 September 2023).
60. Barrenetxe, J.; Villaro, A.C.; Guembe, L.; Pascual, I.; Muñoz-Navas, M.; Barber, A.; Lostao, M.P. Distribution of the long leptin receptor isoform in brush border, basolateral membrane, and cytoplasm of enterocytes. *Gut* **2002**, *50*, 797–802. [CrossRef] [PubMed]
61. Hardwick, J.C.; Brink, G.R.V.D.; Offerhaus, G.; Van Deventer, S.J.; Peppelenbosch, M.P. Leptin is a growth factor for colonic epithelial cells. *Gastroenterology* **2001**, *121*, 79–90. [CrossRef]
62. Lee, Y.Y.; Erdogan, A.; Rao, S.S.C. How to Assess Regional and Whole Gut Transit Time with Wireless Motility Capsule. *J. Neurogastroenterol. Motil.* **2014**, *20*, 265–270. [CrossRef]

pharmaceutics

MDPI

Article

Compaction Properties of Particulate Proteins in Binary Powder Mixtures with Common Excipients

Else Holmfred *,†,‡, Cosima Hirschberg †,§ and Jukka Rantanen *

Department of Pharmacy, Faculty of Health and Medical Sciences, University of Copenhagen, 2100 Copenhagen, Denmark
* Correspondence: holmfred@stanford.edu (E.H.); jukka.rantanen@sund.ku.dk (J.R.)
† These authors contributed equally to this work.
‡ Current address: Earth and Planetary Sciences, Stanford Doerr School of Sustainability, Stanford University, 367 Panama St., Stanford, CA 94305, USA.
§ Current address: BASF A/S, Malmparken 5, 2750 Ballerup, Denmark.

Abstract: The increasing interest in protein- and peptide-based oral pharmaceuticals has culminated in the first protein-based products for oral delivery becoming commercially available. This study investigates the compaction properties of proteins in binary mixtures with common excipients up to 30% (*w*/*w*) of particulate protein. Two model proteins, lysozyme and bovine serum albumin, were compacted with either microcrystalline cellulose, spray-dried lactose monohydrate, or calcium hydrogen phosphate dihydrate at two different compaction pressures. Compared to the compacted pure materials, a significant increase in the tensile strength of the compacts was observed for the binary blends containing lysozyme together with the brittle excipients. This could be attributed to the increased bonding forces between the particles in the blend compared to the pure materials. The use of bovine serum albumin with a larger particle size resulted in a decrease in tensile strength for all the compacts. The change in the tensile strength with an increasing protein content was non-linear for both proteins. This work highlights the importance of considering the particulate properties of protein powders and that protein-based compacts can be designed with similar principles as small-molecules in terms of their mechanical tablet properties.

Keywords: protein; pharmaceutical; tableting; powder properties; compaction

1. Introduction

Oral delivery of proteins has been attempted for almost 100 years, with only a few drugs reaching the market [1,2]. Currently, the interest in oral drug products containing peptides and proteins is increasing [3,4], and culminated in 2019 when the oral glucagon-like peptide 1 (GLP-1) agonist, semaglutide (Rybelsus®), was approved by the Food and Drug Administration [3,5]. The oral route of administration is the most preferred due to its simplicity and convenience for the patients when contrasted with injectables [6,7]. Compared to small molecules, the structure of proteins has several complicating characteristics, e.g., the amino acid sequence and the unique folding that determine their function [7,8]. Although the number of approved medicines containing proteins is increasing, the delivery of proteins remains challenging given the low absorption and related poor bioavailability of peptides and proteins [1,3,9,10].

There is a clear interest in the development of oral protein formulations; however, the manufacturing of tablets involves stress factors like pressure, temperature, and exposure to environmental conditions that potentially can affect the protein structure. The unique protein structure should be maintained during processing, and potential structural changes must affect the functionality of the proteins minimally [7,8]. This has been investigated in several studies in which the activity and structural integrity of proteins after compaction have been analyzed [10–14]. The sensitive protein structure [10,15,16] consequently forces most protein products to be formulated as injectable drugs, either liquid formulations ready for injection or freeze-dried powder formulations, reconstituted right before administration to the patient.

Few studies have investigated the consequence of the compaction of proteins [10,12,14,17], but limited attention has been paid to the particulate properties of peptides and proteins and the related secondary processing. Klukkert et al. (2015) investigated the conformational changes in trypsin due to compaction, where a decrease in the enzymatic activity of trypsin was found with an increasing compaction pressure [10]. Controlling and pre-conditioning the relative humidity of the protein is potentially a critical parameter for protein stability and the level of aggregation before and during compaction. Wei et al. (2019) reported the effect of compaction on the stability of pure lysozyme and BSA and found that both proteins were highly plastic when compressed individually and showed excellent tabletability. The enzymatic activity of lysozyme was unchanged up to a compaction pressure of 300 MPa. BSA was seen to be more sensitive to compaction pressure at a small particle size, and a high compaction pressure showed upon compression a tendency for aggregation in the tablet. The authors found lysozyme and BSA stable after compaction, even when pre-conditioning at elevated humidities [12]. On the contrary, Lu et al. (2021) described how changes in relative humidity storage conditions induced conformational changes and the aggregation of immunoglobin prior to compaction. Immunoglobin was pre-conditioned at 32%, 52%, 75%, or 93% for 1 month, and the level of aggregation increased with increasing relative humidity. The immunoglobin binding activity was unaffected by the aggregation induced by changes in the relative humidity, while compaction pressures (50–350 MPa) did not induce aggregation but changed the binding activity significantly [17]. The studies from Klukkert et al. (2015), Lu et al. (2021), and Wei et al. (2019) focused on the protein stability and aggregation prior to or after compaction but did not investigate the protein as a particulate matter [10,12,17]. A recent study by Pedersen et al. (2023) described the tabletability properties of an oral drug formulation containing insulin, however, placing the focus on improving the often poorly tabletability of formulations containing high doses of permeation enhancers [14]. As permeation enhancers are often expensive, the authors replaced permeation enhancers with maltitol and added maltitol to the spray-drying process of insulin. The tensile strength of the tablets was significantly improved with the use of small-sized insulin–maltitol particles (2.16 µm, Dx50) compared to large-sized insulin–maltitol particles (4.89 µm, Dx50). Incorporating small-sized insulin–maltitol particles into the formulation did not influence the drug release of insulin from the formulation. Focusing mainly on improving the tabletability parameters, the stability of insulin or the binding activity was not addressed [14].

The particulate properties of both the drug and the excipients are of critical importance when designing a solid dosage form. This is well documented in the literature for small-molecule-based oral products and has recently been summarized in the Manufacturing Classification System [18]. Also, extensive work on the compaction of binary powder blends and the impact of different particulate factors on the percolation threshold of a binary blend has been the focus of research [19–23]. Identifying the concentration and the particulate properties of an active ingredient that impacts the downstream processability is crucial to ensure a robust production process.

The aim of this work was therefore to investigate the impact of increasing concentrations of two model proteins, lysozyme and bovine serum albumin (BSA), in binary mixtures containing three different model excipients (spray-dried lactose monohydrate (LacMH), microcrystalline cellulose (MCC), and calcium hydrogen phosphate dihydrate (CaHP)). The excipients used in this work were chosen based on their different particulate properties, leading to diverse behavior during the tableting process, and commercial availability. MCC is one of the most commonly used excipients in direct compression due to its high plasticity and ability to form tablets with high tensile strength [24–26]. LacMH and CaHP are less plastic than MCC [25,27], although they are also commonly used excipients in tablets.

2. Materials and Methods

2.1. Materials

The lysozyme from chicken egg white and bovine serum albumin (BSA) (Sigma-Aldrich, Schnelldorf, Germany), MCC (Avicel PH-102, FMC, Cork, Ireland), CaHP (EM-COMPRESS Premium, JRS Pharm, Rosenberg, Germany), and LacMH (FlowLac 100SD, Meggle, Wasserburg, Germany) were all of analytical grade. The magnesium stearate and potassium carbonate were purchased from Sigma-Aldrich, Schnelldorf, Germany.

2.2. Particle Size Distribution

A laser diffraction particle sizer with a Scirocco dry powder feeder (Mastersizer 2000, Malvern Instruments, Worcestershire, UK) was used to analyze the particle size distribution of the protein powders (n = 3).

2.3. X-ray Powder Diffraction

The X-ray powder diffraction measurements were performed using an X'Pert PANalytical Pro X-ray diffractometer (PANalytical, Almelo, The Netherlands) (CuKα radiation, λ: 1.54187 Å; acceleration voltage: 45kV; current: 40 mA; reflectance mode: 5°–35° 2θ; scan rate: 0.067° 2θ/s; step size: 0.026°). The data were collected and analyzed using the software X'Pert Data Collector version 2.2 (PANalytical, Almelo, The Netherlands).

2.4. Dynamic Vapor Sorption

The dynamic vapor sorption profiles of the proteins were analyzed using a VTI-SA+ instrument (TA-Instruments, New Castle, DE, USA). Approx. 15 mg of the powder sample was used (n = 1). The samples were dried inside the VTI-SA+ at 60 °C for either 180 min or until weight equilibrium (less than 0.0010 wt% change in 5 min) was achieved. Afterward, the temperature was adjusted to 25 °C, and the relative humidity (RH) was increased stepwise to 95% RH. Steps of 10% RH were chosen up to 90% RH, followed by one 5% step to 95%RH. The same steps were used for desorption. The sample was equilibrated at each relative humidity for 180 min or until the weight equilibrium was reached.

2.5. Sample Preparation

The BSA was gently ground using a mortar and pestle to de-aggregate and ensure the proper mixing behavior. Lysozyme and BSA were mixed with MCC, CaHP, and LacMH at three concentrations: 5, 10, and 30% (*w*/*w*) protein content. The sample size was approximately 10 g. All powders were mixed in a Turbula mixer for 3 min at 32 rpm (Type T2F, System Schatz, Willy A Bachhofen AG, Muttenz, Switzerland). All the blends and protein powders were conditioned in a desiccator at 43% RH (saturated potassium carbonate salt solution) for a minimum of 48 h. This condition was selected based on the dynamic vapor sorption analysis. Prior to compaction, 0.5% (*w*/*w*) magnesium stearate was added to the mixtures and mixed for 30 s in the Turbula mixer.

2.6. Compaction

All compactions were performed using a compaction simulator (HB10, Huxley Bertram Engineering Limited, Cambridge, UK). The samples (n = 4) were compacted at two different compaction pressures: 136 MPa and 265 MPa. The chosen compaction pressures reflect the range of compaction pressures used for pre-compression and the main compaction during general tablet manufacturing. Equally, 10 mm flat-faced punches were used for compaction with a compaction speed of 2 mm/s. The maximum load was kept constant for 50 ms. The compaction simulator with Euro B type tooling was set to provide a maximum load of 50 kN with a punch speed of a maximum of 2.5 mm/s. The die filling and compact removal were performed manually.

2.7. Properties of Compacts

The compacts were characterized after 24 h of storage at ambient conditions. The mass of the compact (n = 4) was determined using an analytical balance (Mettler AJ150, Mettler Toledo, Columbus, OH, USA), and the height of the compact (n = 4) was determined using a stage (7007, Mitutoyo Deutschland GmbH, Neuss, Germany) equipped with a digimatic indicator (Type IDF-130; Mitutoyo Deutschland GmbH, Neuss, Germany). The compact diameter and the crushing strength (n = 4) were measured using a Dr. Schleuniger Pharmatron Tablet Tester 8M (SOTAX AG, Aesch, Switzerland). The elastic recovery of the compacts was calculated using Equation (1)

$$ER = \frac{h_{out} - h_{max}}{h_{max}} \quad (1)$$

where h_{max} is the thickness of the compact at maximum compaction pressure (mm) and h_{out} is the out-of-die thickness of the compacts measured after 24 h of relaxation (mm). The tensile strength of the compacts was calculated using Equation (2)

$$\sigma = \frac{2F}{\pi \cdot D \cdot T} \quad (2)$$

where σ describes the tensile strength of the compacts calculated, F is the breaking force of the compacts (N), D is the compact diameter (m), and T is the compact thickness (m). The dependence of the tensile strength and tablet density on the compaction pressure was analyzed.

2.8. Data Analysis and Statistics

MATLAB 2022b (Mathworks, Natick, MA, USA) was used to extract the relevant data from the compaction profiles. The graphs were evaluated and plotted in Origin Pro 2016 (OriginLab Corporation, Northampton, MA, USA). Student's *t*-test (α = 0.05) was used to determine whether the two means differed significantly.

3. Results and Discussion

3.1. Size Distribution of Bovine Serum Albumin and Lysozyme

In this work, BSA and lysozyme are used as model proteins, focusing on their particulate properties. It should be noted that the protein activity after compaction was not evaluated. Particle size is an essential factor influencing the tableting process and, ultimately, the mechanical properties of the compacted product, e.g., the strength of a tablet. For particles to bind and form a compact, interparticulate forces play a crucial role [28]. Therefore, a large surface area of the materials, corresponding to smaller particle sizes, is usually favorable.

One clear difference between the used model protein powders was particle size and protein size. The average particle size of the lysozyme (d50 value) was 13 $\pm$ 0 µm and that of BSA was 226 $\pm$ 29 µm (Figure 1A).

The particle size of lysozyme was significantly smaller than that of BSA, and based on the particle size, it can be expected that lysozyme will form stronger compacts. The X-ray powder diffractograms indicated the amorphous nature of both proteins (Figure 1B). The amorphous nature of the proteins is interlinked with the water sorption behavior, where lysozyme and BSA demonstrated an ability to absorb a high amount of water (Figure 1C). A comparable water sorption behavior was observed for lysozyme and BSA up to a relative humidity of 60%. With an increasing relative humidity, BSA absorbed more water than lysozyme. At 95% relative humidity, BSA absorbed 41% (w/w) water and lysozyme 29% (w/w).

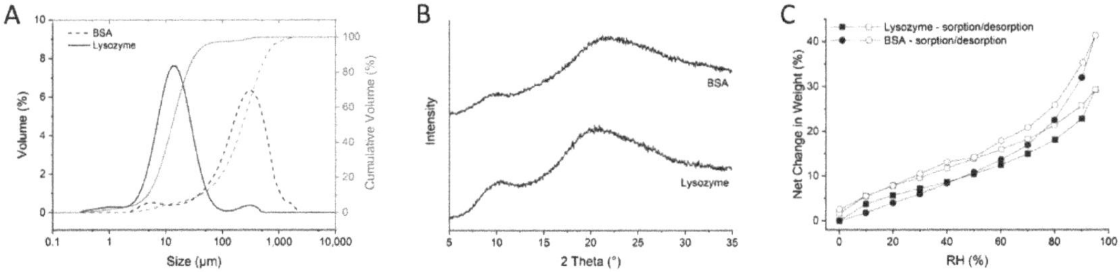

Figure 1. (**A**) Volume-based estimation of the size distribution (black) and cumulative volume-based size distribution (green) of lysozyme (straight line) and bovine serum albumin (BSA) (dashed line) (n = 3, mean). (**B**) X-ray powder diffraction pattern of bovine serum albumin (BSA) and lysozyme (n = 1). (**C**) Vapor sorption (filled symbols) and desorption (open symbols) profiles of lysozyme (squares) and bovine serum albumin (circles) (n = 1).

Properties like the ability to deform due to plastic and/or elastic deformation significantly impact the tabletability of a mixture [26,28]. Wei et al. (2019) investigated the effect of particle size on the compaction behavior of lysozyme and BSA and found that the particle size significantly impacts the tensile strength of compacts made purely from lysozyme, whereas the particle size of BSA had a lower impact on the tensile strength. Wei et al. (2019) further evaluated various standard compaction parameters, including Young's modulus and the contact hardness of the lysozyme and BSA compacts. Lysozyme and BSA demonstrated low Young's modulus values and a contact hardness consistent with their amorphous nature. The low values of contact hardness suggested the plastic deformation of lysozyme and BSA during compaction, favored by an increasing interparticle bonding area [12]. However, adding a second component to the powder matrix, such as excipients, increases the complexity of the formulation and the compaction behavior.

3.2. Binary Blends Containing Bovine Serum Albumin

Physical mixtures of amorphous BSA powder and three common excipients (LacMH, CaHP, and MCC) were prepared at different concentrations of BSA. The tablets were compacted using a compaction simulator at two different compaction pressures (136 MPa and 260 MPa), demonstrating typical low and high compaction pressures in an industrial setting [29]. The characteristic tablet parameters, such as tensile strength and elastic recovery, were monitored with an increasing BSA content (Figure 2A,B). The BSA protein was also compacted as a pure powder to rationalize the effect of BSA in binary blends. It was observed that pure BSA formed coherent compacts, however, with a low tensile strength of 0.3 and 0.6 MPa at the two compaction pressures (136 and 260 MPa) (Figure 2A).

In contrast to our results, Wei et al. (2019) reported that preconditioned (relative humidity 42%) pure BSA compacts (particle size 250–355 µm) had a tensile strength above 2 MPa at a 200 MPa compaction pressure [12]. However, the BSA protein powder quality and grade might differ significantly between this study and the study performed by Wei et al. (2019), which could explain the observed differences in tensile strength.

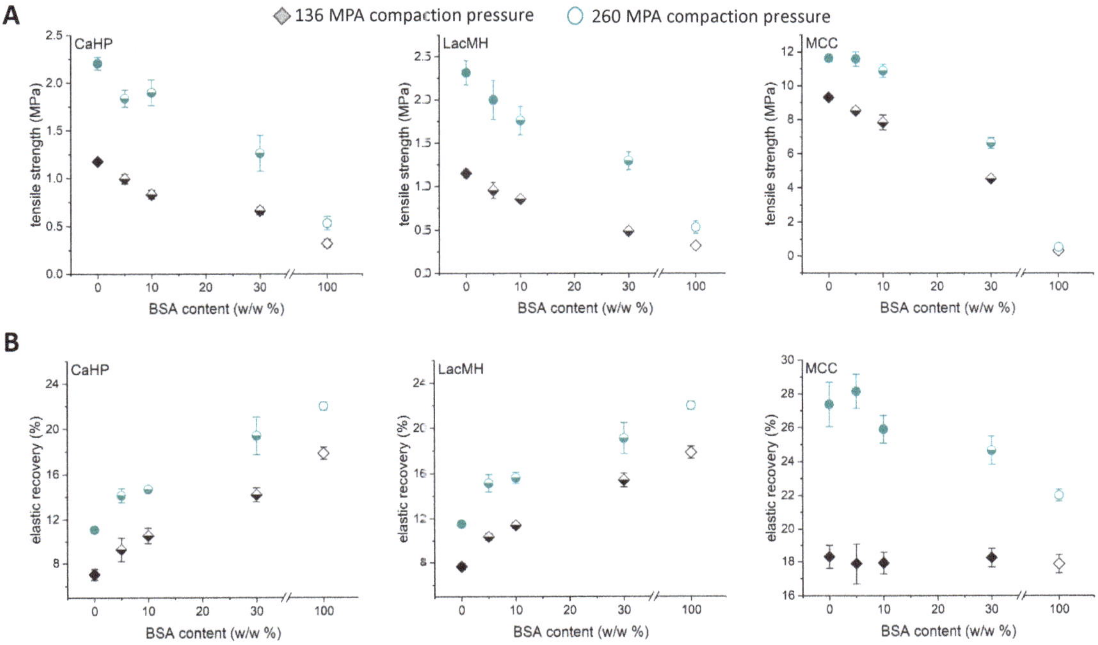

Figure 2. (**A**) Tensile strength of binary blends containing BSA and CaHP, LacMH, and MCC and (**B**) elastic recoveries of binary blends containing BSA and CaHP, LacMH, and MCC. Open symbols: pure protein; filled symbols: pure excipients and binary blends that are not significantly different from pure excipients; half-filled symbols: binary blends that are significantly different from pure excipients (n = 5; mean ± SD). Diamond (♦)—136 MPa compaction pressure; circles (•)—260 MPa compaction pressure.

The excipients showed a higher tensile strength when compacted individually at low and high compaction pressure compared to the binary mixtures. Compacts made of pure CaHP and LacMH had similar tensile strengths, at 1.2 and 2.2 MPa, at compaction pressures of 136 and 260 MPa, respectively. Pure MCC showed the highest tensile strength upon compaction with 9.5 and 11.5 MPa at compaction pressures of 136 and 260 MPa, respectively. Already low amounts of BSA lowered the tensile strength of the used excipient compacts. At 5 w/w% of BSA, the tensile strength of the binary blends containing CaHP was already significantly ($\alpha = 0.05$) decreased, independent of the compaction pressure. For LacMH and MCC, the addition of 5 w/w% of BSA did significantly decrease the tensile strength of the binary blends at a 136 MPa compaction pressure. At a high compaction pressure (260 MPa), 10 w/w% BSA was needed to have a significant impact on the tensile strength, showing that the percolation threshold of this binary blend is dependent on the compaction pressure [19]. It should be noted that acceptable compacts with tensile strengths higher than 2 MPa could be compacted from all BSA binary mixtures and BSA-MCC blends at both compaction pressures. The particle size of BSA might affect the compactability of the protein; however, a decrease in the particle size of BSA is not expected to suddenly increase the tensile strength in binary mixtures, but is expected to be a material-related property of the protein powder, as seen for other materials [26].

Additionally, the elastic recovery (out-of-die) was measured for the compacts (Figure 2B). BSA compacted alone showed an elastic recovery of 18 and 22% at the 136 and 260 MPa compaction pressures, respectively. The elastic recovery of BSA exceeded the elastic recoveries of both LacMH and CaHP (7% at the 136 MPa compaction pressure and 11% at the 260 MPa compaction pressure). It was observed that already 5 w/w% of BSA had a significantly increasing effect ($\alpha = 0.05$) on the elastic recovery. An increase in the BSA weight fraction in the binary blends further increased the elastic recovery. MCC showed an elastic recovery of 27.5% at the 260 MPa compaction pressure, which is higher than the elastic recovery for BSA at that compaction pressure. A significant effect of adding BSA to MCC on the elastic recovery at the 260 MPa compaction pressure was seen after adding 30 w/w% of BSA, indicating that at lower concentrations of BSA, the elastic properties of MCC exceed the effect of BSA. At the 136 MPa compaction pressure, the elastic recovery of both MCC and BSA was around 18%. Adding BSA to MCC showed no effect on the elastic recovery at that compaction pressure.

To the best of our knowledge, no studies have considered the particulate properties of protein binary mixtures, though a few studies have considered the importance of the protein stability upon compaction [10,12,17]. Compacting BSA in binary mixtures of three commonly used excipients was possible, indicating that the general concepts of compacting proteins can be used for the design of oral protein drug delivery. However, the challenges of peptide and protein oral drug delivery, such as poor absorption, gastrointestinal enzymatic digestion, etc. [30] must also be addressed to succeed with oral protein drug delivery. Protein-coating [31], mucus-penetrating agents [32,33], permeation enhancers [14,34], etc. are examples of approaches to overcoming the oral protein formulation challenges, but the strategies are likely a case-to-case-based decision from protein to protein. A common strategy is using permeation enhancers to improve the protein absorption, which may feed new challenges, as permeation enhancers are often poorly compactable [35]. Pedersen et al. (2023) simulated the challenges of compacting poorly compactible permeation enhancers using high concentrations of maltitol in formulations containing insulin. The authors described how the tabletability properties were significantly improved by tailoring the spray-drying process of insulin with maltitol to form small and non-hollow insulin-maltitol particles [14].

3.3. Binary Blends Containing Lysozyme

As a second model protein, amorphous lysozyme powder with a smaller mean particle size than BSA was used (Figure 1). Similarly to the BSA experiments, lysozyme was added into three different excipients (LacMH, CaHP, and MCC) at increasing weight fractions (5, 10, and 30 w/w%). The compaction of lysozyme alone resulted in tablets with a tensile strength of 2.0 MPa at a 136 MPa compaction pressure and 2.3 MPa at a 260 MPa compaction pressure (Figure 3A). These results are in good agreement with Wei et al. (2019), where compacted pure lysozyme had a tensile strength of ~2 MPa at a 150 MPa compaction pressure [12].

Comparing pure lysozyme with pure CaHP indicated that at a 136 MPa compaction pressure, the tensile strength of BSA is lower than that of lysozyme (1.1 MPa). At a 260 MPa compaction pressures, the tensile strengths of CaHP and lysozyme are comparable at 2.2 MPa. Interestingly, a significant increase in the tensile strength of binary blends containing CaHP and lysozyme above the tensile strength of the individual ingredients was observed, indicating that a combination of those components has a higher bonding strength within the tablet than the individual materials at a 260 MPa compaction pressure. A similar behavior was seen for binary blends containing LacMH and lysozyme. Surprisingly, this effect was only observed for the higher compaction pressure (260 MPa). This shows that a certain compaction pressure is needed to see this effect of an increased bonding strength.

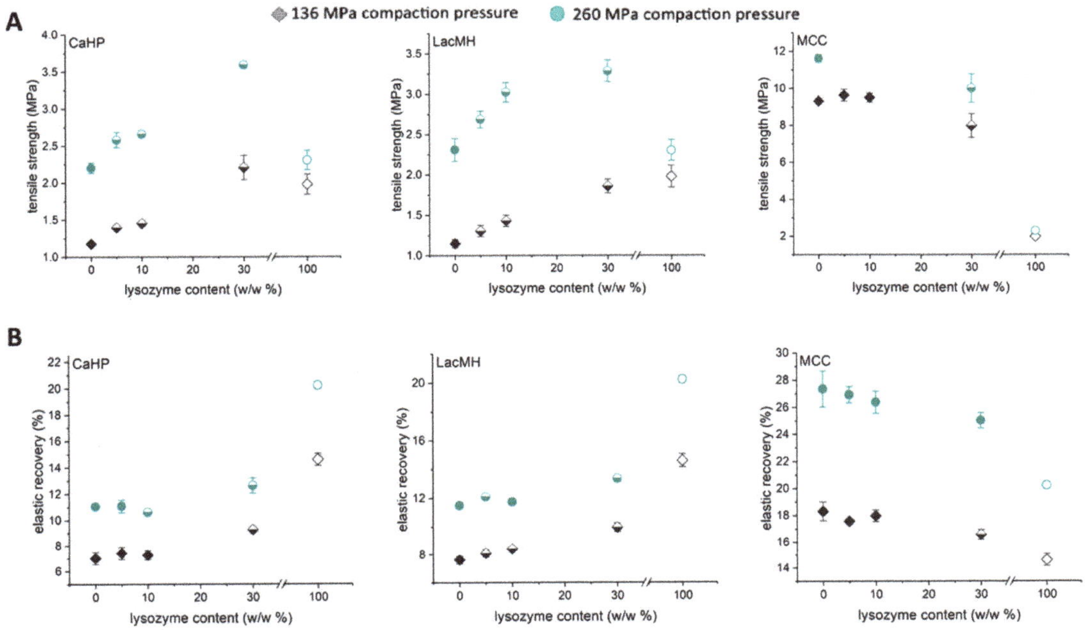

Figure 3. (**A**) Tensile strength of binary blends containing lysozyme and CaHP, LacMH, and MCC. (**B**) Elastic recovers of binary blends containing lysozyme and CaHP, LacMH, and MCC. Open symbols: pure protein; filled symbols: pure excipients and binary blends that are not significantly different from pure excipients; half-filled symbols: binary blends significantly different from pure excipients (n = 5; mean ± SD). Diamond (♦)—136 MPa compaction pressure; circles (•)—260 MPa compaction pressure.

We suggest that lysozyme in combination with LacMH or CaHP increases the bonding strength via the solid bridge formation or increased mechanical interlocking between the two excipients. Lysozyme could hereby show functionality comparable to common dry binders. However, another possible reason for the increased mechanical properties is the moisture introduced into the blend by the lysozyme, inducing surface sintering at the particle surfaces in contact with the excipient particles. The hypothesis of the increased bonding strength between the two materials (in this case, LacMH or CaHP and lysozyme) is supported by the fact that the tablet density was not affected by the addition of lysozyme at high compaction pressures (Figure 3).

For binary blends containing MCC, this effect was not observed. However, it should be noted that MCC alone forms strong tablets [24,26], and a potential increase in tensile strength could not be detected due to the limitations of the tablet strength tester (individual tablets of MCC/5 w/w% and 10 w/w% lysozyme blends). Compared to BSA, lysozyme showed a higher elastic recovery than CaHP and LacMH and a lower elastic recovery than MCC (Figure 3B). Adding 5 w/w% lysozyme affected only the elastic recovery of the blends containing LacMH. At 30 w/w% lysozyme and 260 MPa compaction, all blends except those containing MCC significantly impacted the elastic recovery. The unexpected increased bonding strength between lysozyme and LacMH or CaHP might result from solid bridge formation or increased mechanical interlocking between protein powder and excipients. Lysozyme could hereby show functionality comparable to common dry binders. However, another possible reason for the increased mechanical properties is the moisture introduced to the blend by lysozyme-inducing surface sintering at the particle surfaces in contact with the excipient particles. The hypothesis of increased bonding strength between the two materials (in this case, LacMH or CaHP and lysozyme) is supported by the fact that adding lysozyme at high compaction pressures does not affect the tablet density. However, to fully understand the impact of particle size of the used model proteins, it would be of benefit to use the same protein in different sizes, as reported by Wei et al. (2019) [12]. Conclusions based on the particle sizes between two different proteins cannot be made, as the intrinsic properties of both proteins vary.

In general, a lower impact on the elastic recovery for blends containing lysozyme was seen compared to BSA (Figures 2B and 3B), and it was possible to compact lysozyme with all three excipients. Wei et al. (2019) reported that the compaction of pure BSA and lysozyme did not cause any detectable changes in the secondary or tertiary structure or the thermal stability [12]. The stability of BSA and lysozyme is not expected to be affected in binary mixtures, but this could be evaluated in a future study.

With this study, we have demonstrated that the particulate properties of binary protein–excipient mixtures, in terms of their tablet properties, share similarities with small molecule-based studies. For developing biological oral tablet products, not only the particulate properties but also the protein stability and activity must be in focus.

4. Conclusions

This study showed that compacting up to 30 w/w% of the selected model proteins with commonly used excipients into tablets with a sufficient tensile strength for downstream processing is possible. Especially with MCC, compacts with a tensile strength of more than 4 MPa could be compacted with all the powder blends, which indicates that MCC could be a good choice for tablet-based products containing proteins. With an increasing BSA content, the tensile strength decreased when compared to the tablets with the pure excipient. The change in elastic recovery with an increasing BSA content indicated a strong effect at an already low BSA concentration. The increase in the tensile strength of the mixtures of lysozyme with LacMH and CaHP indicated the formation of stronger bonds between the components in the tablet, suggesting lysozyme acted as a dry binder.

Author Contributions: Conceptualization, E.H., C.H. and J.R.; methodology, E.H. and C.H.; software, E.H. and C.H.; validation, E.H. and C.H.; formal analysis, E.H. and C.H.; investigation, E.H. and C.H.; resources, J.R.; data curation, E.H. and C.H.; writing—original draft preparation, E.H. and C.H.; writing—review and editing, E.H. and J.R.; visualization, E.H. and C.H.; supervision, J.R.; project administration, E.H. and J.R.; funding acquisition, J.R. All authors have read and agreed to the published version of the manuscript.

Funding: This research was funded by Innovation Fund Denmark, project High-Quality Dry Products with Superior Functionality and Stability—Q-Dry, grant number 5150-0024B.

Data Availability Statement: Data are available upon request.

Acknowledgments: The authors would like to acknowledge Claus Cornett, Thomas Rades, and Jørn Sonnergaard from the Department of Pharmacy at the University of Copenhagen, for their valuable scientific discussions during this project.

Conflicts of Interest: The authors declare no conflict of interest. The company had no role in the design of the study; in the collection, analyses, or interpretation of data; in the writing of the manuscript, and in the decision to publish the results.

References

1. Aguirre, T.A.S.; Teijeiro-Osorio, D.; Rosa, M.; Coulter, I.S.; Alonso, M.J.; Brayden, D.J. Current Status of Selected Oral Peptide Technologies in Advanced Preclinical Development and in Clinical Trials. *Adv. Drug Deliv. Rev.* **2016**, *106*, 223–241. [CrossRef] [PubMed]
2. Moroz, E.; Matoori, S.; Leroux, J.C. Oral Delivery of Macromolecular Drugs: Where We Are after Almost 100 Years of Attempts. *Adv. Drug Deliv. Rev.* **2016**, *101*, 108–121. [CrossRef] [PubMed]
3. Walsh, G.; Walsh, E. Biopharmaceutical Benchmarks 2022. *Nat. Biotechnol.* **2022**, *40*, 1722–1760. [CrossRef] [PubMed]
4. Zizzari, A.T.; Pliatsika, D.; Gall, F.M.; Fischer, T.; Riedl, R. New Perspectives in Oral Peptide Delivery. *Drug Discov. Today* **2021**, *26*, 1097–1105. [CrossRef] [PubMed]

5. U.S. Food and Drug Administration FDA Approves First Oral GLP-1 Treatment for Type 2 Diabetes. Available online: https://www.fda.gov/news-events/press-announcements/fda-approves-first-oral-glp-1-treatment-type-2-diabetes (accessed on 1 August 2023).
6. Leonard, T.W.; Lynch, J.; McKenna, M.J.; Brayden, D.J. Promoting Absorption of Drugs in Humans Using Medium-Chain Fatty Acid-Based Solid Dosage Forms: GIPET^{TM}. *Expert Opin. Drug Deliv.* **2006**, *3*, 685–692. [CrossRef] [PubMed]
7. Frokjaer, S.; Otzen, D.E. Protein Drug Stability: A Formulation Challenge. *Nat. Rev. Drug Discov.* **2005**, *4*, 298–306. [CrossRef] [PubMed]
8. Park, K.; Kwon, I.C.; Park, K. Oral Protein Delivery: Current Status and Future Prospect. *React. Funct. Polym.* **2011**, *71*, 280–287. [CrossRef]
9. Walsh, G. Biopharmaceutical Benchmarks 2018. *Nat. Biotechnol.* **2018**, *36*, 1136–1145. [CrossRef]
10. Klukkert, M.; Van De Weert, M.; Fanø, M.; Rades, T.; Leopold, C.S. Influence of Tableting on the Conformation and Thermal Stability of Trypsin as a Model Protein. *J. Pharm. Sci.* **2015**, *104*, 4314–4321. [CrossRef]
11. Picker, K.M. Influence of Tableting on the Enzymatic Activity of Different A-Amylases Using Various Excipients. *Eur. J. Pharm. Biopharm.* **2002**, *53*, 181–185. [CrossRef]
12. Wei, Y.; Wang, C.; Jiang, B.; Sun, C.C.; Middaugh, C.R. Developing Biologics Tablets: The Effects of Compression on the Structure and Stability of Bovine Serum Albumin and Lysozyme. *Mol. Pharm.* **2019**, *16*, 1119–1131. [CrossRef] [PubMed]
13. Wurster, D.E.; Ternik, R.L. Pressure-Induced Activity Loss in Solid State Catalase. *J. Pharm. Sci.* **1994**, *84*, 190–194. [CrossRef]
14. Pedersen, M.D.; Megarry, A.; Naelapää, K.; Rades, T.; Pessi, J. Enhancing Tabletability of High-Dose Tablets by Tailoring Properties of Spray-Dried Insulin Particles. *Int. J. Pharm.* **2023**, *631*, 122526. [CrossRef] [PubMed]
15. Forbes, R.T.; Barry, B.W.; Elkordy, A.A. Preparation and Characterisation of Spray-Dried and Crystallised Trypsin: FT-Raman Study to Detect Protein Denaturation after Thermal Stress. *Eur. J. Pharm. Sci.* **2007**, *30*, 315–323. [CrossRef] [PubMed]
16. Parkins, D.A.; Lashmar, U.T. The Formulation of Biopharmaceutical Products. *Pharm. Sci. Technol. Today* **2000**, *3*, 130–137. [CrossRef] [PubMed]
17. Lu, Y.; Wang, C.; Jiang, B.; Sun, C.C.; Hoag, S.W. Effects of Compaction and Storage Conditions on Stability of Intravenous Immunoglobulin–Implication on Developing Oral Tablets of Biologics. *Int. J. Pharm.* **2021**, *604*, 120737. [CrossRef]
18. Leane, M.; Pitt, K.; Reynolds, G.; Anwar, J.; Charlton, S.; Crean, A.; Creekmore, R.; Davies, C.; DeBeer, T.; De-Matas, M.; et al. A Proposal for a Drug Product Manufacturing Classification System (MCS) for Oral Solid Dosage Forms. *Pharm. Dev. Technol.* **2015**, *20*, 12–21. [CrossRef]
19. Holman, L.E.; Leuenberger, H. The Effect of Varying the Composition of Binary Powder Mixtures and Compacts on Their Properties: A Percolation Phenomenon. *Powder Technol.* **1990**, *60*, 249–258. [CrossRef]
20. Van Veen, B.; Van Der Voort Maarschalk, K.; Bolhuis, G.K.; Frijlink, H.W. Predicting Mechanical Properties of Compacts Containing Two Components. *Powder Technol.* **2004**, *139*, 156–164. [CrossRef]
21. Michrafy, A.; Diarra, H.; Dodds, J.A. Compaction Behavior of Binary Mixtures. *Powder Technol.* **2009**, *190*, 146–151. [CrossRef]
22. Queiroz, A.L.P.; Faisal, W.; Devine, K.; Garvie-Cook, H.; Vucen, S.; Crean, A.M. The Application of Percolation Threshold Theory to Predict Compaction Behaviour of Pharmaceutical Powder Blends. *Powder Technol.* **2019**, *354*, 188–198. [CrossRef]
23. Sun, C.C. A Classification System for Tableting Behaviors of Binary Powder Mixtures. *Asian J. Pharm. Sci.* **2016**, *11*, 486–491. [CrossRef]
24. Doelker, E. Comparative Compaction Properties of Various Microcrystalline Cellulose Types and Generic Products. *Drug Dev. Ind. Pharm.* **1993**, *19*, 2399–2471. [CrossRef]
25. Rehula, M.; Adamek, R.; Spacek, V. Stress Relaxation Study of Fillers for Directly Compressed Tablets. *Powder Technol.* **2012**, *217*, 510–515. [CrossRef] [PubMed]
26. McKenna, A.; McCafferty, D.F. Effect of Particle Size on the Compaction Mechanism and Tensile Strength of Tablets. *J. Pharm. Pharmacol* **1982**, *34*, 347–351. [CrossRef] [PubMed]
27. Tukaram, B.N.; Vidaya Rajagopalan, I.V.; Shartchandra, P.S.I. The Effects of Lactose, Microcrystalline Cellulose and Dicalcium Phosphate on Swelling and Erosion of Compressed HPMC Matrix Tablets: Texture Analyzer. *Iran. J. Pharm. Res.* **2010**, *9*, 349–358.
28. Korhonen, O.; Pohja, S.; Peltonen, S.; Suihko, E.; Vidgren, M.; Paronen, P.; Ketolainen, J. Effects of Physical Properties for Starch Acetate Powders on Tableting. *AAPS PharmSciTech* **2002**, *3*, 34. [CrossRef]
29. Sedlock, R. A Tabletting Tabletability, Compactibility, and Compressibility: What's the Difference? Available online: https://natoli.com/app/uploads/2016/09/TC-Sept-16-Sedlock.pdf (accessed on 1 August 2023).
30. Drucker, D.J. Advances in Oral Peptide Therapeutics. *Nat. Rev. Drug Discov.* **2020**, *19*, 277–289. [CrossRef]
31. Binkley, N.; Bolognese, M.; Sidorowicz-Bialynicka, A.; Vally, T.; Trout, R.; Miller, C.; Buben, C.E.; Gilligan, J.P.; Krause, D.S. A Phase 3 Trial of the Efficacy and Safety of Oral Recombinant Calcitonin: The Oral Calcitonin in Postmenopausal Osteoporosis (ORACAL) Trial. *J. Bone Miner. Res.* **2012**, *27*, 1821–1829. [CrossRef]
32. Sheng, J.; He, H.; Han, L.; Qin, J.; Chen, S.; Ru, G.; Li, R.; Yang, P.; Wang, J.; Yang, V.C. Enhancing Insulin Oral Absorption by Using Mucoadhesive Nanoparticles Loaded with LMWP-Linked Insulin Conjugates. *J. Control. Release* **2016**, *233*, 181–190. [CrossRef]
33. Shan, W.; Zhu, X.; Liu, M.; Li, L.; Zhong, J.; Sun, W.; Zhang, Z.; Huang, Y. Overcoming the Diffusion Barrier of Mucus and Absorption Barrier of Epithelium by Self-Assembled Nanoparticles for Oral Delivery of Insulin. *ACS Nano* **2015**, *9*, 2345–2356. [CrossRef] [PubMed]

34. Twarog, C.; Fattah, S.; Heade, J.; Maher, S.; Fattal, E.; Brayden, D.J. Intestinal Permeation Enhancers for Oral Delivery of Macromolecules: A Comparison between Salcaprozate Sodium (SNAC) and Sodium Caprate (C10). *Pharmaceutics* **2019**, *11*, 78. [CrossRef] [PubMed]
35. Chantraine, F.; Viana, M.; Cazalbou, S.; Brielles, N.; Mondain-Monval, O.; Pouget, C.; Branlard, P.; Rubinstenn, G.; Chulia, D. From Compressibility to Structural Investigation of Sodium Dodecyl Sulphate-Part 1: Powder and Tablet Physico-Chemical Characteristics. *Powder Technol.* **2007**, *177*, 34–40. [CrossRef]

pharmaceutics

MDPI

Review

Research Progress on Peptide Drugs for Type 2 Diabetes and the Possibility of Oral Administration

Xinxin Yang [1,†], Ruiting Lin [1,†], Changzhuo Feng [2], Qiyuan Kang [2], Peng Yu [2], Yongzhi Deng [1,*] and Ye Jin [1,*]

1 School of Pharmacy, Changchun University of Chinese Medicine, Changchun 130117, China; yangxx@ccucm.edu.cn (X.Y.); 23203070208@stu.ccucm.edu.cn (R.L.)

2 College of Traditional Chinese Medicine, Changchun University of Chinese Medicine, Changchun 130117, China; 21203070201@ccucm.edu.cn (C.F.); 2302040121@ccucm.edu.cn (Q.K.); yupeng@ccucm.edu.cn (P.Y.)

* Correspondence: dengyz@ccucm.edu.cn (Y.D.); jinye@ccucm.edu.cn (Y.J.)

† These authors contributed equally to this work.

Abstract: Diabetes is a global disease that can lead to a range of complications. Currently, the treatment of type 2 diabetes focuses on oral hypoglycemic drugs and insulin analogues. Studies have shown that drugs such as oral metformin are useful in the treatment of diabetes but can limit the liver's ability to release sugar. The development of glucose-lowering peptides has provided new options for the treatment of type 2 diabetes. Peptide drugs have low oral utilization due to their easy degradation, short half-life, and difficulty passing through the intestinal mucosa. Therefore, improving the oral utilization of peptide drugs remains an urgent problem. This paper reviews the research progress of peptide drugs in the treatment of diabetes mellitus and proposes that different types of nano-formulation carriers, such as liposomes, self-emulsifying drug delivery systems, and polymer particles, should be combined with peptide drugs for oral administration to improve their absorption in the gastrointestinal tract.

Keywords: oral delivery; nano-formulations; peptide drugs; type 2 diabetes mellitus

1. Introduction

Diabetes is one of the major causes of long-term ill health and a growing global disease. Often leading to severe metabolic disease and a range of serious complications, diabetes is a global disease burden [1]. Diabetes mellitus is classified as type 1 diabetes mellitus (T1DM) and type 2 diabetes mellitus (T2DM). T1DM is characterized by insufficient insulin secretion, which renders pancreatic islet cells incompetent against autoimmune [2]. T2DM is the most prevalent type, with a longer disease course, and is characterized by hyperglycemia due to a decrease in insulin secretion by the pancreas [3]. T2DM also causes complications such as cardiovascular disease and type 2 diabetic nephropathy, as well as an increased risk of hypertension [4,5]. T2DM is characterized by relative insulin deficiency or insulin resistance, in which the muscles and organs, such as the liver, are not sensitive enough to insulin so that blood glucose cannot be used effectively and remains at a high level [6]. In recent years, treatment for T2DM has focused on drugs that increase insulin secretion, sensitize, and reduce hepatic glucose production. Other non-modifiable risk factors include family history and ethnicity [7]. Obesity, disrupted sleep cycles or abnormal circadian rhythms, and a lack of sufficient regular physical activity may have compounding effects [8]. While current treatment strategies can help people with diabetes improve their symptoms, new and effective treatments are needed.

In recent years, peptide drugs synthesized using modern biotechnology have become one of the hotspots of drug research and development and are now widely used in the prevention, diagnosis, and treatment of tumors, hepatitis, diabetes, AIDS, and other diseases due to their wide indications, high safety, and remarkable efficacy, and have a broad development prospect. Some peptide drugs use less dosage, are more selective, have better specificity, and have fewer side effects than small-molecule drugs. Peptide therapeutics are usually administered by injection, but injections are invasive and reduce patient compliance. In addition, injectables increase the complexity and cost of manufacturing and storage. There is a growing interest in the oral delivery of peptides, a technology that could provide a safe and convenient alternative to peptide drug delivery [9]. However, direct delivery of peptides is not feasible. Oral peptides must overcome physiological barriers such as low solubility, permeability, and early degradation to achieve efficient and sustained drug delivery [10].

In exploring technological approaches to achieve efficient oral peptide delivery, drugs combined with nano-formulations are particularly promising due to their wide diversity, good biocompatibility, and ease of modification and thus functionalization [11]. As shown in Figure 1,this paper reviews the current research progress, therapeutic scope, and potential applications of peptide drugs for the treatment of diabetes (Table 1) and lists oral formulations that can be loaded with peptides. It is hoped that combining the two will provide new ideas for the oral delivery of peptide drugs for the treatment of diabetes.

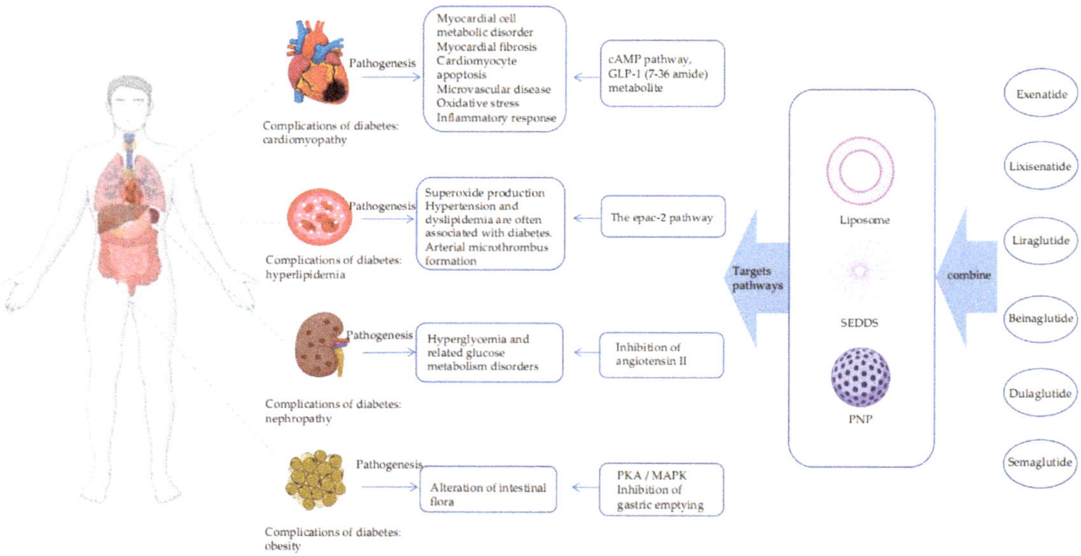

Figure 1. The mechanism/target of the combination of peptide drugs and nano-preparations on diabetic complications.

Table 1. Application of polypeptide drugs in clinical research of type 2 diabetes mellitus.

Type	Molecular Formula	CAS Number	Molecular Weight	Detection Indexes of Type 2 Diabetes Mellitus	Phase	Trial Number	Reference
Exenatide	C184H282N50O60S	141758-74-9	4186.57	Hepatic fat content	Phase 4	NCT01432405	[12]
Lixisenatide	C215H347N61O65S	320367-13-3	4858.49	Blood lipid level	Phase 2	NCT02274740	[13]
Loxenatide	C210H325N55O69S	2420483-82-3	44,212.65	Phase 1	kidney function	NCT02467790	[14]
Liraglutide	C172H265N43O51	204656-20-2	3751.20	Cardiovascular	Phase 4	NCT01761318	[15]
Beinaglutide	C149H225N39O46	123475-27-4	3298.61	Blood sugar	Not Applicable	NCT03829891	[16]
Dulaglutide	C149H221N37O49	923950-08-7	3314.62	Blood pressure, heart rate	Phase 2	NCT01149421	[17]
Semaglutide	C187H291N45O59	910463-68-2	4113.58	Heart disease, cardiovascular	Phase 3	NCT03914326	[18]
Tirzepatide	C225H348N48O68 • XNa	2023788-19-2	4813.45	HbA1c	Phase 4	NCT05706506	[19]

2. Glucagon-like Peptide 1 (GLP-1)

GLP-1 is a peptide derived from the *glucagonogen* (*Gcg*) sequence that shares the same precursor molecule as glucagon but has an opposite effect on blood glucose. GLP-1 is mainly secreted by intestinal L-cells and enters the peripheral circulation after entering the bloodstream, while glucagon preprogenitor neurons in the solitary tract nucleus of the brainstem also secrete GLP-1 and play a role in the central nervous system (CNS) [20,21]. Prohormone convertase 1 (PC1) cleaves *Gcg* in cells, thereby expressing GLP-1 [22–24]. GLP-1 promotes insulin secretion after binding to and activating the glucagon-like peptide-1 receptor (GLP-1R) on the surface of β-cells, and glucose dose-dependently increases the concentration of GLP-1 secreted by L cells. GLP-1 also inhibits β-cell apoptosis and induces β-cell proliferation by stimulating the expression of insulin receptor substrate 2, including mechanisms such as acute proinsulin action and stimulation of second messenger cAMP by activation of the response element binding protein (CREB) (Figure 2) [25,26]. Under conditions of insulin resistance and cellular stress, α-cells can regulate insulin secretion by producing GLP-1, thereby compensating for the increased functional demands of β-cells [27]. In addition, GLP-1 can stimulate growth inhibitor secretion and activate the protein kinase A system (PKA) to inhibit α-cell glucagon secretion [28]. Because GLP-1 is cleaved in vivo by dipeptidyl peptidase-4 (DPP-4) (EC number: 3.4.14.5) and the circulating half-life of GLP-1 in diabetic patients is only 1.5 to 2 min [29], GLP-1 receptor agonists (GLP-1RAs) for the treatment of T2DM are widely developed and used.

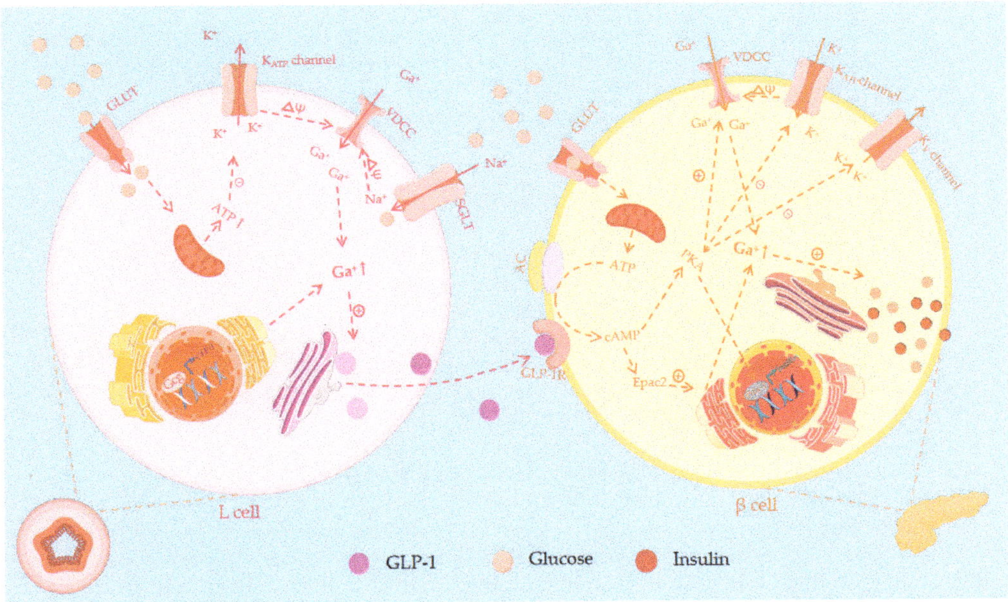

Figure 2. Glucose stimulates GLP-1 secretion from L-cells: Glucose closes ATP-sensitive K^{+} $_{ATP}$ channels and opens Ca^{2+} channel (VDCC) to induce membrane depolarization, and Ca^{2+} inward flow triggers vesicular cytotoxicity and GLP-1 secretion.

GLP-1R is expressed in the heart, brain, kidneys, stomach, and fat cells and ameliorates complications caused by diabetes. GLP-1R is mainly found in cardiac endothelium, coronary arteries, and smooth muscle cells [21,30]. GLP-1 is cardioprotective through the cAMP signaling pathway and DPP-4 degradation of GLP-1 (7–36 amide) to generate GLP-1 (9–36 amide) and its smaller degradation products. Thus, GLP-1RAs increase cardiomyocyte survival and improve endothelial dysfunction [31]. GLP-1 can improve blood pressure by stimulating urinary sodium excretion through epac2-dependent stimulation of atrial natriuretic peptide secretion [32]. Brain GLP-1R activation feeds through PKA/MAPK-induced AMPK inhibition. Peripheral GLP-1 is transmitted via the vagus nerve to the central nervous system to generate electrical signals, and brain-derived GLP-1 is released locally as a neurotransmitter, which together mediate inhibition of gastric motility and reduce the rate of glucose absorption [33,34]. In addition, GLP-1 inhibits gastric emptying through adrenergic signaling and promotes brown remodeling of white fat in a SIRT1-dependent manner, reducing body weight in T2DM patients [35–37]. GLP-1 inhibits angiotensin II and renin and reduces the risk of proteinuria in T2DM patients [38]. Although the exact details of renal regulation by GLP-1 are unknown, it has been found that GLP-1 ameliorates renal injury, fibrosis, and lipid accumulation in diabetic nephropathy rats via the Sirt1/AMPK/PGC1α pathway [39]. In addition, the researchers isolated a GLP-1RAs called Exendin-4 from lizard venom and optimized the structure of GLP-1 and Exendin-4 for the treatment of T2DM [40].

GLP-1 stimulates β cells to secrete insulin. GLP-1-induced elevation of cAMP leads to PKA activation and enhanced signaling via exchange proteins directly activated by cAMP (Epac). cAMP activation of PKA increases the sensitivity of the K^{+}_{ATP} channel to ATP, leading to the closure of the K^{+}_{ATP} channel, depolarization of the cell membrane, and opening of the VDCC channel. Subsequent Ca^{2+} influx promotes cytosolic action of insulin granules and acute secretion of insulin into the circulation. Simultaneously, GLP-1-activated PKA inhibits voltage-gated Kv channels, prevents membrane repolarization, and promotes Ca^{2+} influx by prolonging the opening of the VDCC channel. Epac stimulates the release of Ca^{2+} from the endoplasmic reticulum (ER), increasing insulin secretion by increasing the intracellular pool of Ca^{2+}. cAMP activates Epac 2 by direct binding. Under high glucose conditions, the flow of Ca^{2+} through the VDCC channel into b-cells enhances Ca^{2+} influx, and Epac 2 opens ryanodine receptor Ca^{2+} channels in the ER, further increasing intracellular Ca^{2+} levels and enhancing insulin secretion.

2.1. Exenatide

In April 2005, Exenatide was approved by the US FDA as the first GLP-1RAs for the treatment of T2DM. Exenatide has 50% homology to human GLP-1 and similar affinity for the GLP-1 receptor. It exhibits glucose-regulatory activity similar to that of GLP-1, including enhanced glucose dependence of β-cells in response to insulin secretion, and is accompanied by progressive weight loss. Exenatide reduces the concentration of glucagon in the blood during periods of hyperglycemia. In patients with T2DM, glucagon levels are abnormally high during hyperglycemia, and lowering blood glucagon concentrations during hyperglycemia leads to reduced hepatic glucose output and reduced insulin requirements [41]. In addition, exenatide may also reduce renal dysfunction to a certain extent in patients with diabetic nephropathy, with exenatide significantly reducing proteinuria levels in 26.2% of the patients [42]. Exenatide mediates attenuation of diabetic nephropathy by SIRT1-dependent down-regulation of thioredoxin-interacting protein H3K9ac acetylation and reduces the recruitment of spliced X-box binding protein 1 to the Txnip promoter [43]. Weekly doses of exenatide have also been shown to modestly reduce body weight and systolic blood pressure [44]. Exenatide administered at a dose of 2 mg once a week (QW) showed greater improvements in glycemic control compared to the 10 μg dose taken twice a day (BID), with no increased risk of hypoglycemia and a corresponding reduction in body weight [45]. Compared with other hypoglycemic agents, exenatide significantly improved carotid intima-media thickening, which is associated with cardiovascular probability, and its cardioprotective effects were demonstrated by the inhibition of atrial fibrillation and reduced susceptibility to atrial fibrillation in rats [46,47]. Gastrointestinal adverse events (AEs), including nausea, vomiting, and diarrhea, are common with exenatide during treatment. In 2021, Bydureon, whose main ingredient is exenatide, became the first FDA-approved microsphere formulation for the treatment of T2DM, attenuating gastrointestinal AE. However, subcutaneous nodules can occur at the injection site when the microspheres produce an inflammatory foreign-body reaction in patients treated with exenatide QW [48].

Injection site reactions were more common in the exenatide QW group than in the exenatide BID or non-GLP-1RAs groups. In addition, after the initial release of surface-bound exenatide, the encapsulated peptide was released from the microspheres in approximately two weeks' time [49].

2.2. Loxenatide

Loxenatide, also known as polyethylene glycol loxenatide (PEX-168). It is based on the structure of exenatide and modifies the drug molecule by adding polyethylene glycol, thus extending the half-life of the drug [40]. Clinical trials showed that loxenatide monotherapy significantly improved glycemic control in patients with T2DM, with a safety profile similar to other GLP-RA [14]. A short-term controlled trial with metformin showed that the addition of loxenatide to metformin was superior to the addition of glucagon in improving glycemic control and assessing glycemic variability with continuous glucose monitoring in patients with T2DM [14]. Weight loss was more pronounced in patients given loxenatide subcutaneously once a week compared to metformin, and loxenatide reduced body weight by no more than 20% in purely obese mice irrespective of dose, with some risk of hypoglycemia [50,51]. T2DM can lead to impaired endothelium-dependent vasodilatation and decreased NO expression, manifesting as cardiovascular and endothelial dysfunction. The T2DM patient population with loxenatide showed significant improvements in glycemic lowering indices and inflammation-related indices, as well as significant changes in vascular endothelial cell function-related indices [52]. A controlled trial also demonstrated that loxenatide improved endothelial cell function in patients with T2DM [53]. Loxenatide reduces high glucose-induced ROS production in a concentration-dependent mechanism and inhibits mitochondria-dependent apoptosis of endothelial progenitor cells (EPCs) and mitochondrial membrane depolarization via activation of the sirtuin 3/Foxo3 signaling pathway and enhances mitochondrial respiratory function [54].

2.3. Lixisenatide

Lixisenatide, an Exendin-4 analogue, was approved in the EMA in 2012 for the treatment of T2DM. In preclinical studies, lixisenatide demonstrated high affinity and selectivity for the GLP-1 receptor, binding approximately four times that of natural GLP-1 [55]. Clinical studies have evaluated the efficacy of lixisenatide in combination with oral hypoglycemic agents in the treatment of patients with T2DM, and changes in glycated hemoglobin (HbA1c) demonstrated that the combination of lixisenatide with oral hypoglycemic agents significantly improves the efficacy and safety profile [56]. In an analysis of the results of a phase 3 clinical trial, it was reported that the majority of patients receiving a fixed ratio of glycemic insulin/lixisenatide were no longer experiencing gastrointestinal AE at eight weeks, with a greater potential to achieve target blood glucose compared to those receiving lixisenatide alone [57]. Lixisenatide stimulates insulin secretion when blood glucose is elevated but not when blood glucose is normal, thereby circumventing the risk of hypoglycemia and glucose-dependently inhibiting glucagon secretion [58,59]. The major differences from other GLP-1 RAs are that lixisenatide significantly reduces postprandial glucose immediately after injection and that the delay in gastric emptying is more pronounced with lixisenatide. The increase in intragastric glucose residence time after lixisenatide treatment was associated with a decrease in the systemic oral glucose rate and a decrease in the area under the glycemic curve, and this effect was more pronounced as the duration of dosing increased [60]. Lixisenatide also improves endothelial cell function and inflammation-related markers in T2DM patients [61]. Lixisenatide carries out anti-inflammatory effects by inhibiting the activation of NF-kB signaling in HUVECs cells and inhibiting the adhesion of monocytes and HUVECs [62]. and promotes mitochondrial biogenesis in HUVECs by inducing phosphorylation at the Ser133 site of CREB [63]. Lixisenatide is filtered in the kidney and subsequently degraded in the renal tubules [64]. Lixisenatide dose adjustment is not required in patients with T2DM with mild or moderate renal impairment [65].

2.4. Liraglutide

Liraglutide is based on the natural GLP-1 structure and is 97% homologous to natural GLP-1 [40], chemically modified to extend its half-life to 13 h after subcutaneous injection and to resist DPP-4 degradation [66]. Liraglutide was approved by the FDA in 2010 to improve glycemic control in adult patients with T2DM, and liraglutide is the only GLP-RAs approved for weight loss [67]. Clinical Trial Demonstrates Effectiveness of liraglutide as Monotherapy and Add-on to First-Line Therapy [49]. Liraglutide inhibits oxidative stress and reduces cardiovascular disease while controlling blood glucose [68]. Liraglutide elevated SIRT1 expression, which increased Parkin expression, leading to mitochondrial autophagy activation. Protective mitochondrial autophagy reverses cytosolic adenosine 5′-triphosphate production, reduces cellular oxidative stress and balances redox reactions, maintains mitochondrial homeostasis, and repairs infarcted hearts [69]. Liraglutide inhibits oxidative stress and apoptosis by increasing the concentration of anti-apoptotic proteins and decreasing the levels of pro-apoptotic proteins. Liraglutide treatment is confirmed to reverse microvascular endothelial cell injury [70]. Whereas liraglutide alone reduced pro-inflammatory and pro-atherosclerotic chemokines [71], liraglutide effectively counteracts high glucose-induced dysfunction of HUVECs by inhibiting PINK1/Parkin-dependent mitochondrial autophagy [72]. Together, they validate the vaso-protective effects of liraglutide. In both T2DM and non-T2DM patients, liraglutide reduces the onset and progression of renal disease in addition to conventional therapy [73–75]. Liraglutide protects renal thylakoid cells from hyperglycemia-mediated mitochondrial apoptosis by upregulating SIRT3 expression and activating the ERK-Yap signaling pathway [76]. Liraglutide also inhibits renal cell apoptosis by increasing SIRT1 expression and down-regulating TXNIP expression [72,77]. In addition, liraglutide reduces higher circulating plasma concentrations of dihydroceramide and ceramide, which are positively associated with insulin resistance and hepatic steatosis, in patients with T2DM [13].

2.5. Beinaglutide

Beinaglutide is an amine-free recombinant human GLP-1 (7–36) acid with 100% homology to human GLP-1. It is approved for the treatment of T2DM patients in China [78]. Beinaglutide shows significant weight loss benefits and effective glycemic control in the treatment of T2DM [79] and is more effective than metformin in reducing body weight and fat mass [80,81]. Although safe and effective in reducing visceral fat and body weight in obese T2DM patients, the dose of beinaglutide should be tailored to the individual [82]. Beinaglutide combats high-fat food-induced obesity by targeting the composition of major lipids in adipose tissue and the expression of lipid metabolism genes, e.g., by increasing Acrp30 levels and Akt phosphorylation in adipocytes, thereby ameliorating the associated fatty liver and dyslipidaemia [83]. In addition, serpin E1, leptin, c-reactive protein (CRP), and tumor necrosis factor-alpha (TNF-alpha) were significantly decreased in T2DM patients using beinaglutide, demonstrating that beinaglutide also has an anti-inflammatory effect in T2DM patients [84]. In a model of non-alcoholic steatohepatitis, long-term use of beinaglutide reduced liver weight and hepatic steatosis and improved insulin sensitivity, and increased Sirt1 gene expression levels improved hepatic insulin resistance [78].

2.6. Dulaglutide

Dulaglutide is produced by linking human immunoglobulin IgG-4 heavy chain to GLP-1 modification, which significantly increases its half-life [85]. In 2014, Dulaglutide became the first fragment crystallizable fusion protein to receive FDA approval for T2DM treatment [49]. Dulaglutide results in clinically dose-related reductions in HbA1c and body weight. In the six completed AWARD results, the majority of dulaglutide patients had HbA1c targets <7.0% (53.0 mmol/mol) and ≤6.5% (47.5 mmol/mol), which were superior to the active comparators (Exenatide, Glycine Insulin, Metformin, and Sitagliptin), with the most common adverse events being gastrointestinal AE, the lower rates of hypoglycemia [86–88]. In mouse control experiments, the expression levels of pancreatic beta-cell-related genes, insulin content, and insulin secretion were found to be significantly elevated in the dulaglutide group, and oxidative and endoplasmic reticulum stress, inflammation, fibrosis, and apoptosis were inhibited after treatment. Demonstration of a long-term protective effect of dulaglutide on β-cells [89]. In addition, dulaglutide can inhibit inflammation and oxidative stress by inhibiting the NF-κB signaling pathway and TGF-β/Smad2 signaling pathway, M1 macrophage polarization, and mitochondrial ROS release [90–92]. T2DM patients treated with dulaglutide improved systolic and pulse pressure, although one-third was due to weight loss effects [93]. However, the risk-related indices of urinary albumin/creatinine and HbA1c were reduced by 16.7% and 25.4%, respectively, in patients with adverse cardiovascular events with dulaglutide compared with placebo [94,95]. Dulaglutide may be considered for use in middle-aged and elderly T2DM patients with cardiovascular disease or cardiovascular risk factors [96]. Dulaglutide inhibits high glucose-induced activation of the NLRP3 inflammasome in HUVECs cells by increasing SIRT1 expression and suppressing NLRP3, ASC, and P10 expression. It also attenuated high glucose-induced cellular mitochondrial division in EPCs and significantly ameliorated vascular endothelial tissue damage and inflammation [97,98].

2.7. Semaglutide

Semaglutide is the first GLP-1RAs to have an oral dosage form. Semaglutide is prepared as a tablet in combination with the absorption enhancer sodium N-[8(2-hydroxyben zoyl)amino]octanoate (SNAC) to improve glycemic control in adults with T2DM [99,100]. SNAC binds to semaglutide, elevates local pH to decrease the efficacy of major digestive enzymes, increases the lipophilicity of semaglutide to promote gastric epithelial cell uptake, and facilitates the transit of semaglutide and its entry into the systemic circulation. When semaglutide and SNAC reach the bloodstream, the two molecules readily dissociate, allowing the oral formulation of semaglutide to interact with the body in the same manner as subcutaneous semaglutide [101]. However, the oral formulation of semaglutide has lower bioavailability compared to the subcutaneous formulation. Semaglutide is absorbed in the stomach with a rapid and dose-dependent increase in plasma concentrations, reaching peak concentrations within 15–35 min [102]. Semaglutide oral formulations at doses ≤ 10 mg are significantly less effective than subcutaneously administered forms, and therefore higher doses of semaglutide oral formulations need to be given to achieve the same clinical outcomes as subcutaneous formulations. Because SNAC protects semaglutide from pH-dependent degradation and because eating can lead to an increase in gastric pH, patients should fast prior to dosing and avoid eating for at least 30 min after dosing for optimal results [103,104].

Semaglutide is a favorable option for the treatment of T2DM, both subcutaneously and orally, and several clinical trials have demonstrated the safety and efficacy of semaglutide in the treatment of T2DM [105–108]. Semaglutide has shown significant efficacy in reducing HbA1c and body weight compared to other GLP-1RAs, although semaglutide can cause mild and transient gastrointestinal disturbances that decrease with continuation of treatment and increase the risk of cholelithiasis [109–111]. In controlled trials, 85% of participants taking oral semaglutide lost at least 5% of their body weight and had sustained improvements in obesity-related abnormalities such as hyperglycemia, hypertension, elevated lipids, and high-sensitivity c-reactive protein [112]. And semaglutide has been shown to be effective, safe, and well tolerated in T2DM patients with overweight and atherosclerotic cardiovascular disease [113]. Treatment with semaglutide Significantly Reduces Symptoms and Physical Limitations Associated with Obesity in Heart Failure Patients, Improves Exercise Function, and Reduces Weight [114,115]. Semaglutide ameliorates mitochondrial function and cardiac injury by modulating the PI3K-AKT signaling pathway [116]. Semaglutide avoids oxidative stress and apoptosis in the heart of diabetic mice by activating the Sirt1/AMPK pathway [117]. In a mouse model of HFpEF induced by obesity and T2DM, semaglutide improved cardiometabolic silhouette, cardiac structure, and cardiac function compared to weight loss induced by paired feeding. Transcriptomic and proteomic analyses showed that semaglutide improved left ventricular cytoskeletal function and endothelial function and restored protective immune responses in visceral adipose tissue. Exceeding the weight loss effect of paired feeding [118,119]. Semaglutide is Equally Effective in Glycemic Control and Weight in Patients with Chronic Kidney Disease [120]. Semaglutide directly ameliorates oxidative stress and inflammation-related metabolites such as NAD+ and adenosine in the kidneys of obese mice [121]. In a mouse model of hypertension-accelerated diabetic nephropathy, semaglutide significantly reduced hyperglycemia, hypertension, and proteinuria while significantly improving the severity of glomerulosclerosis and urine/kidney injury molecule-1 (KIM-1) levels [122].

3. Tirzepatide

2022 FDA approval of dual agonists for GLP-1R and glucose-dependent insulinotropic polypeptide receptor (GIPR) tirzepatide to improve glycemic control in adults with T2DM as an adjunct to diet and exercise [123]. Bringing renewed attention to the potential of glucose-dependent insulinotropic polypeptide (GIP) in the treatment of T2DM. GIP is a polypeptide consisting of 42 amino acids, which, along with GLP-1, belongs to the same group of enteric insulin in the human body and is secreted by the K cells of the intestinal mucosa of the duodenum and jejunum in the small intestine. GIP is responsible for most of the body's enteric insulin action; a normal human postprandial GIP level is about 4 times that of GLP-1, which is the most important enteric insulin [124]. Although both GIPR and GLP-1 R are present in β-cells, impaired β-cell function in patients with T2DM affects the regulatory functions of GIP and GLP-1 [125]. In T2DM, GIP has a limited ability to stimulate insulin secretion during hyperglycemia and does not significantly reduce blood glucose concentrations, whereas GLP-1 still significantly regulates blood glucose concentrations in patients with T2DM [126]. Unlike GLP-1, GIP has both glucagon and insulinotropic effects in a glucose-dependent manner, stimulating glucagon secretion under hypoglycemic conditions and insulin secretion under hyperglycemic conditions [127]. GIPRs were abundantly distributed in adipose tissue, and most of the distribution regions of GIPRs and GLP-1Rs in the CNS did not overlap. GIP is involved in the metabolism of adipose tissue carbohydrates and lipids, and it increases lipid storage in white adipose tissue and decreases ectopic storage of fat in the muscle [128]. In contrast, GLP-1 indirectly promotes lipolysis, works with GIP to maintain healthy adipocytes, and increases adipocyte production and secretion of lipocalin to improve insulin sensitivity [129]. GLP-1 synergizes with GIP to promote metabolic homeostasis, prevent hyperglycemia and hypoglycemia, attenuate dyslipidemia, and reduce the risk of cardiovascular disease in patients with T2DM and obesity.

Tirzepatide was injected once weekly, and the pharmacokinetics of tirzepatide were dose-proportional over the dose range studied [130]. In all SURPASS trials, tirzepatide showed a dose-dependent decrease in HbA 1c regardless of background glucose-lowering therapy [19]. The glycemic efficacy of tirzepatide in the treatment of T2DM was found to be due to simultaneous improvements in key components of diabetes pathophysiology, including beta-cell function, insulin sensitivity, and glucagon secretion, in Phase 1 clinical trials [131]. Tirzepatide synergistically activates both GIPR and GLP-1R in T2DM patients. In in vitro studies, tirzepatide elicited significantly higher cAMP responses in human pancreatic beta cell lines than those observed with GLP-1 or GIP alone, and in isolated islets, tirzepatide overcame the effects of GLP-1R to induce a robust increase in glucagon secretion [130,132]. However, the relative activity of tirzepatide at GLP-1 R and GIPR may vary in subjects with and without diabetes and with the degree of hyperglycemia. In SURPASS-2, tirzepatide was associated with dose-dependent weight loss from baseline, with up to 65%, 48%, and 31% of subjects treated with tirzepatide 15 mg/week losing ≥10%, ≥15%, and ≥20% of their body weight, respectively [133]. Tirzepatide provided more significant weight loss compared to selective GLP-1 RA treatment. Preclinical studies demonstrated greater weight loss in obese mice administered tirzepatide than in mice administered selective GLP-1 RA. GIP enhances GLP-1-induced food intake and weight loss by augmenting melanocortin expression and neuronal activation in different neuronal populations in the hypothalamus; thus, co-activation of GIPR and GLP-1R in the brain enhances weight loss efficacy [134,135]. T Therapeutic efficacy and side effects of tirzepatide are similar to those of selective GLP-1RA, with common AEs being gastrointestinal reactions. Tirzepatide effectively slowed the decline in glomerular filtration rate, lowered the urinary albumin/creatinine ratio, and reduced circulating levels of several biomarkers associated with cardiovascular risk, improving cardiovascular risk [136,137].

4. Oral Medications for Type 2 Diabetes

Metformin is considered the best initial therapeutic agent for T2DM. Regarding the mechanism of action of this drug, it may be related to the reduction in hepatic glucose production [125]. In randomized trials of diabetes, metformin was most effective in young, obese subjects. The results showed a decreasing risk of diabetes and long-term weight loss in the subjects [126]. Glipizide, a second-generation sulfonylurea, is a gastrointestinal therapeutic system (GITS) extended-release formulation. Glipizide GITS provides more stable plasma drug concentrations than immediate-release formulations, and the once-daily dosing regimen optimizes patient compliance. In patients with T2DM, the effect of glipizide GITS on fasting blood glucose levels may be greater. Glipizide GITS was shown to reduce the incidence of hypoglycemic symptoms in a 3-year model of type 2 diabetes treatment [123]. Oral repaglinide is a rapid-acting insulinotropic agent that reduces postprandial glucose by targeting early insulin release, and lowering postprandial glucose is considered to be an important factor in the reduction in long-term cardiovascular complications of diabetes. It has a unique binding site on the beta cell membrane, and in in vitro and in vivo studies, alogliptin has been shown to be more potent and faster-acting in terms of insulinotropic effects, but may cause some weight gain [122]. DPP-4 inhibitors are widely used in the treatment of T2DM, which results in intra-insulin release when blood glucose is elevated. After evaluating the patients, the results suggest that DPP-4 inhibitors promote vascular endothelial cell regeneration, but when this effect occurs in the glomerulus, the proliferation of glomerular endothelial cells leads to tma-like lesions, which cause increased proteinuria and a rapid decline in renal function [124]. Miglitol is a second-generation alpha-glucosidase inhibitor that is generally well tolerated and does not cause weight gain or hypoglycemia with monotherapy. The drug is systemically absorbed but not metabolized and is rapidly excreted through the kidneys. Most of the adverse reactions associated with miglitol therapy involve gastrointestinal AE [127]. Pioglitazone is a thiazolidinedione drug that selectively agonizes the peroxisome growth factor-activated receptor PPARγ, which enhances insulin sensitivity in peripheral tissues and the liver and reduces insulin resistance. Pioglitazone significantly improved beta-cell function, liver function, and blood glucose indexes and slowed down the process of atherosclerosis. However, patients taking pioglitazone medication at high doses and for long periods of time may have an increased risk of bladder cancer [138]. Dagliflozin is a sodium-glucose cotransporter protein 2 (SGLT2) inhibitor that lowers blood glucose by inhibiting SGLT-2, reducing glucose reabsorption, and excreting sugar directly from the urine. In addition, dagliflozin can also reduce sodium reabsorption so that plasma volume decreases, achieving an antihypertensive effect and cardiovascular protection. And it reduces blood uric acid and proteinuria, relieves glomerular pressure, restores glomerular filtration rate, and controls the development of diabetic nephropathy [139] (Table 2).

Metformin is currently the first-line hypoglycemic agent of choice for the treatment of diabetes, either alone or as a base agent in various combination regimens, and almost half of patients with T2DM require additional hypoglycemic agents within 1 year of diagnosis. When considering second-line therapy, the central decisions facing providers and patients include safety, efficacy, tolerability, ease of administration, and cost. Several current second-line therapies, including sulfonylureas, glinides, DPP-4 inhibitors, alpha-glucosidase inhibitors, thiazolidinediones, SGLT-2 inhibitors, insulin, and GLP-1RA. Sulfonylureas, thiazolidinediones, and insulin can significantly improve glycemic control, but all three can cause weight gain, and sulfonylureas and insulin analogs can also cause a high risk of hypoglycemia. DPP-4 inhibitors, on the other hand, are less risky but lag behind insulin, sulfonylureas, and thiazolidinediones in glycemic control and are costly. Similar to DPP-4 inhibitors, SGLT-2 inhibitors have been associated with a low risk of hypoglycemia and high costs. However, unlike weight-neutral DPP-4 inhibitors, SGLT-2 inhibitors result in weight loss and lower blood pressure, and some members of this class have specific cardiovascular indications.

Table 2. Comparison of different kinds of oral drugs.

Type	Representative Drug	Function	Advantages	Possible Side Effects	Reference
Polypeptide drugs	Semeglutide	When the blood glucose level rises, it causes the release of insulin It can be used with metformin, basal insulin or sulfonylureas.	It may reduce hunger. May lead to weight loss.	Disgusting. Vomiting. Diarrhoea. Abdominal pain.	[109]
Meglitazone drugs	Reglinet	Triggers pancreas to release insulin	Quick results	Blood sugar levels drop too low, that is, hypoglycemia. Weight gain	[140]
Sulfonylureas	Glipizide	Triggers pancreas to release insulin	low cost. Effectively reduce blood sugar	The blood sugar level dropped too low. Weight gain. Rash. If drinking, there will be nausea or vomiting.	[141]
DPP-4 inhibitors	Saxagliptin	When blood sugar rises, it causes the release of insulin. Limit the ability of the liver to release glucose	Does not lead to weight gain. When used alone or in combination with metformin, it does not cause blood glucose levels to drop too low.	Upper respiratory tract infection. Throat pain. Headache.	[142]
Metformin drug	Metformin	Limit the ability of the liver to release sugar. Improve the sensitivity of cells to insulin	Very effective. May cause a slight weight loss. Low cost.	Nausea. Stomachache. Diarrhoea. In rare cases, there is harmful accumulation of lactic acid in patients with renal or liver failure, that is, lactic acidosis.	[143]
Alpha glucosidase inhibitors	Miglitol	Slow down the body's ability to decompose starch and some sugars	Does not lead to weight gain. Unless taken with insulin or sulfonylureas, it will not cause blood glucose levels to drop too low.	Bloating Stomachache Diarrhoea	[144]
PPARγ agonists	Pioglitazone	Agonizes peroxisome proliferator-activated receptor PPARγ and reduces insulin resistance	Does not stimulate insulin secretion, but exerts its hypoglycemic effect by enhancing tissue sensitivity to insulin. Used alone, it does not cause hypoglycemia.	Increased risk of heart failure. Increased incidence of bladder cancer	[138]
SGLT-2 inhibitor	Dagliflozin	Inhibits SGLT-2, reduces glucose reabsorption, and excretes sugar directly from the urine.	SGLT-2 inhibitors are rarely hypoglycemic and have beneficial effects on improving body weight and blood pressure	May be associated with nasopharyngitis, fungal infections, and genitourinary infections	[139]

The advantage of GLP-1RA is that it has glucose-lowering efficacy similar to that of insulin but without the side effect of weight gain that accompanies insulin therapy. GLP-1RA also provides weight loss and a lower risk of hypoglycemia and has cardiovascular protective properties. Oral small-molecule drugs for GLP-1RA are currently under development and may further alter the use of glucose-lowering drugs.

Orforglipron is a non-peptide oral GLP-1RA biased toward G-protein activation. Orforglipron achieved similar blood glucose-lowering ability to exenatide at low blood concentrations in animal studies, and its G-protein bias may play a role in therapy [145]. Results from phase 2 clinical trials showed that orforglipron at doses of 12 mg or higher significantly reduced HbA1c and body weight compared to placebo or dulaglutide, with AEs similar to other GLP-1RAs [146]. Danuglipron, an oral small molecule GLP-1RA, demonstrated safety with twice-daily danuglipron in an 8-week randomized, double-blind trial, and 24-h mean daily glucose and HbA1c increased proportionally to the danuglipron dose [147]. In clinical trials, danuglipron demonstrated similar glucose-lowering effects to GLP-1RA and slightly reduced blood pressure in patients [148,149]. HRS-7535 is a novel oral small molecule GLP-1RA that significantly improves glucose tolerance, promotes insulin secretion, and reduces food intake without strict food restriction. In phase 1 trials, the pharmacokinetics of HRS-7535 were roughly proportional to the dose, significantly reducing patients' body weight, with nausea and vomiting as common AEs, and its safety has been demonstrated [150]. There are other GLP-1RAs in other stages of development, e.g., Teng Ma et al. synthesized a small-molecule peptide that is a dual agonist of GLP-1R and GIP. It acts similarly to GIP and exendin-4 in a dose-dependent manner. When co-administered with sodium deoxycholate (SDC), SDC increased its bioavailability, and its oral hypoglycemic activity was enhanced. It also significantly improved glucose tolerance and hepatic fibrosis area in mice [151].

5. Oral Strategies for Peptide Drugs

Oral administration holds better promise for the treatment of T2DM than injectable administration. The main limitations of oral delivery of peptides are how to avoid degradation in the digestive system and improve bioavailability. Both the PH environment and digestive enzymes in the gastrointestinal tract greatly reduce the bioactivity of peptides in the GI tract, and the mucus layer and intestinal epithelium in the intestine are major barriers to the entry of peptides into the somatic circulation. Although semaglutide has been successfully prepared for oral administration, this customized approach cannot be directly replicated by other GLP-1Rs. In contrast, nanocarriers can be prepared into oral formulations without altering the structure of GLP-1R, improving bioavailability and prolonging in vivo circulation time through different absorption routes (Figure 3).

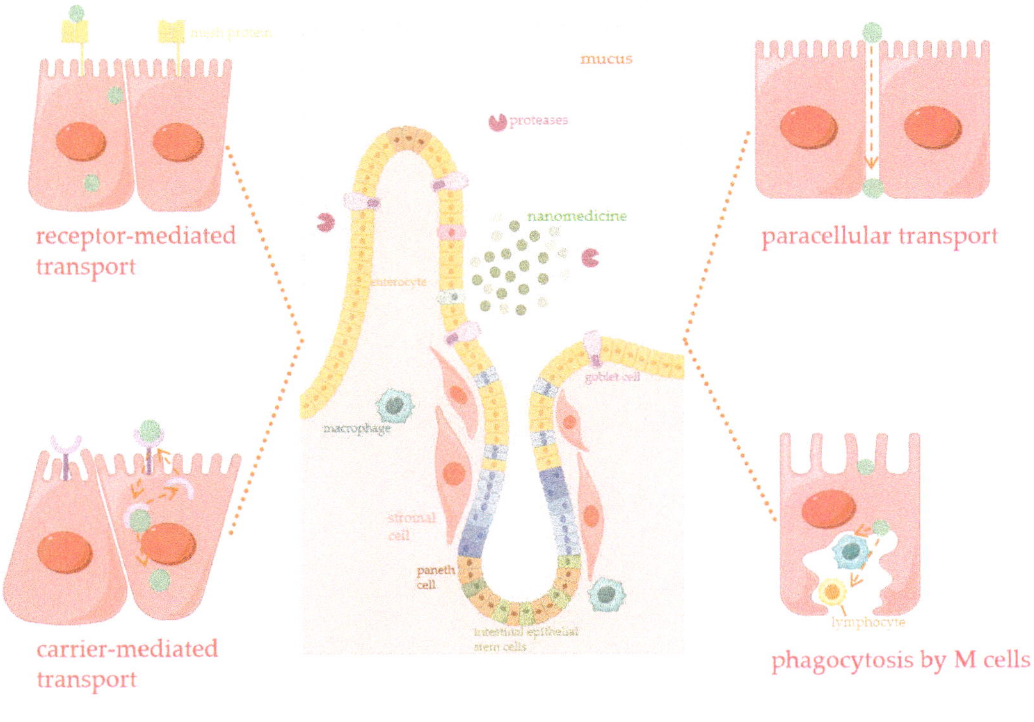

Figure 3. Schematic representation of the transport mechanisms.

5.1. Liposome

Liposomes are spherical vesicles composed of phospholipid bilayers with biological properties similar to those of cell membranes. Intestinal epithelial cells are tightly packed with protein complexes that limit intercellular transport of macromolecules, so liposomes with a structure similar to that of the cell membrane can mediate cellular transport via receptors [152]. In addition, by changing the physical or chemical properties of the liposome surface and thus the nature of the vesicles, different purposes of delivery can be achieved [153,154].

The mucus layer covering the surface of the intestinal epithelial cells is the first physical barrier that prevents drugs from entering the body circulation, rapidly trapping and eliminating larger molecules and pathogens through adhesion, protecting the intestinal tract from pathogen invasion whilst restricting the diffusion of drug absorption. The mucus layer is mainly composed of highly glycosylated mucins, which consist of a protein backbone and oligosaccharide side chains, and the mucus adheres to particles, especially those with positively charged or hydrophobic surfaces, mainly through multivalent adhesion interactions generated by the carboxyl groups of the oligosaccharides and the negative charge of sulphuric acid [155]. Wang and colleagues designed protein-crowned liposomes for insulin delivery by covering cationic liposomes with bovine serum albumin (BSA). Proteins can be adsorbed on the surface of nanoparticles in biological fluids to form a protein envelope, which is known as a protein crown. Hydrophilic and neutrally charged protein crowns promote mucus permeation of protein-crowned liposomes. As protein-crowned liposomes permeate the intestinal mucus, the protein crown is progressively degraded by enzymes, and cationic liposomes interact with anionic cell membranes to achieve trans-epithelial transport of insulin. The results showed that protein-crowned liposomes had an oral bioavailability of up to 11.9% and were effective in lowering blood glucose levels [156]. Ding and colleagues utilized electrostatic interaction forces to cause BSA to form protein crowns on the surface of liposomes and bind to cell-penetrating peptides to load liraglutide, which was used to improve the mucus permeability of the liposomes and enhance their absorption efficiency in the gut. In vitro experiments demonstrated the stability of liraglutide after liposome release. In vivo experiments have demonstrated that liposomes loaded with liraglutide have good intestinal endocytosis, a long intestinal absorption time, and good biosafety [157].

Recombinant microorganisms can be used as natural liposomes loaded with peptides and have unique advantages in biocompatibility. Recombinant microbial drug delivery avoids stimulation by environmental exogenous substances and controls the release of drugs or prodrugs in the body, and specific gene editing of recombinant microbial discourse specifically regulates homeostasis [158]. Fei et al. recombined and loaded *Rhodotorula glutinis* with peptides and insulin for oral administration to Type 2 diabetic mice. The cells of the recombinant strain accumulated more lecithin and fatty acids, which contributed to the loading of the peptide drug. Recombinant strain cells no longer proliferate in mice and slowly release the loaded drug; different levels of insulin were found in serum and tissues and significantly reduced blood glucose levels in mice [159]. Oral drug delivery based on recombinant microorganisms holds great promise, but some of the absorption mechanisms still require in-depth study.

Exosomes are external vesicles secreted by cells that can be released by all kinds of cells, such as human exosomes, plant exosomes, and animal exosomes. Exosomes have low immunogenicity and toxicity and offer advantages in the targeted delivery of therapeutic molecules because of the specific interactions between the surface proteins of these exosomes of different cellular origins and their target cells [160]. Currently the most promising of the oral exosomes are the milk-derived exosomes, which can promote the proliferation of intestinal epithelial cells, enhance intestinal permeability, and have the ability of immunomodulation [161]. Wu et al. prepared milk exosomes and loaded them with insulin for the treatment of Type 1 diabetic mice. Bovine milk exosomes were found to be actively multi-targeted to epithelial cells through active transport, membrane fusion, and niche-mediated transport. In addition, cow's milk exosomes can regulate surface pH during transport to adapt to different environments, avoid endolysosomal restriction, and promote uptake and cytosolization. And subcutaneous insulin has a more sustained glycemic-lowering effect than oral milk exosome-loaded insulin [162]. Xiao and colleagues, on the other hand, utilized the flow and fusion properties of the phospholipid bilayer of the exosome membrane to fuse milk exosomes with modified liposomes. A hybridized vesicle with adaptive surface properties loaded with semaglutide for oral delivery was prepared. Hybridized vesicles contain about 85% of exosomal membrane proteins but encapsulate semaglutide at 2.4 times the rate of natural milk exosomes and are much more hydrophilic, while modified liposomes give hybridized vesicles a neutral surface and are pH-responsive and self-regulating. Hydrophilicity and neutral charge facilitate penetration of the intestinal mucus barrier, and upon reaching the surface of jejunal epithelial cells, the highly retained membrane proteins and positively charged mixed vesicle surfaces effectively overcome the apical barrier, the intracellular transit barrier, and the basolateral cytosolic barrier. Adaptive surface characterization of hybrid vesicles increased the oral bioavailability of semaglutide to 8.7%, significantly improving the pharmacological therapeutic effect [163]. Lactogenic exosomes are widely used in oral delivery, and exosome delivery studies of macromolecules are about to become hot research.

5.2. *Self-Emulsifying Drug Delivery Systems (SEDDS)*

SEDDS are liquid or solid formulations consisting of an oil phase, a nonionic surfactant, and a co-surfactant, which can spontaneously emulsify into emulsions with particle sizes around 100–500 nm by gentle agitation in the gastrointestinal tract or at room temperature. SEDDS are lipid-based formulations that pair hydrophilic molecules such as GLP-1R and proteins with hydrophobic ions of oppositely charged lipophilic auxiliaries to increase their hydrophobicity and improve lipid solubility and can be incorporated into SEDDS for oral administration.

Gastrointestinal hydrolytic enzymes such as pepsin, trypsin, and other peptidases and proteases are insoluble in oily SEDDS droplets but can degrade esters such as triglycerides in SEDDS; therefore, SEDDS loaded with GLP-1R should use a lipolytic stabilizing component to avoid enzymatic degradation. The addition of mucus pro-osmotic agents to SEDDS and a reduction in the size of SEDDS droplets can increase the rate of contact between SEDDS and epithelial cells and improve the amount of drug entering the corpuscular circulation [164,165]. Claudia and coworkers prepared ORAL SEDDS for Exenatide, where a solution of Exenatide was shock-mixed with a solution of the oppositely charged hydrophobic ion docusate, which was paired lipidated and added to the SEDDS. Exenatide interacts with docusate only by inter-ionic forces without structural changes, ensuring the stability and pharmacological effects of exenatide. SEDDS consists of Labrafil 1944, which lacks a triglyceride structure, and Capmul PG-8, whose high HLB value gives SEDDS a smaller droplet size and better mucus permeability. In healthy rats, the SEDDS bioavailability of loaded exenatide was approximately 9% and sustained release for at least 6 h. Healthy rats exhibit better mucus permeability and lower blood glucose levels in vivo, indicating the oral potential of peptides paired with hydrophobic ions in SEDDS [166]. Another hydrophobic ion pairing, n-octadecyl sulfate, was found to pair better with exenatide in SEDDS compared to docusate n-octadecyl sulfate in the study of Thi et al. The molar ratio of n-octadecyl sulfate paired with exenatide is higher than that of docusate paired with exenatide. This means that more n-octadecyl sulfate is required for the same exenatide, which increases the lipophilicity of exenatide and the log P value of exenatide-n-octadecyl sulfate. The ex vivo results showed that the intestinal permeability and bioavailability of n-octadecyl sulfate were 3.5 and 1.3 times higher than those of docusate, respectively [167].

An alternative to hydrophobic ion pairing is to load the peptide into a W/O emulsion, which is then dispersed into SEDDS. Lu et al. used soybean phospholipids to wrap exenatide to form reverse micelles, which were then incorporated into SEDDS. Subsequently, O/W emulsions were prepared on the basis of reverse micelles-SEDDS, the surface of which was positively charged, and finally hyaluronic acid was encapsulated in the outermost layer by electrostatic adsorption. The hyaluronic acid coating adheres to the intestinal mucosa and increases intestinal permeability. Animal experiments showed that exenatide-loaded reverse micelles-SEDDS was more significant in improving the indexes of T2DM rats compared to exenatide-loaded SEDDS. Long-term experiments also showed that long-term administration of exenatide-loaded reverse micelles-SEDDS protects pancreatic β-cells and improves insulin secretion to some extent in T2DM rats [168].

Converting liquid SEDDS to solid SEDDS (S-SEDDS) allows for controlled release of SEDDS. S-SEDDS improves the physicochemical stability and drug loading capacity of SEDDS and offers the advantages of controlled drug release, extended gastric retention time, and reduced production cost. S-SEDDS is prepared by solidifying SEDDS, which is commonly performed by solid carrier adsorption, spray drying, thermosolvent extrusion, and freeze drying [169]. Sun and colleagues prepared cabazitaxel S-SEDDS by solid carrier adsorption, which formed celiac particles into lymphatic transport to avoid the first pass effect, greatly improved the bioavailability of the BCS class IV drug cabazitaxel, and developed more potential formulations of cabazitaxel [170].

5.3. Polymer Nanoparticles (PNP)

Nanoparticles prepared from biocompatible and biodegradable polymers are widely used in oral delivery systems. Polymers are classified into natural and synthetic polymers; natural polymers such as polysaccharides, proteins, and polyamino acids have the advantage of being non-toxic and non-immunogenic in oral delivery. Synthetic polymers allow for the flexible production or modification of materials according to patient needs, such as synthetic polymers, silica, porous coordination polymers, etc. [171].

Chitosan is a cationic polysaccharide derived from naturally occurring chitin and therefore adheres to negatively charged mucus layers and cell surfaces. Intestinal epithelial intercellular channels are restricted by a combination of tightly linked protein complexes, cellular bridges, and adherens junctions, whereas chitosan transiently opens tight junctions to increase penetration of the drug into the paracellular pathway, and this process is reversible [172]. Sodium alginate is a PH-sensitive anionic polysaccharide and is adhesive, interacting with the mucus layer through hydrogen bonding and van der Waals forces [173]. Yang and colleagues prepared chitosan sodium alginate gel nanoparticles loaded with exenatide using sodium tripolyphosphate as a cross-linking agent. Due to the PH sensitivity of sodium alginate and the strong electrostatic interaction with chitosan, the nanoparticles shrink under acidic conditions, thereby protecting the exenatide. In the intestinal tract, sodium alginate adheres to the intestinal mucosa, increasing drug retention time, and chitosan increases the permeability of the nanoparticles. In vivo experiments showed that nanoparticles loaded with exenatide had an oral bioavailability of approximately 9% and significantly and consistently reduced blood glucose concentrations in diabetic rats [174].

Protein carriers are abundant and self-targeting, and the structure of the protein itself gives it the potential to deliver RNA, drugs, vaccines, and other biomolecules at specific sites in the body. However, it should be noted that high concentrations of proteins can be denatured by aggregation, and protein solubility can be improved by adding buffer components or low concentrations of surfactants [175]. Bao et al. used zeinolysin to protect the complex formed by the non-covalent interaction of liglutide with bile acids and added a surface-active glycolipid, rhamnolipid, to improve the stability of zeinolysin nanoparticles. Bile acids, as intestinal mucosal pro-osmotic agents, in combination with liraglutide may improve the oral absorption of liraglutide without affecting its potency. Corn Alcohol Soluble Protein, as a hydrophobic protein, can help its encapsulated material to resist protease degradation, while rhamnolipid prevents its hydrophobic aggregation, thereby reducing the particle size of the nanoparticles. Cellular experiments showed that in contrast to the ligraglutide bile acid complex alone, which is absorbed only via the bile acid transporter protein pathway, zeinolysin particles are absorbed via active transport, lattice proteins, vesicles, and microcellular drinking-mediated endocytosis. In vivo experiments revealed that oral administration of corn alcohol-soluble protein loaded with liraglutide had a bioavailability of 9.6% and significantly reduced blood glucose levels in T2DM mice [176].

The most interesting of the current polyamino acids are the amphoteric amino acid polymers, where the average distribution of oppositely charged groups makes them strongly hydrated, and thus the amphoteric amino acid polymers have the advantage of resisting protein adsorption, interfacial lubrication, facilitating mucus permeation, enhancing the internalization of the nanoparticles in the cell, and also preventing degradation of the proteopeptides in inflammatory and enzymatic environments [177]. The degradation products of poly(lactic-co-glycolic) acid, PLGA, are lactic acid and hydroxyacetic acid, which are also by-products of the human metabolic pathway, so when it is in the body, it is not toxic, except for those with lactose deficiency. PLGAs can also be modified in various ways and are therefore often used in the design and development of nanocarriers for controlled and targeted drug delivery systems. Zhao et al. selected amphoteric sulfobetaine for surface modification of PLGA nanoparticles for loading of liraglutide. Amphoteric sulfobetaine can self-assemble on the surface of PLGA nanoparticles to form hydrophilic and electroneutral coatings and to form protein coronas to resist adsorption to nonspecific proteins. The results showed that the hydrophilicity and electroneutrality of the surface of PLGA particles greatly improved their mucus permeability, and the relative bioavailability of the orally administered nanoparticles was 9.95% of that of the subcutaneously administered group, with a stable blood glucose-lowering effect [178].

Silica has the advantages of easy synthesis, large pore size, large specific surface area, good physical stability, non-toxicity, etc. Silica-skeleton-loaded drugs have better stability under temperature changes, organic solvents, or acidic conditions, making them suitable for use as a drug nanocarrier [179]. Silicon dioxide uptake in the GI tract is related to the size of the nanoparticles; e.g., 250 nm particles can be transported via cellular uptake and cytosis, while 100 nm particles result in a lower rate of cellular transport due to faster degradation. Silica particles smaller than 100 nm in size, on the other hand, improved intestinal osmotic penetration, but when penetrating the mucus layer, the penetration rate of 20 nm particles was much lower than that of 50 nm particles [180]. Therefore the relationship between the size of silica nanoparticles and their absorption in the GI tract still needs to be explored. Silica for the preparation of nanoparticles can be classified into mesoporous and non-porous silica, and mesoporous silica can be used for the delivery of peptide drugs. The ordered nanoscale porous structure in mesoporous silica nanoparticles allows drug molecules to be easily confined and stabilized within the mesopore in an amorphous form, which further enhances the drug dissolution rate [181]. Muhammad and colleagues tried macroporous dendritic silica nanoparticles loaded with exenatide, modified the nanoparticles using phosphonate, and covered the surface with a chitosan coating. The phosphonate enhanced the surface charge and porosity of the nanoparticles, resulting in a more homogeneous dispersion and increased exenatide loading. The stronger electronegativity of phosphonate can form electrostatic adsorption with chitosan, and the chitosan-coated nanoparticles can protect the exenatide leakage in the pores and improve the drug loading capacity. In addition, chitosan coating reduced the burst release of exenatide at acidic and alkaline pH, and increased the permeability of nanoparticles in intestinal epithelial cells [182].

Porous coordination polymers are materials with infinite network structures formed by self-assembly of metal nodes (metal ions or clusters) and organic linkers through coordination bonds, which have the advantages of diverse structures and compositions, designable structures, adjustable pore channels, and easy functionalization [183–185]. The nanocarriers commonly used in porous coordination polymers for loading drugs are metal-organic frameworks, and functional metal-organic framework nanoparticles can protect proteins from the gastric environment and overcome the intestinal barrier, offering the possibility of orally delivering biomolecules. Jun-Jie Zou et al. Encapsulation of insulin using acid-resistant metal-organic framework nanoparticles and modification of its surface with transferrin for efficient transport and targeted release of insulin [186].

The macroporous structure of metal-organic framework nanoparticles allows for up to 33% encapsulation of insulin and its environmental sensitivity for controlled release under phosphorus-rich physiological conditions. Transferrin achieves iron uptake and transport by binding to the transferrin receptor on epithelial cells, which increases the efficiency of insulin transport. The intracellular nanoparticles, due to their strong positive charge and unique membrane switching effect, interact electrostatically with the lysosomal membrane to achieve rapid escape from the lysosome and release from the cellular monolayer. Animal experiments showed that transferrin-modified metal-organic framework nanoparticles rapidly reduced in vivo blood glucose levels in rats to about 30% of the initial level and extended insulin efficacy up to 10 h, achieving a high oral bioavailability of 29.6%, while long-term experiments demonstrated that such orally-administered nanoparticles are well biocompatible. This demonstrates the potential of metal-organic frameworks for loading peptide drugs for oral treatment of diabetes.

6. Conclusions and Outlook

Oral delivery of peptides is one of the major challenges in the field of drug delivery. Currently, the focus of peptide drug formulation research is mainly on protecting the biological activity of peptides and improving bioavailability. Nano-formulations can avoid the inactivation of peptides in the gastrointestinal environment, increase the transmembrane absorption in the small intestinal epithelium, change the distribution of the drug in the body, and improve bioavailability. Therapeutic effects of controlled release and targeted treatment of diseases are achieved by ligand modification, which prolongs retention time at specific absorption sites. In addition, nano-formulations activate cellular transport mechanisms to maximize drug activity, ensuring rapid and stable drug action [187]. This paper contributes to the field of therapeutic diabetes by reviewing the progress of research on peptide drugs for the treatment of diabetes, as well as exploring the possibility of combining peptide drugs with nano-formulations.

Author Contributions: Conceptualization, X.Y. and R.L.; methodology, C.F.; software, Q.K.; validation, Y.D., P.Y. and Y.J.; formal analysis, X.Y.; investigation, R.L.; resources, X.Y.; data curation, C.F.; writing—original draft preparation, R.L.; writing—review and editing, Y.D.; visualization, P.Y.; supervision, X.Y.; project administration, R.L.; funding acquisition, Y.J. All authors have read and agreed to the published version of the manuscript.

Funding: This research was funded by the National Natural Science Foundation of China (Grant No. 82003985); Drug Administration project of Jilin province (Grant No. JLPZGF-2020-107), and the National College Students' innovation and entrepreneurship training program (Grant No. 202310199001 and 202310199051X), Jilin Province Science and Technology Development Project in China (Grant No. 20210204013YY, 20230401062YY, 20230204019YY, 20230401075YY); Jilin Provincial Development and Reform Commission program (Grant No. 2023C027-3); Changchun University of Chinese Medicine postgraduate training innovation demonstration project (Grant No. 2022JP06).

Conflicts of Interest: The authors declare no conflicts of interest.

References

1. Jin, Q.; Ma, R.C.W. Metabolomics in Diabetes and Diabetic Complications: Insights from Epidemiological Studies. *Cells* **2021**, *10*, 2832. [CrossRef] [PubMed]
2. Haak, T.; Gölz, S.; Fritsche, A.; Füchtenbusch, M.; Siegmund, T.; Schnellbächer, E.; Klein, H.H.; Uebel, T.; Droßel, D. Therapy of Type 1 Diabetes. *Exp. Clin. Endocrinol. Diabetes* **2019**, *127*, S27–S38. [CrossRef]
3. Berbudi, A.; Rahmadika, N.; Tjahjadi, A.I.; Ruslami, R. Type 2 Diabetes and its Impact on the Immune System. *Curr. Diabetes Rev.* **2020**, *16*, 442–449. [CrossRef] [PubMed]
4. Pavlou, D.I.; Paschou, S.A.; Anagnostis, P.; Spartalis, M.; Spartalis, E.; Vryonidou, A.; Tentolouris, N.; Siasos, G. Hypertension in patients with type 2 diabetes mellitus: Targets and management. *Maturitas* **2018**, *112*, 71–77. [CrossRef]
5. Alsaadon, H.; Afroz, A.; Karim, A.; Habib, S.H.; Alramadan, M.J.; Billah, B.; Shetty, A.N. Hypertension and its related factors among patients with type 2 diabetes mellitus—A multi-hospital study in Bangladesh. *BMC Public Health* **2022**, *22*, 198. [CrossRef]
6. Wang, Z.J.; Wang, J.Q.; Kahkoska, A.R.; Buse, J.B.; Gu, Z. Developing Insulin Delivery Devices with Glucose Responsiveness. *Trends Pharmacol. Sci.* **2021**, *42*, 31–44. [CrossRef]

7. Goff, L.M. Ethnicity and Type 2 diabetes in the UK. *Diabet. Med.* **2019**, *36*, 927–938. [CrossRef] [PubMed]
8. Cloete, L. Diabetes mellitus: An overview of the types, symptoms, complications and management. *Nurs. Stand.* **2021**, *37*, 61–66. [CrossRef]
9. Rekha, M.R.; Sharma, C.P. Oral delivery of therapeutic protein/peptide for diabetes—Future perspectives. *Int. J. Pharmaceut.* **2013**, *440*, 48–62. [CrossRef]
10. Bhutani, U.; Basu, T.; Majumdar, S. Oral Drug Delivery: Conventional to Long Acting New-Age Designs. *Eur. J. Pharm. Biopharm.* **2021**, *162*, 23–42. [CrossRef]
11. Niu, Z.G.; Conejos-Sánchez, I.; Griffin, B.T.; O'Driscoll, C.M.; Alonso, M.J. Lipid-based nanocarriers for oral peptide delivery. *Adv. Drug Deliv. Rev.* **2016**, *106*, 337–354. [CrossRef] [PubMed]
12. Shaw, J.E.; Gallwitz, B.; Han, J.; Hardy, E.; Schernthaner, G. Variability in and predictors of glycaemic responses after 24 weeks of treatment with exenatide twice daily and exenatide once weekly. *Diabetes Obes. Metab.* **2017**, *19*, 1793–1797. [CrossRef]
13. Denimal, D.; Bergas, V.; Pais-de-Barros, J.-P.; Simoneau, I.; Demizieux, L.; Passilly-Degrace, P.; Bouillet, B.; Petit, J.-M.; Rouland, A.; Bataille, A.; et al. Liraglutide reduces plasma dihydroceramide levels in patients with type 2 diabetes. *Cardiovasc. Diabetol.* **2023**, *22*, 104. [CrossRef] [PubMed]
14. Gao, F.; Lv, X.; Mo, Z.; Ma, J.; Zhang, Q.; Yang, G.; Liu, W.; Li, Q.; Zhou, J.; Bao, Y.; et al. Efficacy and safety of polyethylene glycol loxenatide as add-on to metformin in patients with type 2 diabetes: A multicentre, randomized, double-blind, placebo-controlled, phase 3b trial. *Diabetes Obes. Metab.* **2020**, *22*, 2375–2383. [CrossRef] [PubMed]
15. Tack, C.; Jacob, S.; Desouza, C.; Bain, S.C.; Nauck, M.A.; Petrie, J.; Poulter, N.R.; Pratley, R.E.; Stegmann, H.V.B.K.; Bosch-Traberg, H.; et al. Liraglutide Effects in Insulin-Treated Patients in LEADER. *Diabetes* **2018**, *67*, 438. [CrossRef]
16. Xiangyang, L.; Wenjuan, Y.; Jianrong, L.; Xinxi, H.; Yujie, F.; Jie, M.; Jingbo, L.; Jianfang, F.; Qiuhe, J.; Li, W. The efficacy and safety of beinaglutide alone or in combination with insulin glargine in Chinese patients with type 2 diabetes mellitus who are inadequately controlled with oral antihyperglycemic therapy: A multicenter, open-label, randomized trial. *J. Diabetes* **2023**, *16*, e13483. [CrossRef]
17. Bowe, A.; Poonawalla, I.; Tindal, M.; Meah, Y.A.; Schwab, P. 1428-P: Cardiovascular Outcomes with Dulaglutide vs. Liraglutide. *Diabetes* **2020**, *69*, 1428. [CrossRef]
18. McGuire, D.K.; Busui, R.P.; Deanfield, J.; Inzucchi, S.E.; Mann, J.F.E.; Marx, N.; Mulvagh, S.L.; Poulter, N.; Engelmann, M.D.M.; Hovingh, G.K.; et al. Effects of oral semaglutide on cardiovascular outcomes in individuals with type 2 diabetes and established atherosclerotic cardiovascular disease and/or chronic kidney disease: Design and baseline characteristics of SOUL, a randomized trial. *Diabetes Obes. Metab.* **2023**, *25*, 1932–1941. [CrossRef]
19. Karagiannis, T.; Avgerinos, I.; Liakos, A.; Del Prato, S.; Matthews, D.R.; Tsapas, A.; Bekiari, E. Management of type 2 diabetes with the dual GIP/GLP-1 receptor agonist tirzepatide: A systematic review and meta-analysis. *Diabetologia* **2022**, *65*, 1251–1261. [CrossRef]
20. Drucker, D.J. Mechanisms of Action and Therapeutic Application of Glucagon-like Peptide-1. *Cell Metab.* **2018**, *27*, 740–756. [CrossRef]
21. Müller, T.D.; Finan, B.; Bloom, S.R.; D'Alessio, D.; Drucker, D.J.; Flatt, P.R.; Fritsche, A.; Gribble, F.; Grill, H.J.; Habener, J.F.; et al. Glucagon-like peptide 1 (GLP-1). *Mol. Metab.* **2019**, *30*, 72–130. [CrossRef] [PubMed]
22. Tucker, J.D.; Dhanvantari, S.; Brubaker, P.L. Proglucagon processing in islet and intestinal cell lines. *Regul. Pept.* **1996**, *62*, 29–35. [CrossRef]
23. Reimann, F.; Gribble, F.M. Mechanisms underlying glucose-dependent insulinotropic polypeptide and glucagon-like peptide-1 secretion. *J. Diabetes Investig.* **2016**, *7*, 13–19. [CrossRef] [PubMed]
24. Ezcurra, M.; Reimann, F.; Gribble, F.M.; Emery, E. Molecular mechanisms of incretin hormone secretion. *Curr. Opin. Pharmacol.* **2013**, *13*, 922–927. [CrossRef]
25. Ahrén, B. GLP-1 for type 2 diabetes. *Exp. Cell Res.* **2011**, *317*, 1239–1245. [CrossRef]
26. Nauck, M.A.; Quast, D.R.; Wefers, J.; Meier, J.J. GLP-1 receptor agonists in the treatment of type 2 diabetes—State-of-the-art. *Mol. Metab.* **2020**, *46*, 101102. [CrossRef]
27. Vasu, S.; Moffett, R.C.; Thorens, B.; Flatt, P.R. Role of endogenous GLP-1 and GIP in beta cell compensatory responses to insulin resistance and cellular stress. *PLoS ONE* **2014**, *9*, e101005. [CrossRef] [PubMed]
28. De Marinis, Y.Z.; Salehi, A.; Ward, C.E.; Zhang, Q.; Abdulkader, F.; Bengtsson, M.; Braha, O.; Braun, M.; Ramracheya, R.; Amisten, S.; et al. GLP-1 inhibits and adrenaline stimulates glucagon release by differential modulation of N- and L-type Ca2+ channel-dependent exocytosis. *Cell Metab.* **2010**, *11*, 543–553. [CrossRef]
29. Drucker, D.J.; Habener, J.F.; Holst, J.J. Discovery, characterization, and clinical development of the glucagon-like peptides. *J. Clin. Investig.* **2017**, *127*, 4217–4227. [CrossRef]
30. Baggio, L.L.; Yusta, B.; Mulvihill, E.E.; Cao, X.; Streutker, C.J.; Butany, J.; Cappola, T.P.; Margulies, K.B.; Drucker, D.J. GLP-1 Receptor Expression Within the Human Heart. *Endocrinology* **2018**, *159*, 1570–1584. [CrossRef]
31. Sonne, D.P.; Engstrøm, T.; Treiman, M. Protective effects of GLP-1 analogues exendin-4 and GLP-1(9-36) amide against ischemia-reperfusion injury in rat heart. *Regul. Pept.* **2007**, *146*, 243–249. [CrossRef] [PubMed]
32. Helmstädter, J.; Keppeler, K.; Küster, L.; Münzel, T.; Daiber, A.; Steven, S. Glucagon-like peptide-1 (GLP-1) receptor agonists and their cardiovascular benefits—The role of the GLP-1 receptor. *Br. J. Pharmacol.* **2021**, *179*, 659–676. [CrossRef] [PubMed]

33. Smith, N.K.; Hackett, T.A.; Galli, A.; Flynn, C.R. GLP-1: Molecular mechanisms and outcomes of a complex signaling system. *Neurochem. Int.* **2019**, *128*, 94–105. [CrossRef] [PubMed]
34. Holst, J.J. The physiology of glucagon-like peptide 1. *Physiol. Rev.* **2007**, *87*, 1409–1439. [CrossRef] [PubMed]
35. Trapp, S.; Brierley, D.I. Brain GLP-1 and the regulation of food intake: GLP-1 action in the brain and its implications for GLP-1 receptor agonists in obesity treatment. *Br. J. Pharmacol.* **2021**, *179*, 557–570. [CrossRef]
36. Xu, F.; Lin, B.; Zheng, X.; Chen, Z.; Cao, H.; Xu, H.; Liang, H.; Weng, J. GLP-1 receptor agonist promotes brown remodelling in mouse white adipose tissue through SIRT1. *Diabetologia* **2016**, *59*, 1059–1069. [CrossRef]
37. Giralt, M.; Vergara, P. Sympathetic pathways mediate GLP-1 actions in the gastrointestinal tract of the rat. *Regul. Pept.* **1998**, *74*, 19–25. [CrossRef]
38. Jiménez, D.L.; Babkowski, M.C.; Miramontes González, J.P. GLP-1 and the renin-angiotensin-aldosterone system. *Lancet Diabetes Endocrinol.* **2019**, *7*, 337. [CrossRef]
39. Han, L.; Chen, X.; Wan, D.; Xie, M.; Ouyang, S. One anastomosis gastric bypass ameliorates diabetic nephropathy via regulating the GLP-1-mediated Sirt1/AMPK/PGC1α pathway. *Clin. Exp. Nephrol.* **2024**, *28*, 1051–1061. [CrossRef]
40. Niu, B.; Fang, H.; Chen, Q. The Discovery and Development of Glucagon-Like Peptide-1 Receptor Agonists. *Curr. Med. Chem.* **2023**, *30*, 2921–2943. [CrossRef]
41. Davidson, M.B.; Bate, G.; Kirkpatrick, P. Exenatide. *Nat. Rev. Drug Discov.* **2005**, *4*, 713–714. [CrossRef] [PubMed]
42. Aart-van der Beek, A.B.; Raalte, D.H.; Guja, C.; Hoogenberg, K.; Suchower, L.J.; Hardy, E.; Sjöström, C.D.; Heerspink, H.J.L. Exenatide once weekly decreases urinary albumin excretion in patients with type 2 diabetes and elevated albuminuria: Pooled analysis of randomized active controlled clinical trials. *Diabetes Obes. Metab.* **2020**, *22*, 1556–1566. [CrossRef] [PubMed]
43. Wang, M.-J.; Cai, X.; Liang, R.-Y.; Zhang, E.-M.; Liang, X.-Q.; Liang, H.; Fu, C.; Zhou, A.-D.; Shi, Y.; Xu, F.; et al. SIRT1-dependent deacetylation of Txnip H3K9ac is critical for exenatide-improved diabetic kidney disease. *Biomed. Pharmacother.* **2023**, *167*, 115515. [CrossRef]
44. Tsapas, A.; Karagiannis, T.; Kakotrichi, P.; Avgerinos, I.; Mantsiou, C.; Tousinas, G.; Manolopoulos, A.; Liakos, A.; Malandris, K.; Matthews, D.R.; et al. Comparative efficacy of glucose-lowering medications on body weight and blood pressure in patients with type 2 diabetes: A systematic review and network meta-analysis. *Diabetes Obes. Metab.* **2021**, *23*, 2116–2124. [CrossRef]
45. Drucker, D.J.; Buse, J.B.; Taylor, K.; Kendall, D.M.; Trautmann, M.; Zhuang, D.; Porter, L. Exenatide once weekly versus twice daily for the treatment of type 2 diabetes: A randomised, open-label, non-inferiority study. *Lancet* **2008**, *372*, 1240–1250. [CrossRef]
46. Lv, Q.; Yang, Y.; Lv, Y.; Wu, Q.; Hou, X.; Li, L.; Ye, X.; Yang, C.; Wang, S. Long-term effects of different hypoglycemic drugs on carotid intima-media thickness progression: A systematic review and network meta-analysis. *Front. Endocrinol.* **2024**, *15*, 1403606. [CrossRef]
47. Zhou, Q.; Hao, G.; Xie, W.; Chen, B.; Lu, W.; Wang, G.; Zhong, R.; Chen, J.; Ye, J.; Shen, J.; et al. Exenatide reduces atrial fibrillation susceptibility by inhibiting hKv1.5 and hNav1.5 channels. *J. Biol. Chem.* **2024**, *300*, 107294. [CrossRef] [PubMed]
48. DeYoung, M.B.; MacConell, L.; Sarin, V.; Trautmann, M.; Herbert, P. Encapsulation of exenatide in poly-(D,L-lactide-co-glycolide) microspheres produced an investigational long-acting once-weekly formulation for type 2 diabetes. *Diabetes Technol. Ther.* **2011**, *13*, 1145–1154. [CrossRef] [PubMed]
49. Varanko, A.K.; Chilkoti, A. Molecular and Materials Engineering for Delivery of Peptide Drugs to Treat Type 2 Diabetes. *Adv. Healthc. Mater.* **2019**, *8*, e1801509. [CrossRef]
50. Cai, H.; Chen, Q.; Duan, Y.; Zhao, Y.; Zhang, X. Short-term effect of polyethylene glycol loxenatide on weight loss in overweight or obese patients with type 2 diabetes: An open-label, parallel-arm, randomized, metformin-controlled trial. *Front. Endocrinol.* **2023**, *14*, 1106868. [CrossRef]
51. Wu, Y.; Guo, Z.; Wang, J.; Wang, Y.; Wang, D.; Li, Y.; Zhu, L.; Sun, X. Polyethylene Glycol Loxenatide (PEX-168) Reduces Body Weight and Blood Glucose in Simple Obese Mice. *Int. J. Endocrinol.* **2021**, *2021*, 1–6. [CrossRef] [PubMed]
52. Chen, F.; He, L.; Li, J.; Yang, S.; Zhang, B.; Zhu, D.; Wu, Z.; Zhang, S.; Hou, D.; Ouyang, C.; et al. Polyethylene Glycol Loxenatide Injection (GLP-1) Protects Vascular Endothelial Cell Function in Middle-Aged and Elderly Patients with Type 2 Diabetes by Regulating Gut Microbiota. *Front. Mol. Biosci.* **2022**, *9*, 879294. [CrossRef] [PubMed]
53. Xie, Y.; Kuang, J.; Li, Q.; Hong, T.; Ji, L.; Kong, Y.; Duan, Y.; Chen, L. Impact of polyethylene glycol loxenatide on cardiovascular outcomes in patients with type 2 diabetes: Study protocol for a multicentre, randomised, double-blind, placebo-controlled trial (BALANCE-3). *BMJ Open* **2023**, *13*, e069080. [CrossRef]
54. Yuan, J.; Wang, Y.; Wang, D.; Yan, H.; Wang, N. Loxenatide attenuates ROS-mediated vascular endothelial progenitor cell damage and mitochondrial dysfunction via SIRT3/Foxo3 signaling pathway. *J. Biochem. Mol. Toxicol.* **2023**, *37*, e23452. [CrossRef]
55. Thorkildsen, C.; Neve, S.; Larsen, B.D.; Meier, E.; Petersen, J.S. Glucagon-like peptide 1 receptor agonist ZP10A increases insulin mRNA expression and prevents diabetic progression in db/db mice. *J. Pharmacol. Exp. Ther.* **2003**, *307*, 490–496. [CrossRef]
56. Raccah, D.; Gourdy, P.; Sagnard, L.; Ceriello, A. Lixisenatide as add-on to oral anti-diabetic therapy: An effective treatment for glycaemic control with body weight benefits in type 2 diabetes. *Diabetes Metab. Res.* **2014**, *30*, 742–748. [CrossRef] [PubMed]
57. Trujillo, J.M.; Roberts, M.; Dex, T.; Chao, J.; White, J.; LaSalle, J. Low Incidence of Gastrointestinal Adverse Events Over Time with a Fixed-Ratio Combination of Insulin Glargine and Lixisenatide vs Lixisenatide Alone. *Diabetes Obes. Metab.* **2018**, *20*, 2690–2694. [CrossRef]
58. Scott, L.J. Lixisenatide: A review of its use in patients with type 2 diabetes mellitus. *BioDrugs* **2013**, *27*, 509–523. [CrossRef] [PubMed]

59. Scott, L.J. Insulin Glargine/Lixisenatide: A Review in Type 2 Diabetes. *Drugs* **2017**, *77*, 1353–1362. [CrossRef]
60. Rayner, C.K.; Watson, L.E.; Phillips, L.K.; Lange, K.; Bound, M.J.; Grivell, J.; Wu, T.; Jones, K.L.; Horowitz, M.; Ferrannini, E.; et al. Effects of Sustained Treatment with Lixisenatide on Gastric Emptying and Postprandial Glucose Metabolism in Type 2 Diabetes: A Randomized Controlled Trial. *Diabetes Care* **2020**, *43*, 1813–1821. [CrossRef]
61. Vinué, Á.; Navarro, J.; Herrero-Cervera, A.; García-Cubas, M.; Andrés-Blasco, I.; Martínez-Hervás, S.; Real, J.T.; Ascaso, J.F.; González-Navarro, H. The GLP-1 analogue lixisenatide decreases atherosclerosis in insulin-resistant mice by modulating macrophage phenotype. *Diabetologia* **2017**, *60*, 1801–1812. [CrossRef] [PubMed]
62. Xu, L.; Chen, G.; Zhang, L.; He, A.; Li, Y. Lixisenatide ameliorated lipopolysaccharide (LPS)-induced expression of mucin and inflammation in bronchial epithelial cells. *J. Biochem. Mol. Toxicol.* **2023**, *38*, e23618. [CrossRef]
63. Zhao, Z.; Pu, Y. Lixisenatide enhances mitochondrial biogenesis and function through regulating the CREB/PGC-1α pathway. *Biochem. Biophys. Res. Commun.* **2019**, *508*, 1120–1125. [CrossRef]
64. Christensen, M.; Knop, F.K.; Vilsbøll, T.; Holst, J.J. Lixisenatide for type 2 diabetes mellitus. *Expert Opin. Investig. Drugs* **2011**, *20*, 549–557. [CrossRef] [PubMed]
65. Hanefeld, M.; Arteaga, J.M.; Leiter, L.A.; Marchesini, G.; Nikonova, E.; Shestakova, M.; Stager, W.; Gómez-Huelgas, R. Efficacy and safety of lixisenatide in patients with type 2 diabetes and renal impairment. *Diabetes Obes. Metab.* **2017**, *19*, 1594–1601. [CrossRef]
66. Lin, C.-H.; Shao, L.; Zhang, Y.-M.; Tu, Y.-J.; Zhang, Y.; Tomlinson, B.; Chan, P.; Liu, Z. An evaluation of liraglutide including its efficacy and safety for the treatment of obesity. *Expert Opin. Pharmacother.* **2019**, *21*, 275–285. [CrossRef] [PubMed]
67. Drucker, D.J.; Dritselis, A.; Kirkpatrick, P. Liraglutide. *Nat. Rev. Drug Discov.* **2010**, *9*, 267–268. [CrossRef]
68. Vandemark, C.; Nguyen, J.; Zhao, Z.-Q. Cardiovascular Protection with a Long-Acting GLP-1 Receptor Agonist Liraglutide: An Experimental Update. *Molecules* **2023**, *28*, 1369. [CrossRef]
69. Qiao, H.; Ren, H.; Du, H.; Zhang, M.; Xiong, X.; Lv, R. Liraglutide repairs the infarcted heart: The role of the SIRT1/Parkin/mitophagy pathway. *Mol. Med. Rep.* **2018**, *17*, 3722–3734. [CrossRef]
70. Le, Y.; Wei, R.; Yang, K.; Lang, S.; Gu, L.; Liu, J.; Hong, T.; Yang, J. Liraglutide ameliorates palmitate-induced oxidative injury in islet microvascular endothelial cells through GLP-1 receptor/PKA and GTPCH1/eNOS signaling pathways. *Peptides* **2020**, *124*, 170212. [CrossRef]
71. Mashayekhi, M.; Beckman, J.A.; Nian, H.; Garner, E.M.; Mayfield, D.; Devin, J.K.; Koethe, J.R.; Brown, J.D.; Cahill, K.N.; Yu, C.; et al. Comparative effects of weight loss and incretin-based therapies on vascular endothelial function, fibrinolysis and inflammation in individuals with obesity and prediabetes: A randomized controlled trial. *Diabetes Obes. Metab.* **2022**, *25*, 570–580. [CrossRef] [PubMed]
72. Liang, R.; Wang, M.; Fu, C.; Liang, H.; Deng, H.; Tan, Y.; Xu, F.; Cai, M. Liraglutide protects against high-fat diet-induced kidney injury by ameliorating apoptosis. *Endocr. Connect.* **2020**, *9*, 946–954. [CrossRef]
73. Slomski, A. Liraglutide May Reduce Diabetic Kidney Disease. *JAMA* **2017**, *318*, 1532. [CrossRef] [PubMed]
74. Wronka, M.; Krzemińska, J.; Młynarska, E.; Rysz, J.; Franczyk, B. New Insights into the Use of Liraglutide—Impact on Cardiovascular Risk and Microvascular Outcomes. *Biomedicines* **2023**, *11*, 1159. [CrossRef] [PubMed]
75. Mann, J.F.E.; Ørsted, D.D.; Brown-Frandsen, K.; Marso, S.P.; Poulter, N.R.; Rasmussen, S.; Tornøe, K.; Zinman, B.; Buse, J.B. Liraglutide and Renal Outcomes in Type 2 Diabetes. *N. Engl. J. Med.* **2017**, *377*, 839–848. [CrossRef] [PubMed]
76. Li, J.; Li, N.; Yan, S.; Lu, Y.; Miao, X.; Gu, Z.; Shao, Y. Liraglutide protects renal mesangial cells against hyperglycemia-mediated mitochondrial apoptosis by activating the ERK-Yap signaling pathway and upregulating Sirt3 expression. *Mol. Med. Rep.* **2019**, *19*, 2849–2860. [CrossRef]
77. Liang, R.; Wang, M.; Fu, C.; Xu, F.E.N.; Cai, M. 2032-P: The Effects of Liraglutide on Ameliorating Diabetic Kidney Disease Is via SIRT1/TXNIP Pathway. *Diabetes* **2019**, *68*, 2032. [CrossRef]
78. Fang, X.; Du, Z.; Duan, C.; Zhan, S.; Wang, T.; Zhu, M.; Shi, J.; Meng, J.; Zhang, X.; Yang, M.; et al. Beinaglutide shows significantly beneficial effects in diabetes/obesity-induced nonalcoholic steatohepatitis in ob/ob mouse model. *Life Sci.* **2021**, *270*, 118966. [CrossRef]
79. Zhang, Y.L.; Zhou, C.; Li, X.F.; Yang, M.N.; Tao, L.; Zheng, X.Y.; Jia, Y.S. Beinaglutide showed significant weight-loss benefit and effective glycaemic control for the treatment of type 2 diabetes in a real-world setting: A 3-month, multicentre, observational, retrospective, open-label study. *Obes. Sci. Pract.* **2019**, *5*, 366–375. [CrossRef]
80. Gao, L.; Huang, H.; Zhang, L.; Zhang, N.; Fu, Y.; Zhu, D.; Bi, Y.; Feng, W. Comparison of Beinaglutide Versus Metformin for Weight Loss in Overweight and Obese Non-diabetic Patients. *Exp. Clin. Endocrinol. Diabetes* **2021**, *130*, 358–367. [CrossRef]
81. Wen, Q.; Fang, S.; Liang, Y.; Tian, Y.; Chen, Y.; Yuan, J.; Chen, Q. Short-term effect of beinaglutide combined with metformin versus metformin alone on weight loss and metabolic profiles in obese patients with polycystic ovary syndrome: A pilot randomized trial. *Front. Endocrinol.* **2023**, *14*, 1156521. [CrossRef] [PubMed]
82. Wang, G.-Y.; Wang, H.-Q.; Zhang, F.-J.; Jiao, A.-F.; Li, Y.-Y.; Zhang, J.-M.; Huang, Z.-L.; Gao, Y.-H.; Chi, Y.-J.; Ma, C.-M.; et al. The effect of beinaglutide on visceral fat and bodyweight in obese type 2 diabetic patients. *Arch. Med. Sci.* **2020**. [CrossRef]
83. Zhang, F.; Chen, Z.; Wu, D.; Tian, L.; Chen, Q.; Ye, Y.; Chen, W.; Wu, X.; Wu, P.; Yuan, W.; et al. Recombinant human GLP-1 beinaglutide regulates lipid metabolism of adipose tissues in diet-induced obese mice. *iScience* **2021**, *24*, 103382. [CrossRef]

84. Wang, G.; Wu, P.; Qiu, Y.; Dong, X.; Wang, Y.; Chi, Y.; Zhang, F.; Li, Y.; Zhang, J.; Huang, Z.; et al. Effect of beinaglutide treatment on weight loss in Chinese patients with type 2 diabetes mellitus and overweight/obesity. *Arch. Endocrinol. Metab.* **2021**, *65*, 421–427. [CrossRef]
85. Sanford, M. Dulaglutide: First global approval. *Drugs* **2014**, *74*, 2097–2103. [CrossRef] [PubMed]
86. Jendle, J.; Grunberger, G.; Blevins, T.; Giorgino, F.; Hietpas, R.T.; Botros, F.T. Efficacy and safety of dulaglutide in the treatment of type 2 diabetes: A comprehensive review of the dulaglutide clinical data focusing on the AWARD phase 3 clinical trial program. *Diabetes Metab. Res. Rev.* **2016**, *32*, 776–790. [CrossRef] [PubMed]
87. Scott, L.J. Dulaglutide: A Review in Type 2 Diabetes. *Drugs* **2020**, *80*, 197–208. [CrossRef] [PubMed]
88. Frias, J.P.; Bonora, E.; Nevarez Ruiz, L.; Li, Y.G.; Yu, Z.; Milicevic, Z.; Malik, R.; Bethel, M.A.; Cox, D.A. Efficacy and Safety of Dulaglutide 3.0 mg and 4.5 mg Versus Dulaglutide 1.5 mg in Metformin-Treated Patients with Type 2 Diabetes in a Randomized Controlled Trial (AWARD-11). *Diabetes Care* **2021**, *44*, 765–773. [CrossRef]
89. Kimura, T.; Obata, A.; Shimoda, M.; Hirukawa, H.; Kanda-Kimura, Y.; Nogami, Y.; Kohara, K.; Nakanishi, S.; Mune, T.; Kaku, K.; et al. Durability of protective effect of dulaglutide on pancreatic β-cells in diabetic mice: GLP-1 receptor expression is not reduced despite long-term dulaglutide exposure. *Diabetes Metab.* **2018**, *44*, 250–260. [CrossRef]
90. Zheng, W.; Pan, H.; Wei, L.; Gao, F.; Lin, X. Dulaglutide mitigates inflammatory response in fibroblast-like synoviocytes. *Int. Immunopharmacol.* **2019**, *74*, 105649. [CrossRef]
91. Yifan, W.; Yixiang, W.; Yang, W.; Yiqing, W. Dulaglutide Ameliorates Intrauterine Adhesion by Suppressing Inflammation and Epithelial–Mesenchymal Transition Via Inhibiting the TGF-β/Smad2 Signaling Pathway. *Pharmaceuticals* **2023**, *16*, 964. [CrossRef] [PubMed]
92. Wang, Y.; Deng, F.; Zhong, X.; Du, Y.; Fan, X.; Su, H.; Pan, T. Dulaglutide provides protection against sepsis-induced lung injury in mice by inhibiting inflammation and apoptosis. *Eur. J. Pharmacol.* **2023**, *949*, 175730. [CrossRef] [PubMed]
93. Ferdinand, K.C.; Dunn, J.; Nicolay, C.; Sam, F.; Blue, E.K.; Wang, H. Weight-dependent and weight-independent effects of dulaglutide on blood pressure in patients with type 2 diabetes. *Cardiovasc. Diabetol.* **2023**, *22*, 1–11. [CrossRef]
94. Konig, M.; Riddle, M.C.; Colhoun, H.M.; Branch, K.R.; Atisso, C.M.; Lakshmanan, M.C.; Mody, R.; Raha, S.; Gerstein, H.C. Exploring potential mediators of the cardiovascular benefit of dulaglutide in type 2 diabetes patients in REWIND. *Cardiovasc. Diabetol.* **2021**, *20*, 194. [CrossRef] [PubMed]
95. Hertzel, C.G.; Shun-Fu, L.; Guillaume, P.; Bethel, M.A.; Helen, M.C.; Anastasia, H.; Mark, L.; Yanzhu, L.; Valentino, P.; Hui-Rong, Q.; et al. Biomarker Changes Associated with Both Dulaglutide and Cardiovascular Events in the REWIND Randomized Controlled Trial: A Nested Case-Control Post Hoc Analysis. *Diabetes Care* **2023**, *46*, 1046–1051. [CrossRef]
96. Gerstein, H.C.; Colhoun, H.M.; Dagenais, G.R.; Diaz, R.; Lakshmanan, M.; Pais, P.; Probstfield, J.; Riesmeyer, J.S.; Riddle, M.C.; Rydén, L.; et al. Dulaglutide and cardiovascular outcomes in type 2 diabetes (REWIND): A double-blind, randomised placebo-controlled trial. *Lancet* **2019**, *394*, 121–130. [CrossRef]
97. Luo, X.; Hu, Y.; He, S.; Ye, Q.; Lv, Z.; Liu, J.; Chen, X. Dulaglutide inhibits high glucose- induced endothelial dysfunction and NLRP3 inflammasome activation. *Arch. Biochem. Biophys.* **2019**, *671*, 203–209. [CrossRef]
98. Mei, X.; Li, Y.; Wu, J.; Liao, L.; Lu, D.; Qiu, P.; Yang, H.-l.; Tang, M.-w.; Liang, X.-y.; Liu, D. Dulaglutide restores endothelial progenitor cell levels in diabetic mice and mitigates high glucose-induced endothelial injury through SIRT1-mediated mitochondrial fission. *Biochem. Biophys. Res. Commun.* **2024**, *716*, 15000. [CrossRef]
99. Dhillon, S. Semaglutide: First Global Approval. *Drugs* **2018**, *78*, 275–284. [CrossRef]
100. Bucheit, J.D.; Pamulapati, L.G.; Carter, N.; Malloy, K.; Dixon, D.L.; Sisson, E.M. Oral Semaglutide: A Review of the First Oral Glucagon-Like Peptide 1 Receptor Agonist. *Diabetes Technol. Ther.* **2019**, *22*, 10–18. [CrossRef]
101. Hedrington, M.S.; Davis, S.N. Oral semaglutide for the treatment of type 2 diabetes. *Expert Opin. Pharmacother.* **2018**, *20*, 133–141. [CrossRef] [PubMed]
102. Anderson, S.L.; Beutel, T.R.; Trujillo, J.M. Oral semaglutide in type 2 diabetes. *J. Diabetes Its Complicat.* **2020**, *34*, 107520. [CrossRef] [PubMed]
103. Baekdal, T.A.; Donsmark, M.; Hartoft-Nielsen, M.-L.; Søndergaard, F.L.; Connor, A. Relationship Between Oral Semaglutide Tablet Erosion and Pharmacokinetics: A Pharmacoscintigraphic Study. *Clin. Pharmacol. Drug Dev.* **2021**, *10*, 453–462. [CrossRef] [PubMed]
104. Bækdal, T.A.; Breitschaft, A.; Donsmark, M.; Maarbjerg, S.J.; Søndergaard, F.L.; Borregaard, J. Effect of Various Dosing Conditions on the Pharmacokinetics of Oral Semaglutide, a Human Glucagon-Like Peptide-1 Analogue in a Tablet Formulation. *Diabetes Ther.* **2021**, *12*, 1915–1927. [CrossRef]
105. Gallwitz, B.; Giorgino, F. Clinical Perspectives on the Use of Subcutaneous and Oral Formulations of Semaglutide. *Front. Endocrinol.* **2021**, *12*, 645507. [CrossRef]
106. Li, A.; Su, X.; Hu, S.; Wang, Y. Efficacy and safety of oral semaglutide in type 2 diabetes mellitus: A systematic review and meta-analysis. *Diabetes Res. Clin. Pract.* **2023**, *198*, 110605. [CrossRef]
107. Davies, M.; Pieber, T.R.; Hartoft-Nielsen, M.-L.; Hansen, O.K.H.; Jabbour, S.; Rosenstock, J. Effect of Oral Semaglutide Compared with Placebo and Subcutaneous Semaglutide on Glycemic Control in Patients with Type 2 Diabetes. *JAMA* **2017**, *318*, 1460–1470. [CrossRef]
108. Smits, M.M.; Van Raalte, D.H. Safety of Semaglutide. *Front. Endocrinol.* **2021**, *12*, 645563. [CrossRef] [PubMed]

109. James, A.; Riddhi, P.D.; Joshua, N.; Xi, T.A.N.; Lin, X.I.E.; Cory, L.G.; Mico, G.; Justin, C.; Aaron, A.K. 86-LB: Real-World Impact of Oral Semaglutide on Glycemic Control and Weight Outcomes in Type 2 Diabetes (RELATE–Oral Semaglutide). *Diabetes* **2023**, *72*, 86. [CrossRef]
110. James, A.; Riddhi, P.D.; Joshua, N.; Xi, T.A.N.; Lin, X.I.E.; Cory, L.G.; Mico, G.; Justin, C.; Aaron, A.K. 87-LB: Real-World Impact of Once-Weekly Injectable Semaglutide on Glycemic Control and Weight Outcomes in Type 2 Diabetes (RELATE-OW Injectable Semaglutide). *Diabetes* **2023**, *72*, 87. [CrossRef]
111. Aroda, V.R.; Erhan, U.; Jelnes, P.; Meier, J.J.; Abildlund, M.T.; Pratley, R.; Vilsbøll, T.; Husain, M. Safety and tolerability of semaglutide across the SUSTAIN and PIONEER phase IIIa clinical trial programmes. *Diabetes Obes. Metab.* **2023**, *25*, 1385–1397. [CrossRef] [PubMed]
112. Priya, M.; Arya, M.S. Oral semaglutide: An OASIS from injectables. *Lancet* **2023**, *402*, 670–671. [CrossRef]
113. Selvarajan, R.; Subramanian, R. A Peptide in a Pill—Oral Semaglutide in the Management of Type 2 Diabetes. *Diabetes Metab. Syndr. Obes. Targets Ther.* **2023**, *16*, 1709–1720. [CrossRef]
114. Irene, F.-R. Semaglutide is beneficial in patients with HFpEF and obesity. *Nat. Rev. Cardiol.* **2023**, *20*, 719. [CrossRef]
115. Javed, B.; Steen, Z.A.; Barry, A.B.; Melanie, J.D.; Dalane, W.K.; Mark, C.P.; Sanjiv, J.S.; Subodh, V.; Walter, P.A.; Vijay, C.; et al. Semaglutide Effects According to Ejection Fraction in Heart Failure with Preserved Ejection Fraction and Obesity. *J. Am. Coll. Cardiol.* **2023**, *82*, 2087–2096. [CrossRef]
116. Li, X.; Luo, W.; Tang, Y.; Wu, J.; Zhang, J.; Chen, S.; Zhou, L.; Tao, Y.; Tang, Y.; Wang, F.; et al. Semaglutide attenuates doxorubicin-induced cardiotoxicity by ameliorating BNIP3-Mediated mitochondrial dysfunction. *Redox Biol.* **2024**, *72*, 103129. [CrossRef]
117. Yan, M.; Lin, K.; Huang, D.; Li, J.; Qu, X.; Chen, K. Semaglutide attenuates pathological electrophysiological remodeling in diabetic cardiomyopathy via restoring Cx43 expression. *Endocrine* **2024**, *84*, 969–979. [CrossRef]
118. Coenraad, W.; Laura, M.G.M.; Edgar, E.N.; Schouten, E.M.; Marie, A.S.; Lotte, B.K.; Kristoffer, N.; Christian, T.M.; Annabelle, H.; Gianluca, M.; et al. The Cardioprotective Effects of Semaglutide Exceed Those of Dietary Weight Loss in Mice with HFpEF. *JACC Basic Transl. Sci.* **2023**, *8*, 1298–1314. [CrossRef]
119. Mikhail, N.K.; Steen, Z.A.; Barry, A.B.; Javed, B.; Søren, R.; Melanie, D.; Hovingh, G.K.; Dalane, W.K.; Marie, L.L.; Daniél, V.M.; et al. Semaglutide in Patients with Heart Failure with Preserved Ejection Fraction and Obesity. *N. Engl. J. Med.* **2023**, *115*, 869–875. [CrossRef]
120. Maria Marques, V.; Paula, L.; Paula Sanchez, B.; María Victoria López, I.; Jose, M.P. #6005 Comparison of Semaglutide Oral vs Subcutaneous in Chronic Kidney Disease (CKD). *Nephrol. Dial. Transplant.* **2023**, *38*, gfad063c_6005. [CrossRef]
121. Chen, X.; Chen, S.; Ren, Q.; Niu, S.; Pan, X.; Yue, L.; Li, Z.; Zhu, R.; Jia, Z.; Chen, X.; et al. Metabolomics Provides Insights into Renoprotective Effects of Semaglutide in Obese Mice. *Drug Des. Dev. Ther.* **2022**, *16*, 3893–3913. [CrossRef] [PubMed]
122. Michael, C.; Louise, S.D.; Martin Rønn, M.; Henrik Björk, H.; Rune, I.; Mette Viberg, Ø. #5826 Nephroprotective Effects of Semaglutide in a Mouse Model of Hypertension-Accelerated Diabetic Kidney Disease. *Nephrol. Dial. Transplant.* **2023**, *38*, gfad063c_5826. [CrossRef]
123. Syed, Y.Y. Tirzepatide: First Approval. *Drugs* **2022**, *82*, 1213–1220. [CrossRef]
124. Gasbjerg, L.S.; Bergmann, N.C.; Stensen, S.; Christensen, M.B.; Rosenkilde, M.M.; Holst, J.J.; Nauck, M.; Knop, F.K. Evaluation of the incretin effect in humans using GIP and GLP-1 receptor antagonists. *Peptides* **2019**, *125*, 170183. [CrossRef]
125. Rhodes, R.S.S.; Singh, S.K.; Rajendran, V.M.; Walk, S.T.; Coon, S.D. Regulation of Glucose Insulinotropic Peptide and Intestinal Glucose Transporters in the Diet-Induced Obese Mouse. *J. Diabetes Res.* **2022**, *2022*, 5636499. [CrossRef]
126. Vilsbøll, T.; Knop, F.K.; Krarup, T.; Johansen, A.; Madsbad, S.; Larsen, S.; Hansen, T.; Pedersen, O.; Holst, J.J. The pathophysiology of diabetes involves a defective amplification of the late-phase insulin response to glucose by glucose-dependent insulinotropic polypeptide-regardless of etiology and phenotype. *J. Clin. Endocrinol. Metab.* **2003**, *88*, 4897–4903. [CrossRef]
127. Baggio, L.L.; Drucker, D.J. Glucagon-like Peptide-1 Receptor co-agonists for the treatment of metabolic disease. *Mol. Metab.* **2020**, *46*, 101090. [CrossRef]
128. Holst, J.J.; Rosenkilde, M.M. GIP as a Therapeutic Target in Diabetes and Obesity: Insight from Incretin Co-agonists. *J. Clin. Endocrinol. Metab.* **2020**, *105*, e2710–e2716. [CrossRef] [PubMed]
129. Thomas, M.K.; Nikooienejad, A.; Bray, R.; Cui, X.; Wilson, J.; Duffin, K.; Milicevic, Z.; Haupt, A.; Robins, D.A. Dual GIP and GLP-1 Receptor Agonist Tirzepatide Improves Beta-cell Function and Insulin Sensitivity in Type 2 Diabetes. *J. Clin. Endocrinol. Metab.* **2020**, *106*, 388–396. [CrossRef]
130. Coskun, T.; Sloop, K.W.; Loghin, C.; Alsina-Fernandez, J.; Urva, S.; Bokvist, K.B.; Cui, X.; Briere, D.A.; Cabrera, O.; Roell, W.C.; et al. LY3298176, a novel dual GIP and GLP-1 receptor agonist for the treatment of type 2 diabetes mellitus: From discovery to clinical proof of concept. *Mol. Metab.* **2018**, *18*, 3–14. [CrossRef]
131. Heise, T.; Mari, A.; DeVries, J.H.; Urva, S.; Li, J.; Pratt, E.J.; Coskun, T.; Thomas, M.K.; Mather, K.J.; Haupt, A.; et al. Effects of subcutaneous tirzepatide versus placebo or semaglutide on pancreatic islet function and insulin sensitivity in adults with type 2 diabetes: A multicentre, randomised, double-blind, parallel-arm, phase 1 clinical trial. *Lancet Diabetes Endocrinol.* **2022**, *10*, 418–429. [CrossRef] [PubMed]
132. El, K.; Douros, J.D.; Willard, F.S.; Novikoff, A.; Sargsyan, A.; Perez-Tilve, D.; Wainscott, D.B.; Yang, B.; Chen, A.; Wothe, D.; et al. The incretin co-agonist tirzepatide requires GIPR for hormone secretion from human islets. *Nat. Metab.* **2023**, *5*, 945–954. [CrossRef] [PubMed]

133. Garvey, W.T.; Frias, J.P.; Jastreboff, A.M.; le Roux, C.W.; Sattar, N.; Aizenberg, D.; Mao, H.; Zhang, S.; Ahmad, N.N.; Bunck, M.C.; et al. Tirzepatide once weekly for the treatment of obesity in people with type 2 diabetes (SURMOUNT-2): A double-blind, randomised, multicentre, placebo-controlled, phase 3 trial. *Lancet* **2023**, *402*, 613–626. [CrossRef] [PubMed]
134. NamKoong, C.; Kim, M.S.; Jang, B.-T.; Lee, Y.H.; Cho, Y.-M.; Choi, H.J. Central administration of GLP-1 and GIP decreases feeding in mice. *Biochem. Biophys. Res. Commun.* **2017**, *490*, 247–252. [CrossRef] [PubMed]
135. Zhang, Q.; Delessa, C.T.; Augustin, R.; Bakhti, M.; Colldén, G.; Drucker, D.J.; Feuchtinger, A.; Caceres, C.G.; Grandl, G.; Harger, A.; et al. The glucose-dependent insulinotropic polypeptide (GIP) regulates body weight and food intake via CNS-GIPR signaling. *Cell Metab.* **2021**, *33*, 833–844.e5. [CrossRef]
136. Heerspink, H.J.L.; Sattar, N.; Pavo, I.; Haupt, A.; Duffin, K.L.; Yang, Z.; Wiese, R.J.; Tuttle, K.R.; Cherney, D.Z.I. Effects of tirzepatide versus insulin glargine on kidney outcomes in type 2 diabetes in the SURPASS-4 trial: Post-hoc analysis of an open-label, randomised, phase 3 trial. *Lancet Diabetes Endocrinol.* **2022**, *10*, 774–785. [CrossRef]
137. Wilson, J.M.; Lin, Y.; Considine, G.; Cox, A.L.; Bowsman, L.M.; Robins, D.A.; Riesmeyer, J.S.; Haupt, A.; Duffin, K.; Ruotolo, G. Abstract 13426: The Dual GIP/GLP-1 Receptor Agonist Tirzepatide Improves Cardiovascular Risk Protein Biomarkers in Patients with Type 2 Diabetes. *Circulation* **2020**, *142*, A13426. [CrossRef]
138. Lian, J.; Fu, J. Pioglitazone for NAFLD Patients with Prediabetes or Type 2 Diabetes Mellitus: A Meta-analysis. *Front. Endocrinol.* **2021**, *12*, 615409. [CrossRef]
139. Lukic, N.; Macvanin, M.T.; Gluvic, Z.; Rizzo, M.; Radak, D.; Suri, J.S.; Isenovic, E.R. SGLT-2 Inhibitors: The Next-generation Treatment for Type 2 Diabetes Mellitus. *Curr. Med. Chem.* **2023**, *31*, 4781–4806. [CrossRef]
140. Repaglinide, S.L.J. Repaglinide: A review of its use in type 2 diabetes mellitus (vol 72, pg 249, 2012). *Drugs* **2012**, *72*, 744.
141. Tomlinson, B.; Patil, N.G.; Fok, M.; Chan, P.; Lam, C.W.K. The role of sulfonylureas in the treatment of type 2 diabetes. *Expert Opin. Pharmaco.* **2022**, *23*, 387–403. [CrossRef] [PubMed]
142. Suenaga, A.; Sawa, N.; Oba, Y.; Ikuma, D.; Sekine, A.; Hasegawa, E.; Mizuno, H.; Suwabe, T.; Ikeda, S.; Tsujimoto, T.; et al. Dipeptidyl peptidase-4 inhibitor-related renal disease. *J. Diabetes Complicat.* **2023**, *37*, 108590. [CrossRef] [PubMed]
143. Sanchez-Rangel, E.; Inzucchi, S.E. Metformin: Clinical use in type 2 diabetes. *Diabetologia* **2017**, *60*, 1586–1593. [CrossRef] [PubMed]
144. Mushtaq, A.; Azam, U.; Mehreen, S.; Naseer, M.M. Synthetic α-glucosidase inhibitors as promising anti-diabetic agents: Recent developments and future challenges. *Eur. J. Med. Chem.* **2023**, *249*, 115119. [CrossRef]
145. Kawai, T.; Sun, B.; Yoshino, H.; Feng, D.; Suzuki, Y.; Fukazawa, M.; Nagao, S.; Wainscott, D.B.; Showalter, A.D.; Droz, B.A.; et al. Structural basis for GLP-1 receptor activation by LY3502970, an orally active nonpeptide agonist [Pharmacology]. *Proc. Natl. Acad. Sci. USA* **2020**, *117*, 29959–29967. [CrossRef]
146. Frias, J.P.; Hsia, S.; Eyde, S.; Liu, R.; Ma, X.; Konig, M.; Kazda, C.; Mather, K.J.; Haupt, A.; Pratt, E.; et al. Efficacy and safety of oral orforglipron in patients with type 2 diabetes: A multicentre, randomised, dose-response, phase 2 study. *Lancet* **2023**, *402*, 472–483. [CrossRef]
147. Ono, R.; Furihata, K.; Ichikawa, Y.; Nakazuru, Y.; Bergman, A.; Gorman, D.N.; Saxena, A.R. 339-OR: Oral Small-Molecule GLP-1R Agonist Danuglipron Robustly Reduces Plasma Glucose and Body Weight after Eight Weeks in Japanese Adults with Type 2 Diabetes Mellitus. *Diabetes* **2022**, *71*, 339. [CrossRef]
148. Saxena, A.R.; Gorman, D.N.; Esquejo, R.M.; Bergman, A.; Chidsey, K.; Buckeridge, C.; Griffith, D.A.; Kim, A.M. Danuglipron (PF-06882961) in type 2 diabetes: A randomized, placebo-controlled, multiple ascending-dose phase 1 trial. *Nat. Med.* **2021**, *27*, 1079–1087. [CrossRef] [PubMed]
149. Saxena, A.R.; Frias, J.P.; Brown, L.S.; Gorman, D.N.; Vasas, S.; Tsamandouras, N.; Birnbaum, M.J. Efficacy and Safety of Oral Small Molecule Glucagon-Like Peptide 1 Receptor Agonist Danuglipron for Glycemic Control Among Patients with Type 2 Diabetes: A Randomized Clinical Trial. *JAMA Netw. Open* **2023**, *6*, e2314493. [CrossRef]
150. Wu, J.; Zhou, R.; Zhang, Q.; Zhang, Q.; Qin, H.; Ye, Z.; Xu, Y.; Feng, S.; Shu, C.; Shen, Y.; et al. Safety, pharmacokinetics and pharmacodynamics of HRS-7535, a novel oral small molecule glucagon-like peptide-1 receptor agonist, in healthy participants: A phase 1, randomized, double-blind, placebo-controlled, single- and multiple-ascending dose, and food effect trial. *Diabetes Obes. Metab.* **2023**, *26*, 901–910. [CrossRef]
151. Ma, T.; Lu, W.; Wang, Y.; Qian, P.; Tian, H.; Gao, X.; Yao, W. An oral GLP-1 and GIP dual receptor agonist improves metabolic disorders in high fat-fed mice. *Eur. J. Pharmacol.* **2021**, *914*, 174635. [CrossRef]
152. He, H.; Lu, Y.; Qi, J.; Zhu, Q.; Chen, Z.; Wu, W. Adapting liposomes for oral drug delivery. *Acta Pharm. Sin. B* **2019**, *9*, 36–48. [CrossRef] [PubMed]
153. He, Y.; Huang, Y.; Xu, H.; Yang, X.; Liu, N.; Xu, Y.; Ma, R.; Zhai, J.; Ma, Y.; Guan, S. Aptamer-modified M cell targeting liposomes for oral delivery of macromolecules. *Colloids Surf. B Biointerfaces* **2022**, *222*, 113109. [CrossRef]
154. Cui, J.; Wen, Z.; Zhang, W.; Wu, W. Recent Advances in Oral Peptide or Protein-Based Drug Liposomes. *Pharmaceuticals* **2022**, *15*, 1072. [CrossRef] [PubMed]
155. Yun, Y.; Cho, Y.W.; Park, K. Nanoparticles for oral delivery: Targeted nanoparticles with peptidic ligands for oral protein delivery. *Adv. Drug Deliv. Rev.* **2013**, *65*, 822–832. [CrossRef]
156. Wang, A.; Yang, T.; Fan, W.; Yang, Y.; Zhu, Q.; Guo, S.; Zhu, C.; Yuan, Y.; Zhang, T.; Gan, Y. Protein Corona Liposomes Achieve Efficient Oral Insulin Delivery by Overcoming Mucus and Epithelial Barriers. *Adv. Healthc. Mater.* **2018**, *8*, e1801123. [CrossRef] [PubMed]

157. Ding, R.; Zhao, Z.; He, J.; Tao, Y.; Zhang, H.; Yuan, R.; Sun, K.; Shi, Y. Preparation, Drug Distribution, and In Vivo Evaluation of the Safety of Protein Corona Liposomes for Liraglutide Delivery. *Nanomaterials* **2023**, *13*, 540. [CrossRef]
158. Blanquet, S.; Marol-Bonnin, S.; Beyssac, E.; Pompon, D.; Renaud, M.; Alric, M. The 'biodrug' concept: An innovative approach to therapy. *Trends Biotechnol.* **2001**, *19*, 393–400. [CrossRef]
159. Fei, Z.; Li, S.; Wang, J.; Wang, Y.; Jiang, Z.; Huang, W.; Sun, H. *Rhodotorula glutinis* as a living cell liposome to deliver polypeptide drugs in vivo. *Drug Deliv.* **2019**, *26*, 51–62. [CrossRef]
160. Kimiz-Gebologlu, I.; Oncel, S.S. Exosomes: Large-scale production, isolation, drug loading efficiency, and biodistribution and uptake. *J. Control. Release* **2022**, *347*, 533–543. [CrossRef]
161. Zhong, J.; Xia, B.; Shan, S.; Zheng, A.; Zhang, S.; Chen, J.; Liang, X.-J. High-quality milk exosomes as oral drug delivery system. *Biomaterials* **2021**, *277*, 121126. [CrossRef] [PubMed]
162. Wu, L.; Wang, L.; Liu, X.; Bai, Y.; Wu, R.; Li, X.; Mao, Y.; Zhang, L.; Zheng, Y.; Gong, T.; et al. Milk-derived exosomes exhibit versatile effects for improved oral drug delivery. *Acta Pharm. Sin. B* **2021**, *12*, 2029–2042. [CrossRef] [PubMed]
163. Xiao, P.; Wang, H.; Liu, H.; Yuan, H.; Guo, C.; Feng, Y.; Qi, P.; Yin, T.; Zhang, Y.; He, H.; et al. Milk Exosome–Liposome Hybrid Vesicles with Self-Adapting Surface Properties Overcome the Sequential Absorption Barriers for Oral Delivery of Peptides. *ACS Nano* **2024**, *18*, 21091–21111. [CrossRef] [PubMed]
164. Haddadzadegan, S.; To, D.; Matteo Jörgensen, A.; Wibel, R.; Laffleur, F.; Bernkop-Schnürch, A. Comparative Analysis of PEG-Free and PEG-Based Self-Emulsifying Drug Delivery Systems for Enhanced Oral Bioavailability of Therapeutic (Poly) Peptides. *Small* **2024**, *20*, e2307618. [CrossRef] [PubMed]
165. Mahmood, A.; Bernkop-Schnürch, A. SEDDS: A game changing approach for the oral administration of hydrophilic macromolecular drugs. *Adv. Drug Deliv. Rev.* **2018**, *142*, 91–101. [CrossRef]
166. Menzel, C.; Holzeisen, T.; Laffleur, F.; Zaichik, S.; Abdulkarim, M.; Gumbleton, M.; Bernkop-Schnürch, A. In vivo evaluation of an oral self-emulsifying drug delivery system (SEDDS) for exenatide. *J. Control. Release* **2018**, *277*, 165–172. [CrossRef]
167. Phan, T.N.Q.; Ismail, R.; Le-Vinh, B.; Zaichik, S.; Laffleur, F.; Bernkop-Schnürch, A. The Effect of Counterions in Hydrophobic Ion Pairs on Oral Bioavailability of Exenatide. *ACS Biomater. Sci. Eng.* **2020**, *6*, 5032–5039. [CrossRef]
168. Lu, Y.; Wu, L.; Lin, M.; Bao, X.; Zhong, H.; Ke, P.; Dai, Q.; Yang, Q.; Tang, X.; Xu, W.; et al. Double layer spherical nanoparticles with hyaluronic acid coating to enhance oral delivery of exenatide in T2DM rats. *Eur. J. Pharm. Biopharm.* **2023**, *191*, 205–218. [CrossRef]
169. Maji, I.; Mahajan, S.; Sriram, A.; Medtiya, P.; Vasave, R.; Khatri, D.K.; Kumar, R.; Singh, S.B.; Madan, J.; Singh, P.K. Solid self emulsifying drug delivery system: Superior mode for oral delivery of hydrophobic cargos. *J. Control. Release* **2021**, *337*, 646–660. [CrossRef]
170. Sun, X.; Lv, G.; Xiong, J.; Zhao, J.; Zhao, J.; Wang, Z.; Wang, Y.; Yin, T.; Gou, J.; He, H.; et al. Novel solid self-emulsifying drug delivery system to enhance oral bioavailability of cabazitaxel. *Int. J. Pharm.* **2024**, *654*, 123899. [CrossRef]
171. Yuan, H.; Guo, C.; Liu, L.; Zhao, L.; Zhang, Y.; Yin, T.; He, H.; Gou, J.; Pan, B.; Tang, X. Progress and prospects of polysaccharide-based nanocarriers for oral delivery of proteins/peptides. *Carbohydr. Polym.* **2023**, *312*, 120838. [CrossRef]
172. Wang, Y.; Li, H.; Rasool, A.; Wang, H.; Manzoor, R.; Zhang, G. Polymeric nanoparticles (PNPs) for oral delivery of insulin. *J. Nanobiotechnol.* **2024**, *22*, 1. [CrossRef] [PubMed]
173. Sarah, L.C.; Stephanie, P.B.; Lisa, M.; Jane, K.P.; Vitaliy, V.K. Mucoadhesion: A food perspective. *Food Hydrocoll.* **2017**, *72*, 281–296.
174. Yang, J.-M.; Wu, L.-J.; Lin, M.-T.; Lu, Y.-Y.; Wang, T.-T.; Han, M.; Zhang, B.; Xu, D.-H. Construction and Evaluation of Chitosan-Based Nanoparticles for Oral Administration of Exenatide in Type 2 Diabetic Rats. *Polymers* **2022**, *14*, 2181. [CrossRef] [PubMed]
175. Sadeghi, S.; Lee, W.K.; Kong, S.N.; Shetty, A.; Drum, C.L. Oral administration of protein nanoparticles: An emerging route to disease treatment. *Pharmacol. Res.* **2020**, *158*, 104685. [CrossRef] [PubMed]
176. Bao, X.; Qian, K.; Xu, M.; Chen, Y.; Wang, H.; Pan, T.; Wang, Z.; Yao, P.; Lin, L. Intestinal epithelium penetration of liraglutide via cholic acid pre-complexation and zein/rhamnolipids nanocomposite delivery. *J. Nanobiotechnol.* **2023**, *21*, 16. [CrossRef]
177. Li, Q.; Wen, C.; Yang, J.; Zhou, X.; Zhu, Y.; Zheng, J.; Cheng, G.; Bai, J.; Xu, T.; Ji, J.; et al. Zwitterionic Biomaterials. *Chem. Rev.* **2022**, *122*, 17073–17154. [CrossRef]
178. Zhao, Z.; Ding, R.; Wang, Y.; Yuan, R.; Zhang, H.; Li, T.; Zheng, W.; Chen, E.; Wang, A.; Shi, Y. Sulfobetaine modification of poly (D, L-lactide-co-glycolic acid) nanoparticles enhances mucus permeability and improves bioavailability of orally delivered liraglutide. *J. Drug Deliv. Sci. Technol.* **2024**, *93*, 105437. [CrossRef]
179. Florek, J.; Caillard, R.; Kleitz, F. Evaluation of mesoporous silica nanoparticles for oral drug delivery—Current status and perspective of MSNs drug carriers. *Nanoscale* **2017**, *9*, 15252–15277. [CrossRef]
180. Abeer, M.M.; Rewatkar, P.; Qu, Z.; Talekar, M.; Kleitz, F.; Schmid, R.; Lindén, M.; Kumeria, T.; Popat, A. Silica nanoparticles: A promising platform for enhanced oral delivery of macromolecules. *J. Control. Release* **2020**, *326*, 544–555. [CrossRef]
181. Ehsan, S.; Mahdis, M.; Elahe, M.; Ahmad, K.; Mohammad Reza, S.; Zohreh, S.; Iman, R.; Shahriar, D.; Siyavash, J.; Iraj, S.; et al. Exploring mesoporous silica nanoparticles as oral insulin carriers: In-silico and in vivo evaluation. *Heliyon* **2023**, *9*, e20430. [CrossRef]
182. Abeer, M.M.; Meka, A.K.; Pujara, N.; Kumeria, T.; Strounina, E.; Nunes, R.; Costa, A.; Sarmento, B.; Hasnain, S.Z.; Ross, B.P.; et al. Rationally Designed Dendritic Silica Nanoparticles for Oral Delivery of Exenatide. *Pharmaceutics* **2019**, *11*, 418. [CrossRef]
183. Xia, J.; Xue, Y.; Lei, B.; Xu, L.; Sun, M.; Li, N.; Zhao, H.; Wang, M.; Luo, M.; Zhang, C.; et al. Multimodal channel cancer chemotherapy by 2D functional gadolinium metal–organic framework. *Natl. Sci. Rev.* **2020**, *8*, nwaa221. [CrossRef]

184. Wei, Q.; Wu, Y.; Liu, F.; Cao, J.; Liu, J. Advances in antitumor nanomedicine based on functional metal–organic frameworks beyond drug carriers. *J. Mater. Chem. B* **2021**, *10*, 676–699. [CrossRef] [PubMed]
185. He, L.; Shang, M.; Chen, Z.; Yang, Z. Metal-Organic Frameworks Nanocarriers for Functional Nucleic Acid Delivery in Biomedical Applications. *Chem. Rec.* **2023**, *23*, e202300018. [CrossRef] [PubMed]
186. Zou, J.-J.; Wei, G.; Xiong, C.; Yu, Y.; Li, S.; Hu, L.; Ma, S.; Tian, J. Efficient oral insulin delivery enabled by transferrin-coated acid-resistant metal-organic framework nanoparticles. *Sci. Adv.* **2022**, *8*, eabm4677. [CrossRef]
187. Agrawal, A.; Joshi, A.; Bhattacharya, S. Recent Excavation of Nanoethosomes in Current Drug Delivery. *Curr. Drug Deliv.* **2024**, *21*, 168–183. [CrossRef]

pharmaceutics

Review

Recent Progress of Oral Functional Nanomaterials for Intestinal Microbiota Regulation

Wanneng Li [1], Minle Zhan [2], Yue Wen [1], Yu Chen [1], Zhongchao Zhang [1], Shuhui Wang [1], Dean Tian [1,*] and Sidan Tian [2,3,*]

1 Department of Gastroenterology, Tongji Hospital, Tongji Medical College, Huazhong University of Science and Technology, Wuhan 430074, China; m202276234@hust.edu.cn (W.L.); wenyue@tjh.tjmu.edu.cn (Y.W.); d202181940@hust.edu.cn (Y.C.); tjhzzc@hust.edu.cn (Z.Z.); d202282081@hust.edu.cn (S.W.)
2 National Engineering Research Center for Nanomedicine, College of Life Science and Technology, Huazhong University of Science and Technology, Wuhan 430074, China; m202172338@hust.edu.cn
3 Key Laboratory of Molecular Biophysics of the Ministry of Education, College of Life Science and Technology, Huazhong University of Science and Technology, Wuhan 430074, China
* Correspondence: datian@tjh.tjmu.edu.cn (D.T.); sdtian1616@hust.edu.cn (S.T.)

Abstract: The gut microbiota is closely associated with human health, and alterations in gut microbiota can influence various physiological and pathological activities in the human body. Therefore, microbiota regulation has become an important strategy in current disease treatment, albeit facing numerous challenges. Nanomaterials, owing to their excellent protective properties, drug release capabilities, targeting abilities, and good biocompatibility, have been widely developed and utilized in pharmaceuticals and dietary fields. In recent years, significant progress has been made in research on utilizing nanomaterials to assist in regulating gut microbiota for disease intervention. This review explores the latest advancements in the application of nanomaterials for microbiota regulation and offers insights into the future development of nanomaterials in modulating gut microbiota.

Keywords: nanomaterial; gut microbiota; therapy; immunity; oral administration

1. Introduction

The gut microbiota is a microbial community residing in the human intestinal tract, comprising thousands of different bacterial species, with the number of microorganisms in the human gut ranging from 10^{14} to 10^{15} [1,2]. In the gut, the normal composition of the gut microbiota is crucial for maintaining intestinal functions such as peristalsis and facilitating normal nutrient metabolism [3,4]. Additionally, metabolites produced by the gut microbiota can interact with intestinal mucosal cells to regulate host immune responses [5]. Outside the gut, the vast microbial composition also influences various aspects of human health, including growth and development, aging, regulation of the skeletal system, and balance of the immune system (Figure 1) [6–9]. Some products secreted by the gut microbiota can enter the bloodstream through the intestinal barrier, thereby affecting extraintestinal organs [10]. Therefore, strategies to manipulate the gut microbiota to treat certain diseases have garnered increasing attention from researchers. Currently, the most common interventions for modulating the gut microbiota include the following two major strategies: (1) oral administration of microbiota-modulating drugs and (2) fecal microbiota transplantation. Fecal microbiota transplantation involves transplanting functional microbiota from healthy donors into the patient's gut to restore the composition of the gut microbiota and thus treat diseases. Fecal microbiota transplantation emphasizes the overall role of the gut microbiota rather than specific components. Studies have shown that the cure rate of fecal microbiota transplantation for *Clostridium difficile* infection can reach 90%. However, this treatment method presents many challenges compared to oral probiotics or medication for modulating the gut microbiota, such as gastrointestinal discomfort, mechanical damage, and low patient acceptance [11,12]. Among these, oral administration is undoubtedly the most common and convenient method of delivery, which can be entirely reliant on the patient and thereby enhance patient acceptance and compliance [13]. Oral administration not only has minimal side effects but also can reduce the systemic toxicity of colon-targeted therapy and improve its efficacy [14]. However, oral administration also faces many challenges. Most of the gut microbiota colonize the colon, so when using oral probiotics to intervene in the disease process, probiotics need to pass through the oral cavity, esophagus, stomach, small intestine, and colon [1]. During this process, probiotics undergo prolonged transportation and endure changes in the surrounding environmental pH and damage from digestive fluids, which cannot guarantee the colonization and activity of probiotics, leading to an increase in the effective dose of probiotics [15]. Additionally, many researchers have indicated that oral probiotics are not entirely safe, but currently, there is a lack of research on the safety of oral probiotics [15–17]. Oral antibiotics are currently commonly used to eliminate harmful gut microbiota. However, due to their uncontrollable effects on other normal microbiota, this method is not conducive to maintaining the balance of the gut microbiota [6,18]. Therefore, improving the application of oral administration systems in the regulation of the gut microbiota is currently an urgent issue. The combination of nanomaterials and oral administration systems is a promising strategy. On the one hand, nanoparticles as carriers can transport microbiota-modulating drugs to prevent them from physical and chemical damage from the intestines. Moreover, specific nanomaterials can also help in the controlled release and targeted delivery of drugs by responding to changes in intestinal chemistry. On the other hand, nanomaterials themselves can also participate in microbiota regulation.

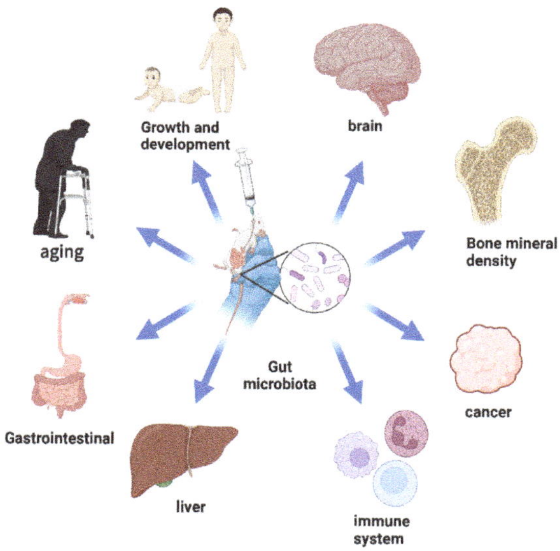

Figure 1. Schematic diagram of the relationship between gut microbiota and human physiology and diseases. (Created with bioRender.com).

Nanomaterials refer to materials where at least one dimension is in the nanoscale range (1–100 nm). The rapid development of nanotechnology has greatly promoted the application of nanomaterials in biomedicine, especially in oral formulations. Compared to other administration methods, oral administration is undoubtedly the most convenient way to administer drugs. However, traditional drugs often have low bioavailability due to the influence of their properties and gastrointestinal environments. However, traditional drugs often have low bioavailability due to the influence of their properties and gastrointestinal environments [19]. Oral nanocarriers carrying microbiota-modulating drugs can protect the drugs from damage by low pH in the stomach and intestinal enzymes, thereby increasing their bioavailability [20]. Furthermore, some nanocarriers can assist in the targeted transport of microbiota-modulating drugs, thereby increasing the concentration and activity of orally administered drugs at the lesion site, reducing the dosage of drugs used, and improving the safety of drugs. For example, materials with pH responsiveness can achieve the colon-targeted release of drugs [21]. Additionally, the combination of nanomaterials and antibiotics can not only maintain the balance of the gut microbiota but also reduce the emergence of drug-resistant bacteria [22]. As mentioned earlier, the influence of the gut microbiota on human health has received increasing attention, and intervention in the gut microbiota through regulation has become a new treatment strategy. However, the regulation of the gut microbiota is constrained by gastrointestinal environments and physiological functions. Fortunately, the application of nanotechnology has greatly increased the feasibility of regulating the gut microbiota. This paper summarizes the regulation of the gut microbiota by nanotechnology as carriers and nanomaterials themselves, the adverse effects of certain nanomaterials on the gut microbiota, and the application of nanotechnology in the treatment of diseases by regulating the gut microbiota, and finally puts forward further prospects for the regulation of the gut microbiota by nanomaterials.

2. Nanomaterials as Drug Carriers to Assist Microbiota Regulation

2.1. Nanomaterials as Carriers for Sustained Release of Microbiota-Modulating Drugs

Nanomaterials can serve as excellent carriers to transport certain microbiota-modulating molecules into the intestine to better exert their regulatory effects (Figure 2A) (Table 1). Polyphenols, compounds found in plant-based foods, have potential health-promoting effects and can interact with targets in the body, exhibiting anti-inflammatory and antioxidant effects [23]. Among them, low-toxicity and health-promoting polyphenolic substances are gradually being explored by researchers as good food additives [24]. These substances can interact with the gut microbiota, and some polyphenols can alter the composition of the gut microbiota, promoting the growth of beneficial bacteria while inhibiting the proliferation of harmful bacteria [25]. Although polyphenolic substances have various excellent biological activities, their low solubility, poor digestibility, and rapid absorption and metabolism during gastrointestinal digestion processes result in their less-than-ideal bioavailability. The sustained-release function of nanomaterials can effectively compensate for the low bioavailability of polyphenols. Wang Luet al. constructed nanoparticles composed of Hohenbuehelia serotina polysaccharides and mucins as carriers to encapsulate polyphenols from *Malus baccata (Linn.) Borkh* (MBP-MC-HSP NPs). This nanocarrier exhibited good sustained-release effects, effectively protecting polyphenols, isolating them from the biological effects of the intestinal tract, and presenting no toxic side effects. Experimental results showed that MBP-MC-HSP NPs indeed promoted intestinal health through microbiota regulation [24]. Similarly, Mejo Kuzhithariel Remanan et al. encapsulated chrysin and rutin (natural polyphenols) using starch nanoparticles formed by the self-assembly of starch from quinoa (Q), maize (M), and waxy maize (WM). Among them, starch nanoparticles formed by quinoa showed sustained release of polyphenols and enhanced the antioxidant activity of polyphenols [26]. Xiaoyu Li et al. reported the design and manufacture of nanoparticles based on Hohenbuehelia serotina polysaccharides (HSP) and bovine serum albumin (BSA) as carriers for delivering polyphenols isolated from the shells of Juglans regia L (BSA-JRP-HSP NPs). BSA-JRP-HSP NPs promoted the growth of probiotics, inhibited the proliferation of harmful bacteria, and significantly increased the content of short-chain fatty acids during colonic fermentation [27]. Additionally, Wenni Tian et al. used nanostructured lipid carriers (6G-NLCs) and NLC-imbedded microcapsules (6G-MCs) loaded with 6-gingerol, respectively. Different delivery materials have distinct biological distributions and release curves, even when loaded with the same 6-gingerol, which can lead to different intervention results on the gut microbiota [28]. The pattern diagrams demonstrate the release of 6G from 6G-NLCs and 6G-MCs in the stimulated gastric fluid (SGF), stimulated intestinal fluid (SIF), and stimulated colon fluid (SCF) in vitro. Among them, the 6G-NLC showed a very small amount of release in the SIF and was completely released in the SCF. However, the 6G-MC only showed release in the SCF (Figure 2B). Meanwhile, Wenni Tian et al. observed the structural evolution of the 6G-MC during in vitro digestion using light microscopy. In the SGF and SIF, the structure of the 6G-MC remained intact. After placing 6G-MCs in the SCF, the figure shows sustained destruction of its structure over a period of 5 h (Figure 2C). According to the authors in the original article, 94.32% of the 6G in the SCF would be released continuously within 20 h [28]. In summary, the use of nanomaterials for delivering polyphenols can significantly improve their bioavailability and assist in their intervention on the gut microbiota. Nanomaterials are not merely delivery tools for polyphenols; the differences in delivery materials can significantly affect the intervention mechanism and efficacy of polyphenolic substances on the gut microbiota. The sustained-release effect of nanomaterials can also be applied to the combination with small-molecule water-soluble drugs. Pengchao Zhao et al. reported a biologically adhesive liquid coacervate assembly based on hydrogen-bond-driven nanoparticles, which enhanced the retention time of Sodium phosphate salt of dexamethasone (small-molecule water-soluble substance) in the intestine, prolonged its action time, reduced the dosage of this drug, and thus reduced its side effects. Additionally, since the balance of intestinal inflammation is complementary to the stability of the gut microbiota, this nanodrug also has a reparative effect on the gut microbiota while exerting anti-inflammatory effects [29].

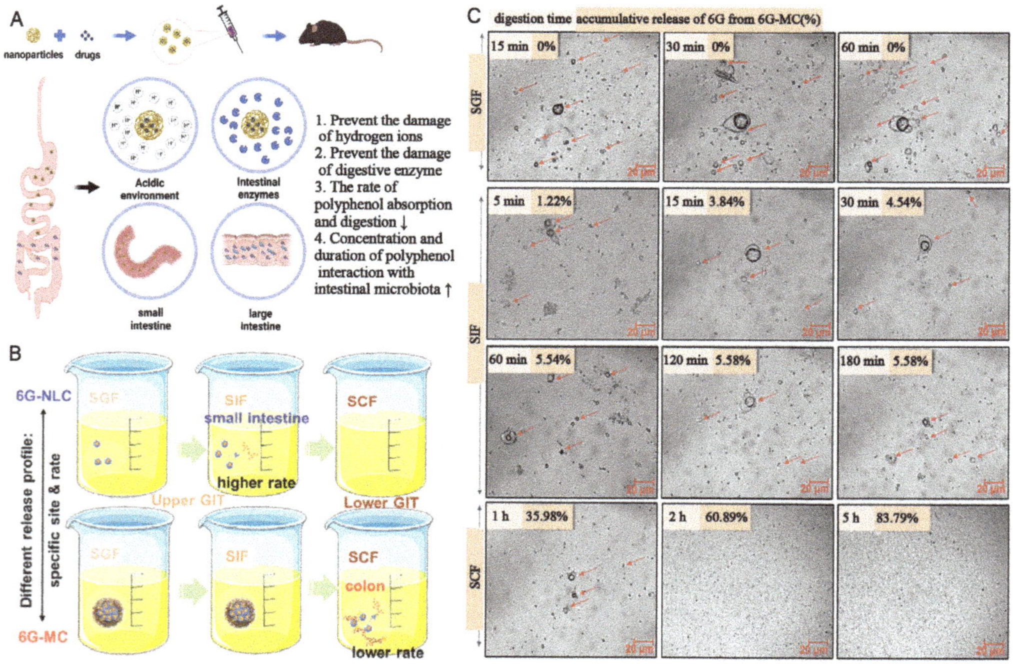

Figure 2. (**A**) Diagram illustrating the protection of drugs by nanomaterials (created with bioRender.com) (**B**) Schematic representation of the release of 6G from 6G-NLC and 6G-MC in different simulated digestive fluids (6G: 6-gingerol, NLC: nanostructured lipid carriers, MC: NLC-imbedded microcapsule, SGF: stimulated gastric fluid, SIF: stimulated intestinal fluid, SCF: stimulated colon fluid, GIT: gastrointestinal tract). The arrows in the figure point to 6G-MC in different states. This figure demonstrates the structural evolution of 6G-MC in different environments (**C**) Observation of the release of 6G from 6G-MC in different simulated digestive fluids under an optical microscope, accompanied by the cumulative release values of 6G at different time points. Adapted with permission from ref. [28]. Copyrights 2022 Elsevier.

2.2. Nanomaterials as Carriers for Controlled Release of Microbiota-Modulating Drugs

The intestinal system is a complex structure, and the effects of oral drugs on the gut microbiota are often influenced by the acidity and enzymatic environment of the digestive tract. The application of nanocarriers can overcome this challenge and, at the same time, control the release of drugs to ensure their action at the damaged sites of diseases as much as possible (Figure 3A) (Table 1) [30,31]. Shangyong Li et al. developed an enzyme-triggered controlled-release system with curcumin-cyclodextrin (CD-Cur) complexes as the core and low-molecular-weight chitosan and unsaturated alginate nanoparticles (CANP) as shells. The pH-sensitive and α-amylase-responsive release characteristics of this nanomaterial endowed it with excellent colon-targeting ability and controlled-release capability. This greatly enhanced the curative effect of curcumin on colitis and promoted the restoration of gut microbiota composition [32]. As shown, the release of curcumin (Cur) from Cur-CD-CANPs varied in response to changes in PH and enzyme environments. In a low PH, α-amylase-free environment such as the SGF, the release of Cur is relatively low, which protects Cur from destruction. On the contrary, at relatively high pH and in the presence of α-amylase, such as the SIF, the release of Cur is significantly increased, which can make Cur better utilized by the body (Figure 3B) [32]. Probiotics are a class of beneficial active microorganisms that colonize the human body and affect human health in a favorable way [33]. As mentioned earlier, although oral probiotics have been confirmed as one of the means to promote health and improve diseases, due to the complex physiological and chemical structure of the intestine, their stable arrival at disease sites cannot be guaranteed. Jiali Chen et al. reported a supramolecular self-assembled nitroreductase (NTR) labile peptidic hydrogel and used it to encapsulate the typical probiotic *Escherichia coli Nissle 1917* (EcN). This nanocomposite not only protected probiotics but also, because of the upregulated nitroreductase in the intestine, which can trigger the decomposition of the hydrogel, enabled the probiotics to be released locally under controlled conditions, significantly improving the treatment of inflammatory bowel disease [34].

2.3. Nanomaterials Assisting in Targeted Microbiota-Modulating Drug Delivery

Nanomaterials can assist drugs in targeting disease sites, enriching drugs at lesion sites, and increasing drug efficacy while reducing side effects (Table 1). Macrophage inflammatory chemotaxis capability can endow nanocomposites with a targeted ability to inflammation sites, increasing drug concentrations at inflammatory sites. Based on this, Meiyu Bao et al. utilized macrophage membranes to encapsulate coupled complexes of polydopamine nanoparticles with mouse cathelicidin-related antimicrobial peptide(mCRAMP), thereby conferring their inflammation-targeting ability. Oral administration of the nanocomplexes significantly reduced colonic inflammation and positively regulated the intestinal microbiota in a mouse model of colitis (Figure 4A) [35]. The PEGylated poly (α lipoic acid) (PEG-PALA) copolymer nanoparticles can achieve antibiotic-targeted delivery in response to hydrogen sulfide released by *Salmonella*, promoting targeted therapy for *Salmonella* infection (Figure 4B). This nanomaterial not only reduces Salmonella colonization in the body but also significantly maintains gut microbial homeostasis [36]. As shown in the figure, in the SGF and SIF, the release of ciprofloxacin (CIP) is low, whereas the addition of NaS significantly promotes the release of CIP and the amount and rate of CIP release increase with increasing concentrations of added NaS (Figure 4D). Meanwhile, the authors treated *Salmonella Typhimurium ATCC 14028, Escherichia Coli ATCC 25922, Klebsiella Pneumoniae ATCC 700603*, and *Enterobacter Cloacae ATCC 13047* in vitro with free CIP and PEG-PALA@CIP, respectively. It was found that PEG-PALA@CIP showed a stronger inhibitory effect on *S. typhimurium ATCC 14028*, which can produce H_2S, than the other bacteria (Figure 4E) [36]. Iron-based ions such as Fe@Fe_3O_4 nanoparticles' self-liver targeting function can assist nanodrugs in targeting liver cancer treatment. Zhigang Ren et al. developed a liver cancer-targeted therapeutic nanomedicine using the coupling of Fe@Fe_3O_4 and ginsenoside Rg3, which can inhibit the development and metastasis of hepatocellular carcinoma by remodeling the imbalanced intestinal microbiota [37]. pH-responsive materials such as rhamnolipid can endow nanomaterials with a colon-targeting ability. Based on this property, Yuxuan Xia et al. developed rhamnolipid (RL)/fullerene (C_{60}) nanocomposites with a colon-targeting ability, which significantly alleviated the inflammation in a mouse model of colitis while restoring the intestinal microbes to near-normal levels in mice [21]. Xiaochen Su et al. developed a highly cross-linked polyphosphazene nanodrug that not only enhanced the bioavailability of polyphenolic substances like curcumin but also achieved targeted release of curcumin for inflammation, alleviating acute lung injury [38]. Oral silicon hydrogen nanoparticles can be adsorbed onto the inflamed epithelium of the colon by electrostatic action to target the site of colonic inflammation and alleviate inflammatory bowel disease by scavenging reactive oxygen species (ROS) at the site of the lesion as well as positively regulating the intestinal microbiota (Figure 4C) [39].

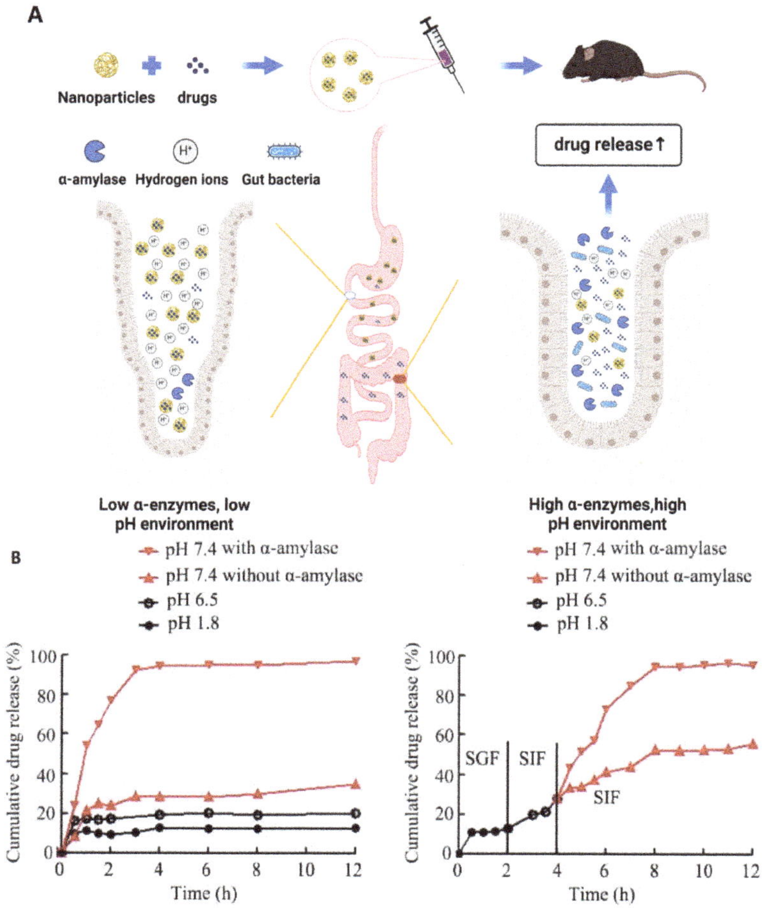

Figure 3. (**A**) Schematic representation of nanomaterial-controlled drug release. (created with bioRender.com) (**B**) pH-dependent and enzyme-responsive drug release curves of CD-Cur-CAMP (an enzyme-triggered controlled-release system with curcumin-cyclodextrin (CD-Cur) complexes as the core and low-molecular-weight chitosan and unsaturated alginate nanoparticles (CANP) as shells) in vitro. Adapted with permission from ref. [32]. Copyright 2021 Informa Healthcare.

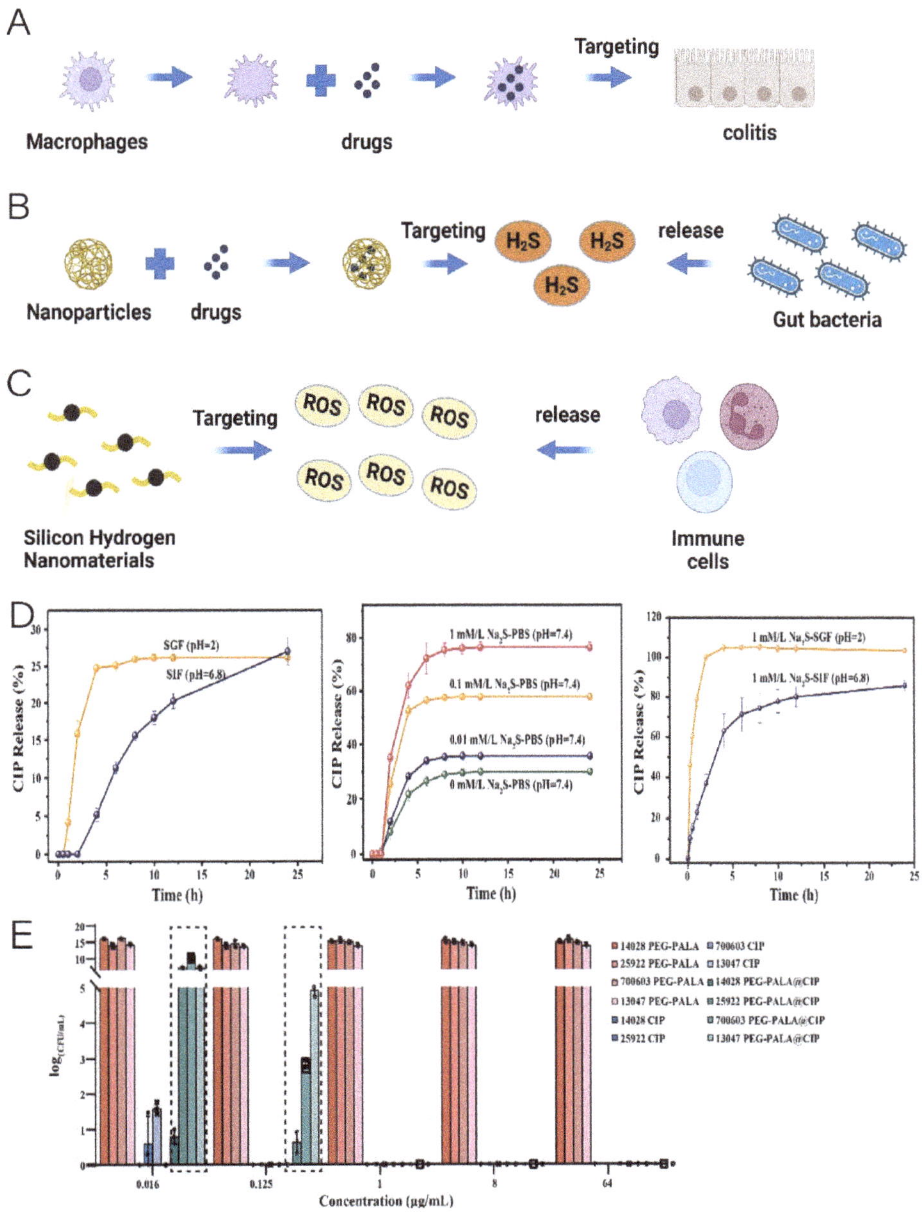

Figure 4. (**A**) Schematic representation of macrophage membrane-assisted drug targeting in colitis. (**B**) Schematic representation of nanomaterial targeting of H_2S released by intestinal bacteria. (**C**) Schematic representation of silicon-based nanomaterial targeting of ROS released by immune cells. (created with bioRender.com) (**D**) Time-dependent release curves of ciprofloxacin under different conditions (CIP: ciprofloxacin, SGF: stimulated gastric fluid, SIF: stimulated intestinal fluid). (**E**) Bactericidal effect of encapsulated ciprofloxacin and free ciprofloxacin under different conditions (PEG-PALA: PEGylated poly (α lipoic acid), PEG-PALA@CIP: PEG-PALA nanoparticles encapsulated with ciprofloxacin). Adapted with permission from ref. [36]. Copyright 2022 Elsevier.

Table 1. Summary of strategies for nanomaterials as carriers to assist in drug modulation of intestinal microbiota.

Target	Material	Drugs	Therapeutic Effects	References
Sustained release	Nanoparticles based on Hohenbuehelia serotina polysaccharides and mucin	Polyphenols from *Malus baccata* (Linn.) Borkh	1. Improve and maintain intestinal health 2. Optimizing the composition of gut microbiota.	[24]
	Self-assembled starch nanoparticles derived from quinoa, maize, and waxy maize starches	Chrysin and rutin (natural polyphenols)	1. Sustain the release of natural polyphenols 2. Antioxidant activity	[26]
	Nanoparticles based on bovine serum albumin and Hohenbuehelia serotina polysaccharides	Polyphenols isolated from the shells of *Juglans regia* L.	1. Modulate the composition of gut microbiota 2. Promote the production of short-chain fatty acids	[27]
	Nanostructured lipid carriers and nanostructured lipid carriers imbedded microcapsule	6-gingerol (polyphenols)	1. Antioxidant 2. Anti-inflammatory 3. Modulate the composition of gut microbiota 4. Promote the intestinal barrier function	[28]
	A bioadhesive liquid coacervate based on bidentate hydrogen bonding-driven nanoparticle assembly	A water-soluble sodium phosphate salt of dexamethasone	1. Significantly mitigate the symptoms of inflammatory bowel disease 2. Restore the diversity of gut microbiota 3. Reduce systemic drug exposure 4. Improve the therapeutic efficacy	[29]
Controlled release	Low molecular weight chitosan and unsaturated alginate resulting nanoparticles	Curcumin–cyclodextrin inclusion complex	1. Promote colonic epithelial barrier integrity 2. Modulate the production of inflammatory cytokines 3. Reshape the gut microbiota	[32]
	A novel nitroreductase labile peptidic hydrogel based on supramolecular self-assembly	*Escherichia coli* Nissle 1917 (probiotic)	1. Downregulate proinflammatory cytokines 2. Repair the intestinal barrier 3. Increase the diversity and abundance of indigenous probiotics	[34]
Targeted delivery	Encapsulation of nanocomplexes formed by the coupling of polydopamine nanoparticles with mCRAMP (mouse cathelicidin-related antimicrobial peptide) using macrophage membrane	mCRAMP (an antimicrobial peptide)	1. Reduce the secretion of pro-inflammatory cytokines 2. Elevate the expression of anti-inflammatory cytokine 3. Positive regulation of intestinal microbiota	[35]
	The PEGylated poly (α lipoic acid) (PEG-PALA) copolymer nanoparticles	Ciprofloxacin	1. Reduce the *Salmonella* colonization 2. Prolong ciprofloxacin persistence in the intestine 3. Keep the gut microbiota homeostasis	[36]

Table 1. *Cont.*

Target	Material	Drugs	Therapeutic Effects	References
Targeted delivery	$Fe@Fe_3O_4$ nanoparticles	Ginsenoside Rg3	1. Significantly inhibit hepatocellular carcinoma (HCC) development and eliminate HCC metastasis to the lung 2. Correct tumor-dominant metabolomics 3. Regulate the composition of the intestinal microbiota	[37]
	Rhamnolipid	Fullerene	1. Promote the colonization of intestinal probiotics 2. Suppress the biofilm formation of pathogenic bacteria 3. Improve the organismal immune system	[21]
	Highly cross-linked polyphosphazene nanodrug developed by copolymerisation of curcumin and acid-sensitive units (4-hydroxy-benzoic acid (4-hydroxy-benzylidene)-hydrazide) with hexachlorotripolyphosph-onitrile	Curcumin	Downregulate several critical inflammatory cytokines (TNF-α, IL-1β, and IL-8)	[38]

2.4. Protective Effect of Nanomaterials on Gut Microbiota

It is well known that the targeted use of antibiotics to inhibit the proliferation of harmful bacteria in the gut is an important means of maintaining intestinal health. However, the use of antibiotics is not conducive to maintaining the balance of gut microbiota and can increase the formation and selection of antibiotic-resistant bacteria [40]. The use of nanomaterials can prevent disruption of the gut microbiota by antibiotics (Figure 5A). Positively charged polymeric nanoparticles with a glucosylated surface carrying antibiotics can improve the utilization of antibiotics in the small intestine, prevent antibiotics from contacting the gut microbiota, and thus maintain the stability of the gut microbiota [41]. Microbial infiltration in tumors is related to the development and treatment of tumors. Self-assembly of an amphiphilic small molecule, metronidazole-fluorouracil into nanomaterials can target tumors, not only killing bacteria in tumors but also preventing disruption of intestinal microbiota by antibiotics [42]. Chunxiao Gao et al. collected feces from treated mice with colorectal cancer and conducted 16S rDNA sequencing. The results of Shannon, Ace, Sobs, Chao, and Simpson indices were analyzed as shown in Figure 5B. The community diversity and abundance of the MTI (metronidazole) group and the MTI and FDU (fluorouridine) co-administration group were significantly lower than that of the control group, whereas there was no significant change in the community diversity and abundance in the MTI–FDU nanomedicine group (Figure 5B). Principal coordinates analysis (PCoA) showed that the difference between the nanomedicine group and the control group was significantly smaller (Figure 5C). The results of community composition analyses showed a significant decrease in bacterial composition changes in the MTI–FDU nanomedicine group (Figure 5D) [42]. Drug-loaded electro-spun nanofibers can carry Streptomycin for delivery to the colon, reducing the risk of resistance and interference with the gut microbiota by antibiotics [22]. Lu Han et al. reported that the PEGylated poly (α lipoic acid) copolymer nanoparticles prolonged the retention time of drugs in the intestine through targeted delivery of antibiotics, thus significantly preventing disruption of intestinal microbiota stability by antibiotics [36].

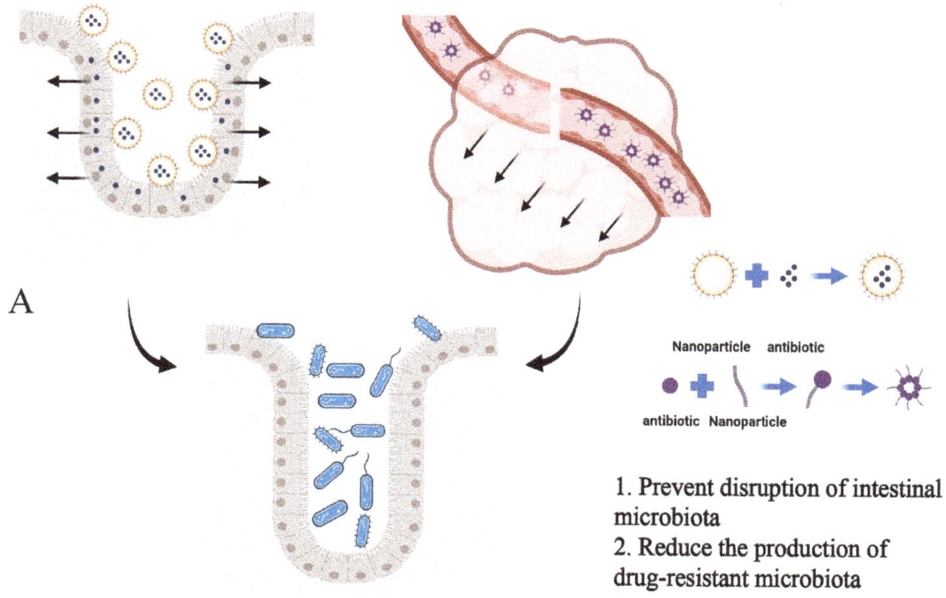

Figure 5. *Cont.*

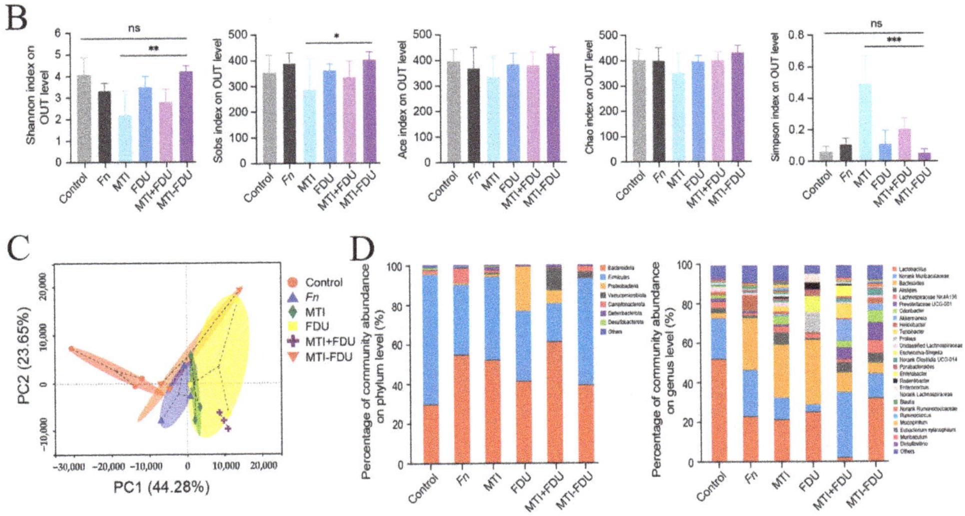

Figure 5. (**A**) Schematic representation of nanomaterials maintaining the stability of intestinal microbiota. (Created with bioRender.com) (**B**) Analysis of alpha diversity coefficients, Shannon index, Sobs index, Ace index, Chao index, and Simpson index of intestinal microbiota through 16S rDNA sequencing (Fn: *Fusobacterium nucleatum*, MTI: metronidazole, FDU: fluorouridine). (**C**) Principal coordinates analysis (PCoA) for beta diversity analysis. (**D**) Stacked bar plots showing the relative abundance of bacterial communities at the phylum and genus levels in samples from mice subjected to different treatments. Adapted with permission from ref. [42]. Copyright 2023 American Chemical Society.

3. Nanomaterials Regulate Intestinal Microbiota

In addition to serving as carriers, some nanomedicines can themselves intervene in disease processes by modulating the gut microbiota (Figure 6A). Yonghyun Lee et al. reported a nanosynthetic drug composed of hyaluronic acid and bilirubin, which enriches the diversity of gut microbiota and significantly increases the abundance of probiotic strains such as *Akkermansia muciniphila* and *Clostridium XIVα*, thereby alleviating inflammatory bowel disease (IBD) [43]. Yonghyun Lee et al. collected treated colitis mice fecal samples and analyzed them by 16s rRNA sequencing. The results of the analyses showed that HABN treatment significantly improved the diversity and composition of the intestinal microbiota of the mice (Figure 6B–D). Further analysis at the phylum/family level showed that HABN (hyaluronic acid-bilirubin nanomedicine) treatment significantly increased the relative abundance of probiotics such as *Akkermansia muciniphila*, *Clostridium XIVα*, and *Lactobacillus* (Figure 6E) [43]. Diwei Zheng et al. developed a biotic–abiotic hybrid nanosystem consisting of bacteriophages covalently linked to dextran nanoparticles encapsulated with irinotecan, which improved chemotherapy for colorectal cancer. This hybrid nanosystem not only inhibits the proliferation of *Enterococcus faecalis* in the gut but also promotes the growth of endogenous butyrate-producing bacteria [44]. Selenium (Se) nanoparticles can decrease the *Firmicutes/Bacteroidetes* ratio and increase the abundance of beneficial bacteria (e.g., *Akkermansia*, *Muribaculaceae*, *Bacteroides*, and *Parabacteroides*), thus protecting against acute toxicity induced by herbicide [45]. Hydrogen nanoparticles synthesized by encapsulating ammonia borane into hollow mesoporous silica nanoparticles can increase the abundance of *Akkermansia muciniphila* and reshape the gut microbiota, thereby improving metabolic disorders associated with fatty liver disease [46]. Rhamnolipid/fullerene-60 nanomaterials can promote the proliferation of probiotic bacteria such as *Lactobacillus*, *Bifidobacterium*, and *Enterococcus* in the gut while inhibiting the formation of biofilms by pathogenic bacteria such as *Escherichia coli* and *Shigella*, thereby alleviating ulcerative colitis [21]. Oral administration of silica-hydrogen nanoparticles can restore gut dysbiosis induced by dextran sulfate sodium (DSS), increasing the relative abundance of the beneficial bacteria *Muribaculaceae* and *Lachnospiraceae_NK4A136_group* while decreasing *Enterobacteriaceae* abundance [39]. Surface-deacetylated chitin nanofibers (SDACNF) can increase the abundance of beneficial bacteria from the genus *Blautia* while reducing the abundance of harmful bacteria from the genera *Morganella* and *Prevotella* in spontaneously hypertensive rats [47].

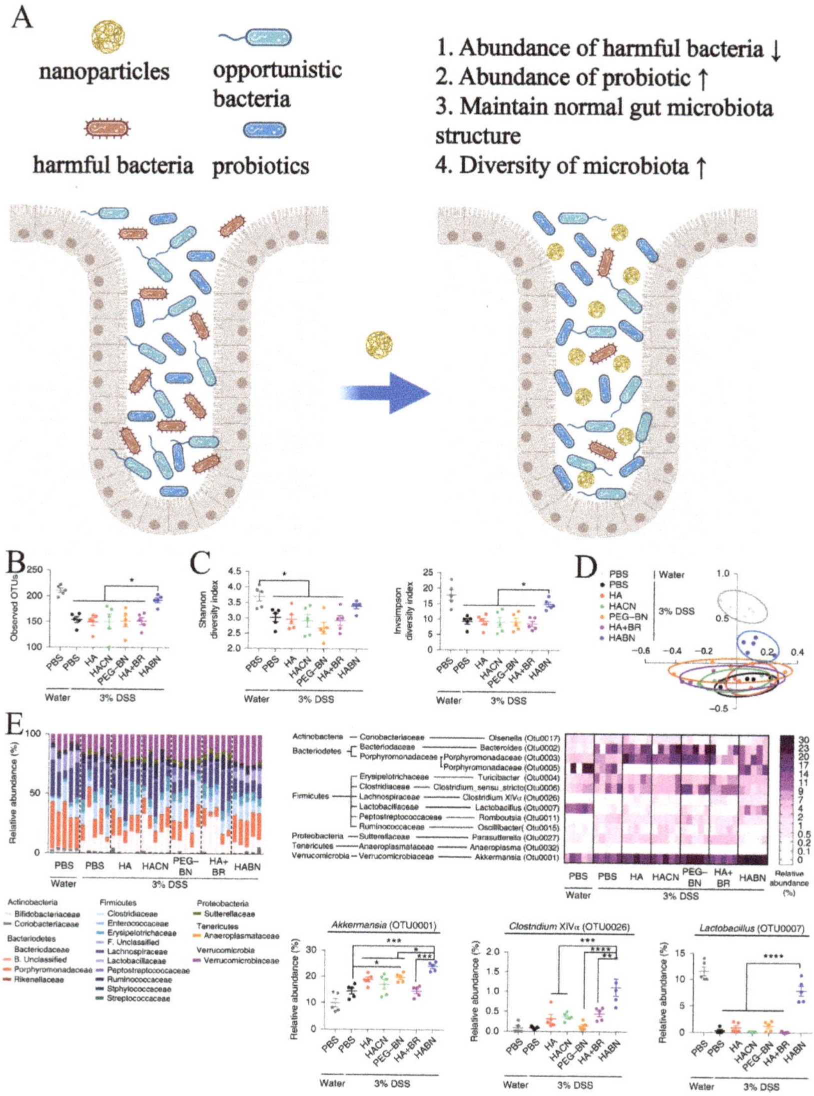

Figure 6. (**A**) Schematic representation of nanomaterials modulating intestinal microbiota (created with bioRender.com). (**B–E**) 16S rRNA sequencing analysis of mouse gut microbiota (HA: Hyaluronic acid, HACN: HA-cholesterol conjugates, PEG-BN: PEGylated bilirubin nanoparticles, HA + BR: HA and bilirubin, HABN: hyaluronic acid-bilirubin nanomedicine). (**B**) Abundance of operational taxonomic units (OTUs) in microbial communities. (**C**) Estimation of alpha diversity. (**D**) Beta diversity of gut microbiota. (**E**) Relative abundance of gut microbiota. Adapted from ref. [43] Copyright 2019 Nature Publishing Group. * $p < 0.05$, ** $p < 0.01$, *** $p < 0.001$, **** $p < 0.0001$, analyzed by one-way ANOVA with Tukey's HSD multiple comparison post hoc test.

Furthermore, polyphenols, in addition to acting as drug carriers, can also serve as components of nanomaterials to help regulate the gut microbiota. Polyphenols, proteins, and nucleic acids have self-assembly capabilities. Bing Hu et al. assembled proteins into flexible biocolloids, and amyloid fibrils with high aspect ratios, which support the deposition of polyphenols and self-assemble with polyphenols into hybrid nanofibers. These hybrid nanofibers ultimately form functional macroscopic hydrogels. This hydrogel enhances the stability of polyphenols and, when orally administered, can remain in the colon, where the gut microbiota is most abundant, promoting intestinal barrier function, modulating the composition of gut microbiota, and alleviating metabolic disorders associated with colitis [48]. Resveratrol is a polyphenol. The resveratrol-selenium-peptide nanocomposite can regulate the dysbiosis of gut microbiota induced by Alzheimer's disease, particularly oxidative stress and inflammation-related bacteria [49]. Artificial probiotics constructed by Jiaqi Xu et al. can increase the diversity of gut microbiota and regulate the microbial spectrum of the gut, thereby correcting dysbiosis in a colitis model [50]. Nanoparticles self-assembled from berberine and baicalin, traditional Chinese medicines, can reduce the abundance of *Bacteroidia, Deferribacteres, Verrucomicrobia, Candidatus_Saccharibacteria,* and *Cyanobacteria* in the gut of a diarrhea-predominant irritable bowel syndrome model [51].

Exosomes are natural nanovesicles secreted by cells, plants, and microorganisms, containing small molecules that contribute to human health maintenance. Exosomes derived from *Portulaca oleracea L* can promote the growth of *Lactobacillus reuteri* in the gut of dextran sulfate sodium (DSS)-induced colitis mice models [52]. Extracellular vesicles derived from *Clostridium butyricum* can significantly reduce the abundance of pathogenic bacteria such as *Escherichia coli* and *Shigella flexneri,* thereby alleviating ulcerative colitis in mice [53]. Pectins and modified pectins derived from marine microalgae and Spirulina maxima can increase the abundance of *Bacteroidetes* in the gut while reducing the abundance of *Firmicutes* [54].

4. The Dual-Edged Sword Effect of Nanomaterials on Gut Microbiota

Nanomaterials, due to their numerous advantages, have been increasingly utilized in various fields. However, with the growing exposure of nanomaterials in the living environment, scholars have become aware that nanomaterials are not flawless, particularly in their disruption of the human gut microbiota (Figure 7A). Exposure to graphene materials can significantly alter the human gut microbiota and disrupted gut microbiota, unfavorable for maintaining intestinal homeostasis, can further lead to adverse conditions [55]. Microplastics or nanoplastics are present in food and food packaging and are often ingested by humans through ingestion or inhalation. In mouse models, ingestion of microplastics or nanoplastics can lead to gut dysbiosis and immune imbalance. Although evidence of their toxicity in humans is currently lacking, we should remain vigilant about their potential risks to human health [56]. Studies have shown that nanoplastic ingestion can lead to gut microbiota and metabolic disorders, resulting in neurotoxicity via the gut–brain axis [57]. Furthermore, anxiety-like behaviors induced in mice by nanoplastic and microplastic exposure are also associated with gut microbiota dysbiosis [58]. To verify this finding, Xuebing Chen et al. exposed mice to PS-NPs (polystyrene nanoparticles) and PS-MPs (polystyrene microparticles) for 30 and 60 days and then performed open field tests (OFTs) and elevated plus maze tests (EPMs). The results showed that the PS-NPs and PS-MPs groups exhibited increased anxiety behavior compared to the control group (Figure 7B,C) [58].

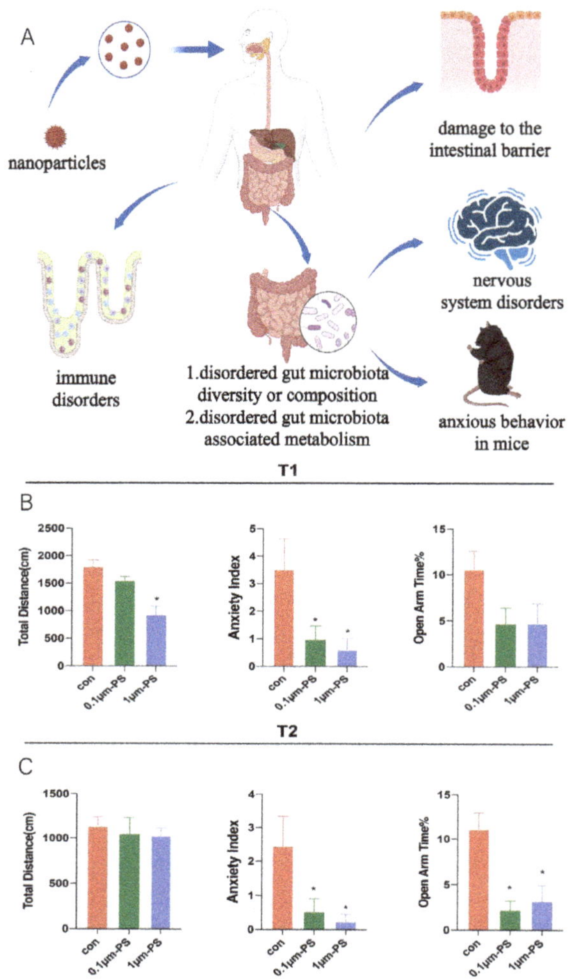

Figure 7. (**A**) Schematic representation of nanomaterials disrupting intestinal microbiota leading to disease (created with bioRender.com). (**B**,**C**) PS-MPs and PS-NPs induced anxiety in the adult mice (PS-MPs: polystyrene-microplastics, PS-NPs: polystyrene-nanoplastics). (**B**) Open field test (OFT) and elevated plus maze test (EPM) results for 30 days. (**C**) OFT and EPM results for 60 days. Adapted from ref. [58]. Copyright 2023 Academic Press Inc. Elsevier Science. * indicates a significant difference among the three groups (* $p < 0.05$).

Engineered nanomaterials, such as titanium dioxide (TiO_2), silver (Ag), zinc oxide, and silica nanoparticles, are increasingly used in food and food packaging. Ingestion of nanomaterials entering the gut through accidental ingestion causes disruption of the gut microbiota, inhibition of probiotic proliferation, and alteration of the *Firmicutes/Bacteroidetes* ratio [59–61]. Robert Landsiedel et al. demonstrated that oral administration of silver nanoparticles significantly reduced the abundance of *Akkermansia* (a probiotic) in the gut and plasma levels of indole-3-acetic acid derived from gut microbes [62]. Moreover, when the gut microbiota composition is already compromised, such as by antibiotic use, it further exacerbates the intestinal damage caused by silver nanoparticles [63]. Exposure to zinc oxide nanoparticles reduces the abundance and diversity of intestinal microbiota and the ratio of probiotic to pathogenic bacteria [64]. Ingestion of food-grade titanium dioxide by young mice leads to dynamic changes in the gut microbiota (including the abundance of *Bacteroidetes, Lactobacillus, Bifidobacterium,* and *Prevotella*), which is one of the important reasons for titanium-dioxide-induced gut toxicity [65]. Only minor effects on the intestinal microbiota were observed with short-term (48 h) exposure to TiO_2 nanoparticles; however, toxic effects on the intestinal microbiota were clearly observed with prolonged (28 days) exposure to TiO_2 nanoparticles, such as an increase in the abundance of *Actinobacteria* and *Proteobacteria* as well as a decrease in the proportions of *Bacteroidetes* and *Firmicutes* [66]. NanoAl_2O_3 disrupts the gut microbiota in a colon simulator, reduces microbial metabolism, and increases pathways related to human gut microbiota and disease [67]. Dalel Askri et al. showed that oral administration of iron oxide nanoparticles did not affect the overall health of the animals, but showed a decrease in the relative weights of organs such as the brain, kidneys, lungs, and stomach, which may reflect the potential toxicity of iron oxide nanoparticles to humans [68].

Carbon nanotubes are novel nanomaterial that may induce immune toxicity. Inhalation of carbon nanotubes disrupts the composition of gut microbiota, increases the *Firmicutes/Bacteroidetes* ratio, and promotes inflammation. Exposure to both carbon nanotubes and cigarette smoke exhibits an additive effect on disrupting gut microbiota and promoting inflammation [69]. Furthermore, it has been shown that repeated exposure to multiwalled carbon nanotubes does not cause changes in the intestinal microbiota of mice [70]. On the contrary, multi-walled carbon nanotubes exacerbated the doxorubicin-induced changes in the intestinal microbiota [71]. High-dose injection of biomimetic mesoporous polydopamine nanoparticles disrupts gut microbiota, immune balance, and oxidative stress damage [72]. Poly(lactic-co-glycolic acid) (PLGA) nanoparticles used for scaffold implants can induce cecal acidification, reduce *Firmicutes* and *Bacteroidetes*, and disrupt microbial composition [73]. Ingestion of nanoparticles of polyethylene terephthalate (PET) also disturbs gut microbiota and intestinal metabolism [74]. Careful selection of nanomaterials and greater use of low-toxic or non-toxic nanomedicines can greatly advance the application of nanotechnology in regulating gut microbiota.

5. Nanomaterials Treat Diseases by Regulating the Intestinal Microbiota

5.1. Gastrointestinal Tract

5.1.1. Immune Diseases

Inflammatory bowel disease (IBD) refers to a group of nonspecific chronic gastrointestinal inflammatory diseases of unknown etiology, including ulcerative colitis, Crohn's disease, and indeterminate colitis. The incidence and prevalence of IBD are rapidly increasing worldwide, particularly in emerging industrialized regions such as East Asia [75]. Among these, East Asia has experienced the largest increase in disease burden, with the highest incidence of IBD occurring in the 30–34 age group and the peak prevalence in the 45–49 age group [76]. Additionally, in most countries worldwide, the incidence and prevalence of IBD in children continue to rise [77]. IBD is commonly associated with genetic susceptibility, impaired intestinal barrier function, dysbiosis of gut microbiota, and immune dysregulation (Figure 8) [78]. The combination of these factors contributes to the occurrence of IBD, although none of them individually are sufficient to cause colitis. IBD is a lifelong inflammatory disease, necessitating long-term medication to prevent disease progression [78]. The primary treatment for IBD is medication, with current conventional therapies including anti-tumor necrosis factor agents, 5-aminosalicylic acid (5-ASA), corticosteroids, and immunomodulators. Other medications include some novel small molecule drugs and biologics, such as selective Janus kinase inhibitors, PDE4 inhibitors, and IL-12/IL-23 inhibitors [79].

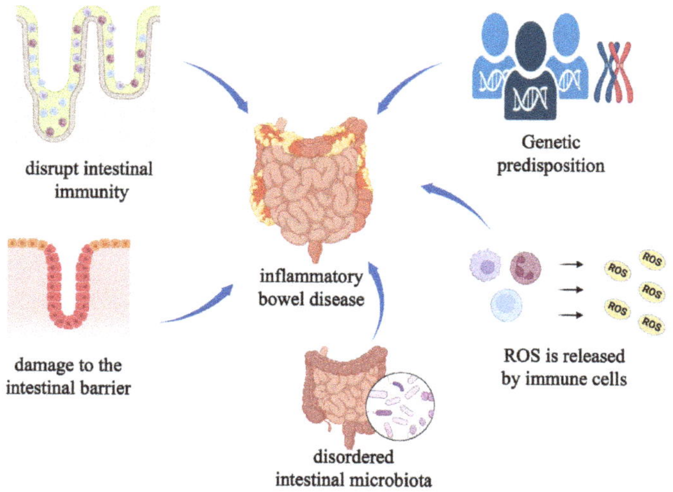

Figure 8. Schematic representation of factors associated with inflammatory bowel disease. (created with bioRender.com).

Although there is a lack of corresponding research results to demonstrate the causality between disrupted gut microbiota composition and IBD, there is indeed a correlation between the two [80]. Patients with IBD often exhibit changes in gut microbiota, including reduced microbial diversity, decreased stability of microbial composition, decreased abundance of *Firmicutes*, and proliferation of *Proteobacteria* [81]. Current research on gut microbiota mainly comes from the analysis of microbial changes in feces. Dari Shalon et al. developed an ingestible device that can sample from different parts of the intestine. They used this device to collect intestinal samples from healthy individuals for multi-omics analysis, demonstrating significant differences in bacteria, phages, host proteins, and metabolism between the intestine and feces [82]. However, studies have also shown that there are changes in microbial communities in the mucosa of the intestines with and without inflammation in the same IBD patients, as well as in mucosal biopsies of CD (Crohn's disease) patients with and without damage [80]. In summary, there is a close relationship between IBD and dysbiosis of gut microbiota, and rebuilding the homeostasis of gut microbiota is a new strategy for alleviating IBD. New methods such as fecal microbiota transplantation, antibiotics, probiotics, and microbial metabolite inhibitors have been proposed. However, these treatments either have side effects or cannot achieve complete clinical relief when used alone [83].

One major challenge in the treatment of gastrointestinal inflammatory diseases is how to make drugs remain in the intestine for a long time to exert their therapeutic effects. The effective application of specific nanomaterials has overcome this challenge, and oral intervention with nanomaterials to modulate gut microbiota and alleviate IBD may have become a new treatment modality. Pengchao Zhao et al. reported a hydrogen-bond-driven nanoparticle-assembled bio-adhesive liquid coacervate, which exhibited significant structural stability and prolonged release of preloaded water-soluble small molecules for over two days. Compared to simple oral administration, orally administered drug-loaded nanoparticles significantly restored microbial diversity and alleviated symptoms of IBD [29]. Similarly, the use of nanomaterials has also greatly facilitated the use of polyphenols to intervene in IBD because nanomaterials significantly enhance the utilization of polyphenolic substances in the intestine. Wenni Tian et al. developed a 6-gingerol-loaded delivery system in the form of nanostructured lipid carriers (NLCs) or NLC-imbedded microcapsules (6G-MCs). 6G-NLCs alleviate colitis by modulating the *Firmicutes/Bacteroidetes* ratio, while

6G-MCs continuously release near the colonic lesion site and treat colitis by maintaining gut microbiota composition and diversity [28].

Furthermore, metabolic products of inflammatory cells such as ROS can damage intestinal cells and reduce their antioxidant capacity, which is also associated with the formation of IBD [21]. Yuxuan Xia et al. reported a therapeutic strategy for colitis using orally administered low-dose rhamnolipid (RL)/fullerene (C_{60}) nanocomposite materials. The significant pH responsiveness endowed this material with excellent colon-targeting ability. The ROS scavenging ability of the C_{60} component effectively restored the anti-inflammatory capacity of colonic cells. Additionally, low-dose oral (RL)/C_{60} exhibited a remarkable ability to reconstruct the abnormal gut microbiota composition in colitic mice [21]. Similarly, Meiyu Bao et al. conjugated polydopamine nanoparticles with the antimicrobial peptide mCRAMP and encapsulated them with macrophage membranes to design a ROS-clearing and inflammation-targeting nanomedicine. This medicine not only regulated the gut microbiota of IBD patients and improved inflammatory responses but also demonstrated significant targeting effects in local inflammatory tissues due to macrophage membrane encapsulation [35]. Other studies have shown that clearing ROS can effectively improve intestinal inflammation in IBD. Importantly, ROS-targeting materials endowed nanocompounds with excellent lesion-targeting abilities, allowing drugs to accumulate at the lesion site [39,84–86]. Additionally, reactive nitrogen species produced in active mucosa can damage intestinal mucosa and barriers, accelerating the occurrence of IBD. Modified bismuth selenide polyvinylpyrrolidone (PVP) nanosheets, a multifunctional nanozyme based on 2D nanomaterials, can alleviate intestinal inflammation by clearing various reactive oxygen and nitrogen species [87].

By using probiotics, prebiotics can easily alter the structural composition of gut microbiota. Using nanomaterials to deliver probiotic products for disease treatment can not only enhance the activity and viability of probiotics reaching the target site but also promote targeted delivery of probiotics. Therefore, incorporating prebiotics or probiotics into nanomaterials has become a new treatment strategy for diseases [88–90]. Abdullah Glil Alkushi et al. combined dietary nanosupplements with *Bacillus* strains to intervene in colitis models, and their results showed that compared to free Bacillus spores, nanomaterial-loaded *Bacillus* significantly improved the therapeutic effect on colitis [90]. To further explore the feasibility of nanomaterial-combined probiotic strategies, Abdullah Glil Alkushi et al. integrated multispecies probiotics into nanomaterials and applied them to colitis model mice, ultimately demonstrating a better therapeutic effect on colitis than free multispecies probiotics [89]. Similarly, polydopamine nanoparticles can also encapsulate probiotics, which, when administered orally, can regulate gut microbiota and alleviate colitis [91]. Additionally, probiotic membranes are also promising nanomaterials. Jiaqi Xu et al. constructed artificial probiotics by using *Escherichia coli Nissle 1917* membrane (EM) as the surface and the biodegradable diselenide-bridged mesoporous silica nanoparticles bridged by disulfides (SeM) as the core. This nanomedicine can regulate the oxidative stress and inflammatory balance in the intestines of IBD mice, increase gut microbiota diversity, and modulate microbial spectrum [50].

Extracellular vesicles (EVs) are double-layered vesicular nanoparticles with a size ranging from 20 to 300 nm, encapsulating exosomes and micro vesicles, containing various small molecules, including proteins, lipids, and nucleic acids [53,92,93]. Human cells can secrete EVs, which can be extracted from various human body fluids, such as serum, urine, and cerebrospinal fluid. Additionally, the gut microbiota in humans and plants can also produce EVs [53,93,94]. EVs from various sources participate in the interaction and communication between intestinal epithelial cells, immune cells, and gut microbiota, thereby regulating intestinal inflammation and homeostasis (Figure 9A) [94]. EVs from different sources can affect the progression of IBD to some extent through different mechanisms. *Clostridium butyricum* has been shown to have a protective effect on intestinal inflammation. Research by Lingyan Ma et al. further demonstrated that the EVs secreted by these probiotics utilize the contained microRNA to inhibit inflammatory signaling pathways in the intestine. Additionally, these EVs can repair the dysbiosis caused by IBD, reduce the abundance of bacterial pathogens, and regulate tryptophan metabolism [53]. EVs secreted by other probiotics can also alleviate IBD. For example, EVs secreted by *Lactobacillus plantarum Q7* can alleviate IBD by modulating gut microbiota [95]. EVs derived from the symbiotic bacterium *F. prausnitzii* can alleviate IBD by regulating intestinal barrier function and immune function [96]. EVs derived from *Bacteroides thetaiotaomicron* can affect intestinal immune cells through different targets in healthy individuals and IBD patients [97]. Furthermore, EVs secreted by human mesenchymal stem cells can inhibit lipid peroxidation and iron death by targeting acyl-CoA synthetase long-chain family member 4 (ACSL4) and *miR-129-5p*, reducing intestinal inflammatory damage [98]. *Turmeric*-derived nanoparticles can inhibit intestinal inflammation, repair colonic damage, and possess colon-targeting ability to prevent and alleviate colitis [99]. An attenuation of DSS-induced inflammatory signaling in colitis was clearly observed after turmeric-derived nanoparticles ($TDNP_S2$) intervention in mice, as shown by the results of chemiluminescent imaging (Figure 9B). In addition, MPO (myeloperoxidase) levels and expression of inflammatory factors, such as TNF-α, IL-6, and IL-1β, were reduced in colonic tissues, whereas the expression of oxidative stress-related protein HO-1 (heme oxygenase-1) was elevated. All these results showed the alleviating effect of $TDNP_S2$ on colitis in mice (Figure 9C) [99]. Oral administration of edible mulberry bark-derived nanoparticles can activate the aryl hydrocarbon receptor/Constitutive Photomorphogenic Homolog Subunit 8 (AhR/COPS8) pathway mediated by plant heat shock protein heat shock protein family A (Hsp70) member 8 (HSPA8) to prevent DSS-induced colitis and promote the repair of intestinal microbiota composition [100]. Exosomes derived from *Portulaca oleracea L* can alleviate DSS-induced mouse models by reprogramming CD4+ T cells into CD4CD8 double-positive T cells, increasing levels of intestinal probiotics and indole derivatives [52]. In summary, EVs from different sources, including effector molecules, can affect the progression of IBD. Their protective ability, targeting ability, and low toxicity make them a natural nanocarrier, and EVs are more advantageous than other nanomaterials in terms of high yield and easy extraction [94,99]. More importantly, this natural nanocarrier has made oral nucleic acid therapy a reality. Yunyue Zhang et al. applied EVs carrying anti-TNF-α siRNA to an IBD rat model, significantly alleviating intestinal inflammation in the rat model [101]. In addition to carrying nucleic acids, EVs can also carry protein substances such as interleukin 10 and interleukin 27, which can be used to alleviate intestinal inflammation in IBD models [102,103]. Furthermore, Jiawei Guo et al. used exosomes inserted with Golgi Glycoprotein 1 to carry Wnt agonist 1. After injecting them into IBD mice, due to the targeting effect of Golgi Glycoprotein 1, this nanocomposite successfully accumulated in the bones and successfully alleviated bone loss in the IBD mouse model by upregulating the Wnt/β-catenin pathway in bone marrow mesenchymal stem cells [104].

In addition to the above, nanocomposites formed by aggregation of hyaluronic acid and bilirubin can increase the overall richness and diversity of gut microbiota in IBD mice and significantly promote the proliferation of *Akkermansia muciniphila* and *Clostridium XIVα* [43]. Yu Xu et al. reported pH- and redox-responsive Angelica sinensis polysaccharide nanoparticles, which significantly improved the stability of intestinal microbiota and the level of short-chain fatty acids in ulcerative colitis (UC) mice. The dual responsiveness endowed them with excellent colon-targeting ability, increasing their concentration at inflammatory sites [105]. Yaping Liu et al. developed an oral radioprotector, ergothioneine hyaluronate gel, which can prevent radiation-induced gastrointestinal syndrome by regulating oxidative stress, inflammation, and gut microbiota [106]. Novel nanoparticles self-assembled from denatured human serum albumin and selenite salts can alleviate cisplatin-induced intestinal mucositis by restoring anti-inflammatory bacteria and reducing pro-inflammatory bacteria [107].

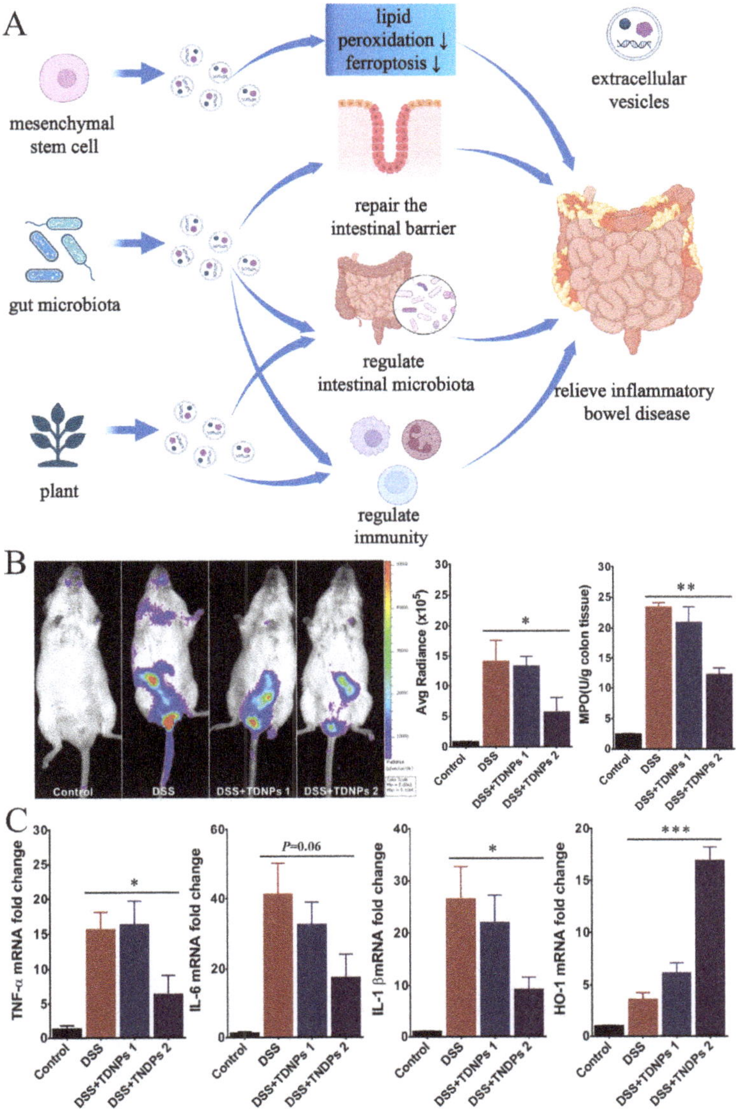

Figure 9. (**A**) Schematic representation of intervention of inflammatory bowel disease by extracellular vesicles from different sources. (created with bioRender.com) (**B**) Colon inflammation was monitored by XenoLight RediJect inflammation probe via chemiluminescence imaging (DSS: dextran sulfate sodium, TDNP: turmeric-derived nanoparticles, band 1 from the sucrose gradient interfaces of 8/30% was named TNDPs 1, and band 2 from the sucrose gradient interfaces of 30/45% was named TNDPs 2). (**C**) Real-time PCR to quantify miRNA. Adapted from ref. [99] Copyright 2022 BioMed Central Ltd. * $p < 0.05$, ** $p < 0.01$, *** $p < 0.001$ and ns represent no significant difference.

5.1.2. Cancer

The discovery of the relationship between microbiota and cancer can be traced back thousands of years, and recent studies have delved deeper into the connection between the two [108]. Numerous studies have indicated the close association between gut microbiota and the occurrence, development, diagnosis, and treatment of tumors [109–111]. For instance, *Lactobacillus gallinarum* and *Akkermansia muciniphila* can prevent the occurrence of intestinal tumors, while *Lactobacillus rhamnosus* can enhance the efficacy of anti-tumor therapy [111–113]. Additionally, some metabolites related to gut microbiota contribute to the detection of colorectal cancer [110]. Therefore, modulating the gut microbiota has emerged as a novel strategy to improve cancer treatment outcomes. For example, Pien Tze Huang can prevent colorectal cancer by regulating the gut microbiota and metabolites [114]. Ginseng polysaccharides can enhance the efficacy of anti-tumor therapy by modulating the gut microbiota and tryptophan metabolism [115]. At the same time, nanomaterials serve as excellent media for modulating the gut microbiota, and their good intervention ability in the gut microbiota can significantly improve cancer treatment outcomes (Figure 10A) [116]. Utilizing a bio-inorganic hybrid system formed by bacteriophage and dextran nanoparticles to carry irinotecan can enhance the efficacy of first-line chemotherapy for colorectal cancer by modulating the proliferation of harmful bacteria and probiotics in the intestine, thus reducing the side effects of chemotherapy [44]. Tianqun Lang et al. constructed nanoparticles using a prebiotic xylan–stearic acid conjugate, which not only increases the intra-tumoral drug concentration by encapsulating capecitabine but also enhances chemotherapy efficacy by promoting probiotic proliferation and short-chain fatty acid production [117]. Qunlang Tian et al. performed in vivo bioluminescence imaging using an in vivo imaging system (IVIS) to demonstrate tumor formation in treated mice (Figure 10B). The results of variation in relative tumor volumes calculated according to the amount of photons showed that applying SCXN (a Cap-loaded nanoparticle using the prebiotic xylan–stearic acid conjugate) to colorectal cancer mice had a higher rate of tumor suppression compared to other groups (Figure 10C) [117]. Zhigang Ren et al. constructed a nanodrug using $Fe@Fe_3O_4$ coupled with ginsenoside Rg3, which increased the abundance of *Bacteroidetes* and *Verrucomicrobia*, reduced the abundance of *Firmicutes*, and significantly prolonged the survival time of mice with hepatocellular carcinoma [37]. Moreover, electrostatic assembly of silver nanoparticles (AgNP) onto the surface capsid protein of M13 bacteriophage(M13@Ag), which specifically binds to *Fusobacterium nucleatum* (Fn), can achieve specific clearance of Fn and reshape the tumor immune microenvironment. This nanocomplex, when used in combination with immune checkpoint inhibitors (α-PD1) or chemotherapy drugs, can significantly improve the overall survival of mice with primary colorectal cancer [118].

5.1.3. Other Disease

Modulation of intestinal microbiota by orally administered nanomaterials can also be used as a therapeutic strategy for other gastrointestinal disorders. Nanocrystalline cellulose can promote the metabolism of bile acids, fatty acids, and amino acids by improving the composition of the gut microbiota, thereby alleviating constipation [119]. Exosome-like nanoparticles derived from broccoli can alleviate loperamide-induced constipation by restoring gut microbiota dysbiosis and regulating short-chain fatty acid and tryptophan metabolism [120]. Nanoparticles self-assembled from berberine and baicalin, traditional Chinese medicine components, can alleviate diarrhea-predominant irritable bowel syndrome in mice by regulating the composition of the gut microbiota [51]. Nanoparticles formed by gold nanostars and acid-sensitive cis-aconitic anhydride conjugates modified with anti-*Helicobacter pylori* polyclonal antibodies can be used for the diagnosis and treatment of *H. pylori* infection. Treatment doses of oral gold nanostars@H. pylori-antibodies nanoprobes (GNS@Ab) can target and eradicate *Helicobacter pylori* without disrupting the balance of intestinal microbiota [121]. Nanomaterial fullerol can inhibit bacterial translocation and neutrophil infiltration in mice undergoing ischemia-reperfusion, reducing intestinal damage caused by ischemia-reperfusion and delaying or reducing mortality [122]. In a weaned pig model, dietary supplementation with different concentrations of coated nano-zinc oxide (Cnz) can modulate the core composition of fecal bacteria and improve intestinal mucosal barrier function [123]. Low doses of Chitosan nanoparticles–microcin J25 (CNM) significantly increase the weight of mice infected with *Escherichia coli O157:H7* and have beneficial effects on lifespan or clinical symptoms, while significantly improving intestinal health [124]. Green carbon dots derived from Atractylodes macrocephala can effectively alleviate alcohol-induced gastric ulcers by regulating immunity, oxidative stress, gastric enzyme activity, and intestinal microbiota [125].

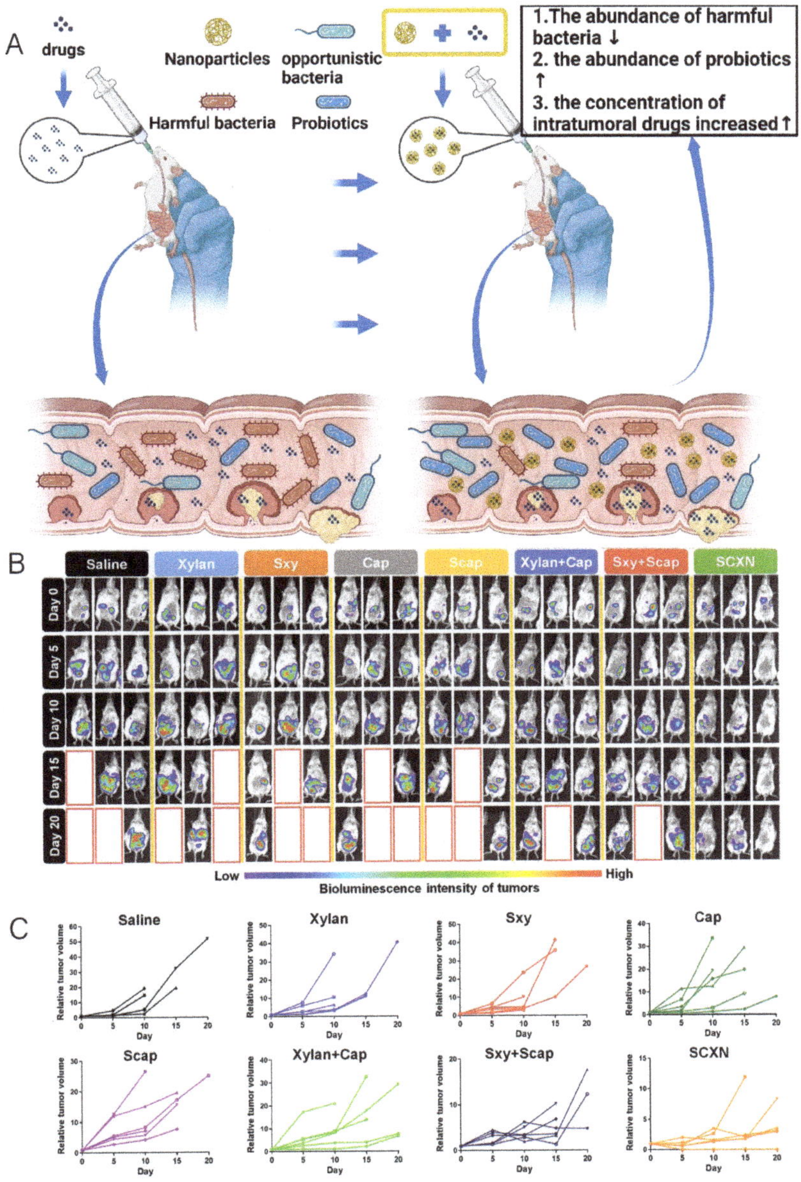

Figure 10. (**A**) Schematic representation of nanomaterial-assisted drug therapy for tumors (created with bioRender.com). (**B**) In vivo bioluminescence imaging using an in vivo imaging system (IVIS) (Cap: Capecitabine, Sxy: amphiphilic derivatives of stearic acid (Sa) and xylan, Scap: amphiphilic derivatives of stearic acid (Sa) and Cap, SCXN: a Cap-loaded nanoparticle using the prebiotic xylan-stearic acid conjugate). (**C**) Change in relative tumor volume calculated based on photon flux during the treatment period. Adapted from ref. [117]. Copyright 2023 Nature Publishing Group.

5.2. Extra-Intestinal Gastrointestinal Tract

5.2.1. Immune-Related Diseases

The interaction between the digestive tract and the intestinal microbiota is essential for maintaining normal function and homeostasis of the gastrointestinal tract. In addition, intestinal bacteria and secretory products can pass through the gastrointestinal tract into the bloodstream to affect various organs of the body. Inflammation of extra-intestinal organs is often accompanied by abnormalities in the intestinal microbiota, so the regulation of the microbiota can to a certain extent alleviate inflammation in other parts of the body outside the gastrointestinal tract. Yuan Li et al. reported that ultrasmall cortex moutan nanoclusters can effectively treat infectious pneumonia and colitis [126]. Polyphenol-containing nanoparticles of curcumin polyphosphonate can treat acute lung injury and improve functional recovery after spinal cord injury [38,127]. Surface-deacetylated chitin nanofibers (SDACNF) can exert hepatoprotective and antioxidative effects by adsorbing lipid substances and regulating gut microbiota [47]. Nel-like Molecule Type 1 Combined with Gold Nanoparticles can treat periodontitis by modulating macrophage polarization and osteoclast activity and improving the periodontal microbiota. However, this medication disrupts the normal composition of the intestinal microbiota [128]. Dietary supplementation of chitosan nanoparticles in the diet can regulate the growth performance and immune status of weaned pigs as well as modulate the ratio of beneficial bacteria to harmful bacteria in the gut [129]. Licong Yang et al. utilized dihydromyricetin-encapsulated selenium nanoparticles to construct dihydromyricetin@ selenium nanoparticles (DMY@SeNPs), and further modified them stepwise with chitosan (CS/DMY@SeNPs) and blood-brain barrier (BBB)-targeting peptide Tg (TGNYKALHPHNG) to obtain Tg-CS/DMY@SeNPs. This nanomaterial can ameliorate neuroinflammation via the gut microbiota-NLRP3(nucleotide-binding oligomerization domain leucine-rich repeat and pyrin domain-containing protein 3) inflammasome-brain axis [130]. Sahar Y. Al-Okbi et al. found that the administration of basil essential oil nanoemulsion (BNO) and its parent basil essential oil (BO) in rats can improve liver lipid and histopathological changes in non-alcoholic fatty liver disease [131]. Obesity can induce chronic inflammation (including neuroinflammation) via the brain–gut axis. Kumaran Sundaram et al. discovered that garlic exosome-like nanoparticles can suppress systemic and cerebral inflammatory activity, and reverse obesity induced by a high-fat diet in mice [132].

5.2.2. Metabolic-Related Diseases

Past studies have shown that the stability of the gut microbiota is likely to be closely related to the metabolic health of the body and that abnormalities in the gut microbiota are likely to be involved in the development of metabolic diseases such as obesity and alcoholic fatty liver disease. Currently, nanomaterials that intervene in the gut microbiota to improve metabolic health are a novel response to metabolic disorders (Figure 11). Amyloid β (Aβ) is a key protein in the pathogenesis of Alzheimer's disease (AD), and the abnormal accumulation of Aβ in brain tissue is one of the important contributors to the development of AD. Resveratrol-selenium-peptide nanocomposites can alleviate Alzheimer's disease in mice by inhibiting β-amyloid aggregation in the hippocampus, exerting antioxidative effects, maintaining neuronal homeostasis, and regulating gut microbiota [49]. Chiral Au nanoparticles can modulate the gut microbiota of Alzheimer's disease model mice, increase indole-3-acetic acid in the intestines, and thus alleviate cognitive impairment in mice [133]. Mesoporous silica nanoparticle-encapsulated *Bifidobacterium* not only can suppress intestinal inflammation and reduce brain Aβ burden but also can enhance olfactory sensitivity in mice [134]. The pathology of Alzheimer's disease (AD) is highly associated with obesity-induced insulin resistance. Licong Yang et al. utilized chitosan (CS) and sodium tripolyphosphate (TPP) to carry low water solubility Res to construct Res-loaded CS/TPP nanoparticles. After oral administration, these nanoparticles can alleviate lipid-deposition-induced insulin resistance, reduce the level of Aβ aggregation, and modulate the gut microbiota to improve cognitive impairment in obesity-related Alzheimer's disease mice [135]. Gold nanospheres can mitigate estrogen deficiency-induced bone loss by regulating gut microbiota homeostasis and reducing trimethylamine-N-oxide (TMAO) metabolism [136]. TMAO is formed by the hepatic conversion of trimethylamine (TMA) derived from nutrient metabolism by intestinal microbiota, and its elevated concentration may lead to serious cardiovascular events [137]. Dietary supplementation with selenium nanoparticles can alleviate acute toxicity induced by diquat via modulating gut microbiota and its metabolism [45]. Zhaokui Jin et al. synthesized hydrogen nanoparticles by encapsulating ammonia borane into hollow mesoporous silica nanoparticles, which continuously release hydrogen gas in the intestine, reshaping gut microbiota and alleviating metabolic dysfunction-associated fatty liver disease [46]. Ginger nanoparticles can prevent insulin resistance in high-fat diet (HFD) mice by restoring the stability of intestinal epithelial *Foxa2*-mediated signaling [138].

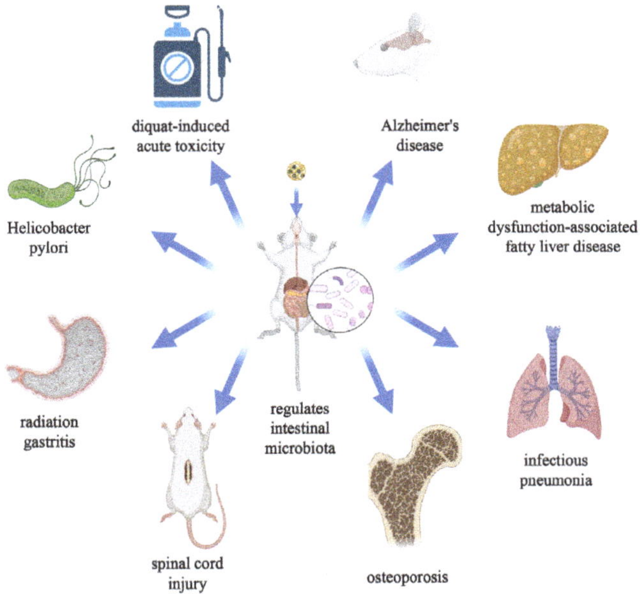

Figure 11. Schematic representation of nanomaterial-mediated alleviation of diseases by modulating gut microbiota. (created with bioRender.com).

6. Discussion and Outlook

As described in this paper, an increasing number of scholars recognize the importance of the gut microbiota in human health. Changes in the gut microbiota not only affect intestinal function but also impact various organs throughout the body through different pathways, such as the gut–brain axis, gut–bone axis, and gut–liver axis [133,136,139]. Treating diseases by influencing the gut microbiota has gradually become a novel therapeutic strategy. Conventional interventions targeting the gut microbiota mainly involve drugs, probiotics and prebiotics, and fecal microbiota transplantation, but these measures often have drawbacks. The use of drugs and probiotics/prebiotics is often limited by the intestinal structure and environment, while fecal microbiota transplantation may lead to many side effects, such as mechanical damage to the intestines, and may not be well accepted by patients. The use of nanotechnology can effectively overcome the shortcomings of microbiota-regulating drugs. Nanomaterials, as carriers, not only protect microbiota-regulating drugs from enzymatic and gastrointestinal degradation but also achieve controlled release and targeted delivery of drugs through responsiveness to pH, reactive oxygen species (ROS), or intestinal enzymes. Additionally, some substances themselves can serve as constituents of nanomaterials, and the resulting nanodrugs often exhibit superior effects compared to their individual components [48]. The combination of nanomaterials with microbiota-regulating drugs can greatly advance the development of gut microbiota-related therapies, such as those for inflammatory bowel disease (IBD), tumors, Alzheimer's disease, etc.

Certainly, there are certain limitations to using nanomaterials to regulate gut microbiota. The biosafety of most existing nanomaterials for in vivo applications remains unclear, which poses significant challenges for the clinical translation of these materials. Meanwhile, we have also noticed that due to the continuous invention of numerous new materials, there is still a lack of research methods and evaluation criteria for the in vivo metabolic behavior of these new materials. When the human body is in a diseased state, it is often the result of various factors, and changes in gut microbiota are typically complex, involving disruptions in microbiota composition, metabolism, and other aspects. However, current research on using nanotechnology to regulate gut microbiota and alleviate diseases often only addresses a partial disruption to achieve the desired therapeutic effect. For example, using nanocarriers to deliver probiotics or antibiotics, or carrying other microbiota-modulating molecules. While such therapeutic strategies can indeed alleviate diseases, combining nanotechnology with multiple treatment methods to comprehensively regulate gut microbiota may achieve better therapeutic outcomes. Therefore, utilizing nanomaterials as a hub and incorporating various microbiota-regulating components as elements to construct nanocomplexes capable of comprehensively modulating gut microbiota for disease treatment may become one of the future research directions. However, compared to the former approach, the latter imposes higher demands on the performance of nanomaterials.

Author Contributions: Writing—original draft preparation, W.L.; review and editing, M.Z., Y.W., Y.C., Z.Z. and S.W.; funding acquisition, S.T. and D.T. All authors have read and agreed to the published version of the manuscript.

Funding: This work is supported by the National Natural Science Foundation of China (22107032, 82270558), and the National Natural Science Foundation of China (81974071).

Conflicts of Interest: The authors declare no conflict of interest.

References

1. Sender, R.; Fuchs, S.; Milo, R. Revised Estimates for the Number of Human and Bacteria Cells in the Body. *PLoS Biol.* **2016**, *14*, e1002533. [CrossRef] [PubMed]
2. Smirnova, D.V.; Zalomova, L.V.; Zagainova, A.V.; Makarov, V.V.; Mezhevikina, L.M.; Fesenko, E.E.; Yudin, S.M. Cryopreservation of the Human Gut Microbiota: Current State and Perspectives. *Int. J. Med. Microbiol.* **2019**, *309*, 259–269. [CrossRef] [PubMed]
3. Brun, P.; Giron, M.C.; Qesari, M.; Porzionato, A.; Caputi, V.; Zoppellaro, C.; Banzato, S.; Grillo, A.R.; Spagnol, L.; De Caro, R.; et al. Toll-Like Receptor 2 Regulates Intestinal Inflammation by Controlling Integrity of the Enteric Nervous System. *Gastroenterology* **2013**, *145*, 1323–1333. [CrossRef] [PubMed]
4. Canfora, E.E.; Meex, R.C.R.; Venema, K.; Blaak, E.E. Gut Microbial Metabolites in Obesity, NAFLD and T2DM. *Nat. Rev. Endocrinol.* **2019**, *15*, 261–273. [CrossRef] [PubMed]
5. Gasaly, N.; De Vos, P.; Hermoso, M.A. Impact of Bacterial Metabolites on Gut Barrier Function and Host Immunity: A Focus on Bacterial Metabolism and Its Relevance for Intestinal Inflammation. *Front. Immunol.* **2021**, *12*, 658354. [CrossRef]
6. Ronan, V.; Yeasin, R.; Claud, E.C. Childhood Development and the Microbiome—The Intestinal Microbiota in Maintenance of Health and Development of Disease During Childhood Development. *Gastroenterology* **2021**, *160*, 495–506. [CrossRef] [PubMed]
7. Boyajian, J.L.; Ghebretatios, M.; Schaly, S.; Islam, P.; Prakash, S. Microbiome and Human Aging: Probiotic and Prebiotic Potentials in Longevity, Skin Health and Cellular Senescence. *Nutrients* **2021**, *13*, 4550. [CrossRef]
8. Zaiss, M.M.; Jones, R.M.; Schett, G.; Pacifici, R. The Gut-Bone Axis: How Bacterial Metabolites Bridge the Distance. *J. Clin. Investig.* **2019**, *129*, 3018–3028. [CrossRef]
9. Shao, T.; Hsu, R.; Rafizadeh, D.L.; Wang, L.; Bowlus, C.L.; Kumar, N.; Mishra, J.; Timilsina, S.; Ridgway, W.M.; Gershwin, M.E.; et al. The Gut Ecosystem and Immune Tolerance. *J. Autoimmun.* **2023**, *141*, 103114. [CrossRef]
10. Hong, M.; Li, Z.; Liu, H.; Zheng, S.; Zhang, F.; Zhu, J.; Shi, H.; Ye, H.; Chou, Z.; Gao, L.; et al. *Fusobacterium Nucleatum* Aggravates Rheumatoid Arthritis through FadA-Containing Outer Membrane Vesicles. *Cell Host Microbe* **2023**, *31*, 798–810.e7. [CrossRef]
11. Antushevich, H. Fecal Microbiota Transplantation in Disease Therapy. *Clin. Chim. Acta* **2020**, *503*, 90–98. [CrossRef] [PubMed]
12. Wang, J.W.; Kuo, C.H.; Kuo, F.C.; Wang, Y.K.; Hsu, W.H.; Yu, F.J.; Hu, H.M.; Hsu, P.I.; Wang, J.Y.; Wu, D.C. Fecal Microbiota Transplantation: Review and Update. *J. Formos. Med. Assoc.* **2019**, *118*, S23–S31. [CrossRef] [PubMed]

13. Vela Ramirez, J.E.; Sharpe, L.A.; Peppas, N.A. Current State and Challenges in Developing Oral Vaccines. *Adv. Drug Deliv. Rev.* **2017**, *114*, 116–131. [CrossRef]
14. Laffleur, F.; Mayer, A.H. Oral Nanoparticulate Drug Delivery Systems for the Treatment of Intestinal Bowel Disease and Colorectal Cancer. *Expert Opin. Drug Deliv.* **2023**, *20*, 1595–1607. [CrossRef] [PubMed]
15. Rao, S.S.C.; Rehman, A.; Yu, S.; De Andino, N.M. Brain Fogginess, Gas and Bloating: A Link between SIBO, Probiotics and Metabolic Acidosis. *Clin. Transl. Gastroenterol.* **2018**, *9*, e162. [CrossRef] [PubMed]
16. Merenstein, D.; Pot, B.; Leyer, G.; Ouwehand, A.C.; Preidis, G.A.; Elkins, C.A.; Hill, C.; Lewis, Z.T.; Shane, A.L.; Zmora, N.; et al. Emerging Issues in Probiotic Safety: 2023 Perspectives. *Gut Microbes* **2023**, *15*, 2185034. [CrossRef] [PubMed]
17. Nabavi-Rad, A.; Sadeghi, A.; Asadzadeh Aghdaei, H.; Yadegar, A.; Smith, S.M.; Zali, M.R. The Double-Edged Sword of Probiotic Supplementation on Gut Microbiota Structure in *Helicobacter Pylori* Management. *Gut Microbes* **2022**, *14*, 2108655. [CrossRef] [PubMed]
18. Becattini, S.; Taur, Y.; Pamer, E.G. Antibiotic-Induced Changes in the Intestinal Microbiota and Disease. *Trends Mol. Med.* **2016**, *22*, 458–478. [CrossRef] [PubMed]
19. Reinholz, J.; Landfester, K.; Mailänder, V. The Challenges of Oral Drug Delivery via Nanocarriers. *Drug Deliv.* **2018**, *25*, 1694–1705. [CrossRef]
20. Grabska-Kobyłecka, I.; Szpakowski, P.; Król, A.; Książek-Winiarek, D.; Kobyłecki, A.; Głąbiński, A.; Nowak, D. Polyphenols and Their Impact on the Prevention of Neurodegenerative Diseases and Development. *Nutrients* **2023**, *15*, 3454. [CrossRef]
21. Xia, Y.; Hong, L.; Zheng, J.; Lu, Z.; Zhang, Q.; Chen, S.; Pang, Z.; Li, L.; Qiao, S.; Wang, Q.; et al. Ulcerative Colitis Alleviation of Colon-Specific Delivered Rhamnolipid/Fullerene Nanocomposites *via* Dual Modulation in Oxidative Stress and Intestinal Microbiome. *J. Mater. Chem. B* **2023**, *11*, 5882–5897. [CrossRef]
22. Guerra, P.R.; Ajalloueian, F.; Wei, S.; Kristensen, K.A.; Bahl, M.I.; Boisen, A.; Licht, T.R. Delivery of Streptomycin to the Rat Colon by Use of Electrospun Nanofibers. *Sci. Rep.* **2022**, *12*, 21503. [CrossRef] [PubMed]
23. Cassini, C.; Zatti, P.H.; Angeli, V.W.; Branco, C.S.; Salvador, M. Mutual Effects of Free and Nanoencapsulated Phenolic Compoundson Human Microbiota. *Curr. Med. Chem.* **2022**, *29*, 3160–3178. [CrossRef]
24. Wang, L.; Li, Z.; An, S.; Zhu, H.; Li, X.; Gao, D. Malus Baccata (Linn.) Borkh Polyphenols-Loaded Nanoparticles Ameliorate Intestinal Health by Modulating Intestinal Function and Gut Microbiota. *Int. J. Biol. Macromol.* **2023**, *252*, 126233. [CrossRef] [PubMed]
25. Fraga, C.G.; Croft, K.D.; Kennedy, D.O.; Tomás-Barberán, F.A. The Effects of Polyphenols and Other Bioactives on Human Health. *Food Funct.* **2019**, *10*, 514–528. [CrossRef] [PubMed]
26. Remanan, M.K.; Zhu, F. Encapsulation of Chrysin and Rutin Using Self-Assembled Nanoparticles of Debranched Quinoa, Maize, and Waxy Maize Starches. *Carbohydr. Polym.* **2024**, *337*, 122118. [CrossRef]
27. Li, X.; Feng, R.; Zhou, P.; Wang, L.; Luo, Z.; An, S. Construction and Characterization of *Juglans Regia* L. Polyphenols Nanoparticles Based on Bovine Serum Albumin and *Hohenbuehelia Serotina* Polysaccharides, and Their Gastrointestinal Digestion and Colonic Fermentation in Vitro. *Food Funct.* **2021**, *12*, 10397–10410. [CrossRef]
28. Tian, W.; Wang, H.; Zhu, Y.; Wang, Q.; Song, M.; Cao, Y.; Xiao, J. Intervention Effects of Delivery Vehicles on the Therapeutic Efficacy of 6-Gingerol on Colitis. *J. Controlled Release* **2022**, *349*, 51–66. [CrossRef]
29. Zhao, P.; Xia, X.; Xu, X.; Leung, K.K.C.; Rai, A.; Deng, Y.; Yang, B.; Lai, H.; Peng, X.; Shi, P.; et al. Nanoparticle-Assembled Bioadhesive Coacervate Coating with Prolonged Gastrointestinal Retention for Inflammatory Bowel Disease Therapy. *Nat. Commun.* **2021**, *12*, 7162. [CrossRef]
30. Adepu, S.; Ramakrishna, S. Controlled Drug Delivery Systems: Current Status and Future Directions. *Molecules* **2021**, *26*, 5905. [CrossRef]
31. Marabada, D.; Li, J.; Wei, S.; Huang, Q.; Wang, Z. Cyclodextrin Based Nanoparticles for Smart Drug Delivery in Colorectal Cancer. *Chem. Biol. Drug Des.* **2023**, *102*, 1618–1631. [CrossRef] [PubMed]
32. Li, S.; Jin, M.; Wu, Y.; Jung, S.; Li, D.; He, N.; Lee, M. An Efficient Enzyme-Triggered Controlled Release System for Colon-Targeted Oral Delivery to Combat Dextran Sodium Sulfate (DSS)-Induced Colitis in Mice. *Drug Deliv.* **2021**, *28*, 1120–1131. [CrossRef] [PubMed]
33. Al-Sadi, R.; Dharmaprakash, V.; Nighot, P.; Guo, S.; Nighot, M.; Do, T.; Ma, T.Y. *Bifidobacterium Bifidum* Enhances the Intestinal Epithelial Tight Junction Barrier and Protects against Intestinal Inflammation by Targeting the Toll-like Receptor-2 Pathway in an NF-κB-Independent Manner. *Int. J. Mol. Sci.* **2021**, *22*, 8070. [CrossRef] [PubMed]
34. Chen, J.; Zhang, P.; Wu, C.; Yao, Q.; Cha, R.; Gao, Y. Reductase-Labile Peptidic Supramolecular Hydrogels Aided in Oral Delivery of Probiotics. *ACS Appl. Mater. Interfaces* **2023**, *15*, 31214–31223. [CrossRef] [PubMed]
35. Bao, M.; Wang, K.; Li, J.; Li, Y.; Zhu, H.; Lu, M.; Zhang, Y.; Fan, Q.; Han, L.; Wang, K.; et al. ROS Scavenging and Inflammation-Directed Polydopamine Nanoparticles Regulate Gut Immunity and Flora Therapy in Inflammatory Bowel Disease. *Acta Biomater.* **2023**, *161*, 250–264. [CrossRef] [PubMed]
36. Han, L.; Liu, X.W.; Zang, T.; Ren, H.; Liang, D.S.; Bai, S.C.; Li, C.; Liao, X.P.; Liu, Y.H.; Zhang, C.; et al. H_2S Responsive PEGylated Poly (Lipoic Acid) with Ciprofloxacin for Targeted Therapy of *Salmonella*. *J. Controlled Release* **2022**, *351*, 896–906. [CrossRef] [PubMed]
37. Ren, Z.; Chen, X.; Hong, L.; Zhao, X.; Cui, G.; Li, A.; Liu, Y.; Zhou, L.; Sun, R.; Shen, S.; et al. Nanoparticle Conjugation of Ginsenoside Rg3 Inhibits Hepatocellular Carcinoma Development and Metastasis. *Small* **2020**, *16*, 1905233. [CrossRef] [PubMed]

38. Su, X.; Jing, X.; Jiang, W.; Li, M.; Liu, K.; Teng, M.; Ma, Y.; Wang, D.; Meng, L.; Zhang, Y.; et al. Polyphosphazene Nanodrugs for Targeting Delivery and Inflammation Responsive Release of Curcumin to Treat Acute Lung Injury by Effectively Inhibiting Cytokine Storms. *Colloids Surf. B Biointerfaces* **2023**, *229*, 113446. [CrossRef] [PubMed]
39. Wei, K.; Gong, F.; Wu, J.; Tang, W.; Liao, F.; Han, Z.; Pei, Z.; Lei, H.; Wang, L.; Shao, M.; et al. Orally Administered Silicon Hydrogen Nanomaterials as Target Therapy to Treat Intestinal Diseases. *ACS Nano* **2023**, *17*, 21539–21552. [CrossRef]
40. Patangia, D.V.; Anthony Ryan, C.; Dempsey, E.; Paul Ross, R.; Stanton, C. Impact of Antibiotics on the Human Microbiome and Consequences for Host Health. *MicrobiologyOpen* **2022**, *11*, e1260. [CrossRef]
41. Zhang, G.; Wang, Q.; Tao, W.; Jiang, W.; Elinav, E.; Wang, Y.; Zhu, S. Glucosylated Nanoparticles for the Oral Delivery of Antibiotics to the Proximal Small Intestine Protect Mice from Gut Dysbiosis. *Nat. Biomed. Eng.* **2022**, *6*, 867–881. [CrossRef] [PubMed]
42. Gao, C.; Wang, X.; Yang, B.; Yuan, W.; Huang, W.; Wu, G.; Ma, J. Synergistic Target of Intratumoral Microbiome and Tumor by Metronidazole–Fluorouridine Nanoparticles. *ACS Nano* **2023**, *17*, 7335–7351. [CrossRef] [PubMed]
43. Lee, Y.; Sugihara, K.; Gillilland, M.G.; Jon, S.; Kamada, N.; Moon, J.J. Hyaluronic Acid–Bilirubin Nanomedicine for Targeted Modulation of Dysregulated Intestinal Barrier, Microbiome and Immune Responses in Colitis. *Nat. Mater.* **2020**, *19*, 118–126. [CrossRef] [PubMed]
44. Zheng, D.W.; Dong, X.; Pan, P.; Chen, K.W.; Fan, J.X.; Cheng, S.X.; Zhang, X.Z. PhageGuided Modulation of the Gut Microbiota of Mouse Models of Colorectal Cancer Augments Their Responses to Chemotherapy. *Nat. Biomed. Eng.* **2019**, *3*, 717–728. [CrossRef]
45. Qiao, L.; Dou, X.; Song, X.; Chang, J.; Pi, S.; Zhang, X.; Zhu, L.; Zeng, X.; Xu, C. Protective Effect of Biogenic Selenium Nanoparticles against Diquat-Induced Acute Toxicity via Regulation of Gut Microbiota and Its Metabolites. *Food Chem. Toxicol.* **2022**, *170*, 113480. [CrossRef] [PubMed]
46. Jin, Z.; Sun, Y.; Yang, T.; Tan, L.; Lv, P.; Xu, Q.; Tao, G.; Qin, S.; Lu, X.; He, Q. Nanocapsule-Mediated Sustained H2 Release in the Gut Ameliorates Metabolic Dysfunction-Associated Fatty Liver Disease. *Biomaterials* **2021**, *276*, 121030. [CrossRef] [PubMed]
47. Goto, M.; Iohara, D.; Michihara, A.; Ifuku, S.; Azuma, K.; Kadowaki, D.; Maruyama, T.; Otagiri, M.; Hirayama, F.; Anraku, M. Effects of Surface-Deacetylated Chitin Nanofibers on Non-Alcoholic Steatohepatitis Model Rats and Their Gut Microbiota. *Int. J. Biol. Macromol.* **2020**, *164*, 659–666. [CrossRef] [PubMed]
48. Hu, B.; Yu, S.; Shi, C.; Gu, J.; Shao, Y.; Chen, Q.; Li, Y.; Mezzenga, R. Amyloid–Polyphenol Hybrid Nanofilaments Mitigate Colitis and Regulate Gut Microbial Dysbiosis. *ACS Nano* **2020**, *14*, 2760–2776. [CrossRef] [PubMed]
49. Li, C.; Wang, N.; Zheng, G.; Yang, L. Oral Administration of Resveratrol-Selenium-Peptide Nanocomposites Alleviates Alzheimer's Disease-like Pathogenesis by Inhibiting Aβ Aggregation and Regulating Gut Microbiota. *ACS Appl. Mater. Interfaces* **2021**, *13*, 46406–46420. [CrossRef]
50. Xu, J.; Xu, J.; Shi, T.; Zhang, Y.; Chen, F.; Yang, C.; Guo, X.; Liu, G.; Shao, D.; Leong, K.W.; et al. Probiotic-Inspired Nanomedicine Restores Intestinal Homeostasis in Colitis by Regulating Redox Balance, Immune Responses, and the Gut Microbiome. *Adv. Mater.* **2023**, *35*, 2207890. [CrossRef]
51. Li, L.; Cui, H.; Li, T.; Qi, J.; Chen, H.; Gao, F.; Tian, X.; Mu, Y.; He, R.; Lv, S.; et al. Synergistic Effect of Berberine-Based Chinese Medicine Assembled Nanostructures on Diarrhea-Predominant Irritable Bowel Syndrome In Vivo. *Front. Pharmacol.* **2020**, *11*, 1210. [CrossRef] [PubMed]
52. Zhu, M.; Xu, H.; Liang, Y.; Xu, J.; Yue, N.; Zhang, Y.; Tian, C.; Yao, J.; Wang, L.; Nie, Y.; et al. Edible Exosome-like Nanoparticles from Portulaca Oleracea L Mitigate DSS-Induced Colitis via Facilitating Double-Positive CD4+CD8+T Cells Expansion. *J. Nanobiotechnol.* **2023**, *21*, 309. [CrossRef]
53. Ma, L.; Lyu, W.; Song, Y.; Chen, K.; Lv, L.; Yang, H.; Wang, W.; Xiao, Y. Anti-Inflammatory Effect of *Clostridium Butyricum* -Derived Extracellular Vesicles in Ulcerative Colitis: Impact on Host microRNAs Expressions and Gut Microbiome Profiles. *Mol. Nutr. Food Res.* **2023**, *67*, 2200884. [CrossRef]
54. Chandrarathna, H.P.S.U.; Liyanage, T.D.; Edirisinghe, S.L.; Dananjaya, S.H.S.; Thulshan, E.H.T.; Nikapitiya, C.; Oh, C.; Kang, D.H.; De Zoysa, M. Marine Microalgae, Spirulina Maxima-Derived Modified Pectin and Modified Pectin Nanoparticles Modulate the Gut Microbiota and Trigger Immune Responses in Mice. *Mar. Drugs* **2020**, *18*, 175. [CrossRef]
55. Bantun, F.; Singh, R.; Alkhanani, M.F.; Almalki, A.H.; Alshammary, F.; Khan, S.; Haque, S.; Srivastava, M. Gut Microbiome Interactions with Graphene Based Nanomaterials: Challenges and Opportunities. *Sci. Total Environ.* **2022**, *830*, 154789. [CrossRef]
56. Yong, C.; Valiyaveettil, S.; Tang, B. Toxicity of Microplastics and Nanoplastics in Mammalian Systems. *Int. J. Environ. Res. Public Health* **2020**, *17*, 1509. [CrossRef]
57. Bazeli, J.; Banikazemi, Z.; Hamblin, M.R.; Sharafati Chaleshtori, R. Could Probiotics Protect against Human Toxicity Caused by Polystyrene Nanoplastics and Microplastics? *Front. Nutr.* **2023**, *10*, 1186724. [CrossRef]
58. Chen, X.; Xu, L.; Chen, Q.; Su, S.; Zhuang, J.; Qiao, D. Polystyrene Micro- and Nanoparticles Exposure Induced Anxiety-like Behaviors, Gut Microbiota Dysbiosis and Metabolism Disorder in Adult Mice. *Ecotoxicol. Environ. Saf.* **2023**, *259*, 115000. [CrossRef]
59. Scarcello, E.; Sofranko, A.; Wahle, T.; Schins, R.P.F. Neurotoxicity of Engineered Nanomaterials: Testing Considerations. *Front. Public Health* **2022**, *10*, 904544. [CrossRef] [PubMed]
60. Bianchi, M.G.; Chiu, M.; Taurino, G.; Bergamaschi, E.; Turroni, F.; Mancabelli, L.; Longhi, G.; Ventura, M.; Bussolati, O. Amorphous Silica Nanoparticles and the Human Gut Microbiota: A Relationship with Multiple Implications. *J. Nanobiotechnol.* **2024**, *22*, 45. [CrossRef] [PubMed]

61. Ghebretatios, M.; Schaly, S.; Prakash, S. Nanoparticles in the Food Industry and Their Impact on Human Gut Microbiome and Diseases. *Int. J. Mol. Sci.* **2021**, *22*, 1942. [CrossRef] [PubMed]
62. Landsiedel, R.; Hahn, D.; Ossig, R.; Ritz, S.; Sauer, L.; Buesen, R.; Rehm, S.; Wohlleben, W.; Groeters, S.; Strauss, V.; et al. Gut Microbiome and Plasma Metabolome Changes in Rats after Oral Gavage of Nanoparticles: Sensitive Indicators of Possible Adverse Health Effects. *Part. Fibre Toxicol.* **2022**, *19*, 21. [CrossRef]
63. Meier, M.J.; Nguyen, K.C.; Crosthwait, J.; Kawata, A.; Rigden, M.; Leingartner, K.; Wong, A.; Holloway, A.; Shwed, P.S.; Beaudette, L.; et al. Low Dose Antibiotic Ingestion Potentiates Systemic and Microbiome Changes Induced by Silver Nanoparticles. *NanoImpact* **2021**, *23*, 100343. [CrossRef]
64. Muhammad, A.; He, J.; Yu, T.; Sun, C.; Shi, D.; Jiang, Y.; Xianyu, Y.; Shao, Y. Dietary exposure of copper and zinc oxides nanoparticles affect the fitness, enzyme activity, and microbial community of the model insect, silkworm Bombyx mori. *Sci. Total Environ.* **2022**, *813*, 152608. [CrossRef]
65. Yan, J.; Chen, Q.; Tian, L.; Li, K.; Lai, W.; Bian, L.; Han, J.; Jia, R.; Liu, X.; Xi, Z. Intestinal Toxicity of Micro- and Nano-Particles of Foodborne Titanium Dioxide in Juvenile Mice: Disorders of Gut Microbiota–Host Co-Metabolites and Intestinal Barrier Damage. *Sci. Total Environ.* **2022**, *821*, 153279. [CrossRef] [PubMed]
66. Lamas, B.; Evariste, L.; Houdeau, E. Dysregulation along the Gut Microbiota-Immune System Axis after Oral Exposure to Titanium Dioxide Nanoparticles: A Possible Environmental Factor Promoting Obesity-Related Metabolic Disorders. *Environ. Pollut.* **2023**, *330*, 121795. [CrossRef]
67. Zhang, T.; Li, D.; Zhu, X.; Zhang, M.; Guo, J.; Chen, J. Nano-Al_2O_3 Particles Affect Gut Microbiome and Resistome in an in Vitro Simulator of the Human Colon Microbial Ecosystem. *J. Hazard. Mater.* **2022**, *439*, 129513. [CrossRef]
68. Askri, D.; Ouni, S.; Galai, S.; Chovelon, B.; Arnaud, J.; Sturm, N.; Lehmann, S.G.; Sakly, M.; Amara, S.; Sève, M. Nanoparticles in Foods? A Multiscale Physiopathological Investigation of Iron Oxide Nanoparticle Effects on Rats after an Acute Oral Exposure: Trace Element Biodistribution and Cognitive Capacities. *Food Chem. Toxicol.* **2019**, *127*, 173–181. [CrossRef]
69. Bhattacharya, S.S.; Yadav, B.; Rosen, L.; Nagpal, R.; Yadav, H.; Yadav, J.S. Crosstalk between Gut Microbiota and Lung Inflammation in Murine Toxicity Models of Respiratory Exposure or Co-Exposure to Carbon Nanotube Particles and Cigarette Smoke Extract. *Toxicol. Appl. Pharmacol.* **2022**, *447*, 116066. [CrossRef] [PubMed]
70. Christophersen, D.V.; Jacobsen, N.R.; Andersen, M.H.G.; Connell, S.P.; Barfod, K.K.; Thomsen, M.B.; Miller, M.R.; Duffin, R.; Lykkesfeldt, J.; Vogel, U.; et al. Cardiovascular Health Effects of Oral and Pulmonary Exposure to Multi-Walled Carbon Nanotubes in ApoE-Deficient Mice. *Toxicology* **2016**, *371*, 29–40. [CrossRef] [PubMed]
71. Liu, X.; Liu, Y.; Chen, X.; Wang, C.; Chen, X.; Liu, W.; Huang, K.; Chen, H.; Yang, J. Multi-Walled Carbon Nanotubes Exacerbate Doxorubicin-Induced Cardiotoxicity by Altering Gut Microbiota and Pulmonary and Colonic Macrophage Phenotype in Mice. *Toxicology* **2020**, *435*, 152410. [CrossRef] [PubMed]
72. Chen, B.Y.; Hong, S.Y.; Wang, H.M.; Shi, Y.; Wang, P.; Wang, X.J.; Jiang, Q.Y.; Yang, K.D.; Chen, W.; Xu, X.L. The Subacute Toxicity and Underlying Mechanisms of Biomimetic Mesoporous Polydopamine Nanoparticles. *Part. Fibre Toxicol.* **2023**, *20*, 38. [CrossRef]
73. Chaplin, A.; Gao, H.; Asase, C.; Rengasamy, P.; Park, B.; Skander, D.; Bebek, G.; Rajagopalan, S.; Maiseyeu, A. Systemically-Delivered Biodegradable PLGA Alters Gut Microbiota and Induces Transcriptomic Reprogramming in the Liver in an Obesity Mouse Model. *Sci. Rep.* **2020**, *10*, 13786. [CrossRef]
74. Lin, X.; Xie, H.; Zhang, Y.; Tian, X.; Cui, L.; Shi, N.; Wang, L.; Zhao, J.; An, L.; Wang, J.; et al. The Toxicity of Nano Polyethylene Terephthalate to Mice: Intestinal Obstruction, Growth Retardant, Gut Microbiota Dysbiosis and Lipid Metabolism Disorders. *Food Chem. Toxicol.* **2023**, *172*, 113585. [CrossRef]
75. Aniwan, S.; Santiago, P.; Loftus, E.V.; Park, S.H. The Epidemiology of Inflammatory Bowel Disease in Asia and Asian Immigrants to Western Countries. *United Eur. Gastroenterol. J.* **2022**, *10*, 1063–1076. [CrossRef]
76. Chen, X.; Xiang, X.; Xia, W.; Li, X.; Wang, S.; Ye, S.; Tian, L.; Zhao, L.; Ai, F.; Shen, Z.; et al. Evolving Trends and Burden of Inflammatory Bowel Disease in Asia, 1990–2019: A Comprehensive Analysis Based on the Global Burden of Disease Study. *J. Epidemiol. Glob. Health* **2023**, *13*, 725–739. [CrossRef]
77. Kuenzig, M.E.; Fung, S.G.; Marderfeld, L.; Mak, J.W.Y.; Kaplan, G.G.; Ng, S.C.; Wilson, D.C.; Cameron, F.; Henderson, P.; Kotze, P.G.; et al. Twenty-First Century Trends in the Global Epidemiology of Pediatric-Onset Inflammatory Bowel Disease: Systematic Review. *Gastroenterology* **2022**, *162*, 1147–1159.e4. [CrossRef]
78. Le Berre, C.; Honap, S.; Peyrin-Biroulet, L. Ulcerative Colitis. *Lancet* **2023**, *402*, 571–584. [CrossRef]
79. Liu, J.; Di, B.; Xu, L. Recent Advances in the Treatment of IBD: Targets, Mechanisms and Related Therapies. *Cytokine Growth Factor Rev.* **2023**, *71–72*, 1–12. [CrossRef] [PubMed]
80. Shan, Y.; Lee, M.; Chang, E.B. The Gut Microbiome and Inflammatory Bowel Diseases. *Annu. Rev. Med.* **2022**, *73*, 455–468. [CrossRef] [PubMed]
81. Lee, M.; Chang, E.B. Inflammatory Bowel Diseases (IBD) and the Microbiome—Searching the Crime Scene for Clues. *Gastroenterology* **2021**, *160*, 524–537. [CrossRef] [PubMed]
82. Shalon, D.; Culver, R.N.; Grembi, J.A.; Folz, J.; Treit, P.V.; Shi, H.; Rosenberger, F.A.; Dethlefsen, L.; Meng, X.; Yaffe, E.; et al. Profiling the Human Intestinal Environment under Physiological Conditions. *Nature* **2023**, *617*, 581–591. [CrossRef] [PubMed]
83. Luo, H.; Cao, G.; Luo, C.; Tan, D.; Vong, C.T.; Xu, Y.; Wang, S.; Lu, H.; Wang, Y.; Jing, W. Emerging Pharmacotherapy for Inflammatory Bowel Diseases. *Pharmacol. Res.* **2022**, *178*, 106146. [CrossRef] [PubMed]

84. Mohajeri, S.; Moayedi, S.; Mohajeri, S.; Yadegar, A.; Haririan, I. Targeting Pathophysiological Changes Using Biomaterials-Based Drug Delivery Systems: A Key to Managing Inflammatory Bowel Disease. *Front. Pharmacol.* **2022**, *13*, 1045575. [CrossRef] [PubMed]
85. Yin, M.; Chen, Y.; Liu, X.; Tian, S.; Zhao, L.; Bai, Y.; Wang, H.; Lin, J.; Jiang, D.; Lei, Z.; et al. Targeted Computed Tomography Visualization and Healing of Inflammatory Bowel Disease by Orally Delivered Bacterial-Flagella-Inspired Polydiiododiacetylene Nanofibers. *ACS Nano* **2023**, *17*, 3873–3888. [CrossRef] [PubMed]
86. Zhang, X.; Zhao, X.; Hua, Z.; Xing, S.; Li, J.; Fei, S.; Tan, M. ROS-Triggered Self-Disintegrating and pH-Responsive Astaxanthin Nanoparticles for Regulating the Intestinal Barrier and Colitis. *Biomaterials* **2023**, *292*, 121937. [CrossRef] [PubMed]
87. Zhang, C.; Li, Q.; Shan, J.; Xing, J.; Liu, X.; Ma, Y.; Qian, H.; Chen, X.; Wang, X.; Wu, L.M.; et al. Multifunctional Two-Dimensional Bi2Se3 Nanodiscs for Anti-Inflammatory Therapy of Inflammatory Bowel Diseases. *Acta Biomater.* **2023**, *160*, 252–264. [CrossRef] [PubMed]
88. Martyniak, A.; Medyńska-Przęczek, A.; Wędrychowicz, A.; Skoczeń, S.; Tomasik, P.J. Prebiotics, Probiotics, Synbiotics, Paraprobiotics and Postbiotic Compounds in IBD. *Biomolecules* **2021**, *11*, 1903. [CrossRef] [PubMed]
89. Alkushi, A.G.; Elazab, S.T.; Abdelfattah-Hassan, A.; Mahfouz, H.; Salem, G.A.; Sheraiba, N.I.; Mohamed, E.A.A.; Attia, M.S.; El-Shetry, E.S.; Saleh, A.A.; et al. Multi-Strain-Probiotic-Loaded Nanoparticles Reduced Colon Inflammation and Orchestrated the Expressions of Tight Junction, NLRP3 Inflammasome and Caspase-1 Genes in DSS-Induced Colitis Model. *Pharmaceutics* **2022**, *14*, 1183. [CrossRef]
90. Alkushi, A.G.; Abdelfattah-Hassan, A.; Eldoumani, H.; Elazab, S.T.; Mohamed, S.A.M.; Metwally, A.S.; El-Shetry, E.S.; Saleh, A.A.; ElSawy, N.A.; Ibrahim, D. Probiotics-Loaded Nanoparticles Attenuated Colon Inflammation, Oxidative Stress, and Apoptosis in Colitis. *Sci. Rep.* **2022**, *12*, 5116. [CrossRef]
91. Li, J.; Hou, W.; Lin, S.; Wang, L.; Pan, C.; Wu, F.; Liu, J. Polydopamine Nanoparticle-Mediated Dopaminergic Immunoregulation in Colitis. *Adv. Sci.* **2022**, *9*, 2104006. [CrossRef]
92. Jeppesen, D.K.; Zhang, Q.; Franklin, J.L.; Coffey, R.J. Extracellular Vesicles and Nanoparticles: Emerging Complexities. *Trends Cell Biol.* **2023**, *33*, 667–681. [CrossRef]
93. Hill, A.F. Extracellular Vesicles and Neurodegenerative Diseases. *J. Neurosci.* **2019**, *39*, 9269–9273. [CrossRef]
94. Li, D.; Yang, M.; Xu, J.; Xu, H.; Zhu, M.; Liang, Y.; Zhang, Y.; Tian, C.; Nie, Y.; Shi, R.; et al. Extracellular Vesicles: The Next Generation Theranostic Nanomedicine for Inflammatory Bowel Disease. *Int. J. Nanomed.* **2022**, *17*, 3893–3911. [CrossRef]
95. Kim, S.H.; Keum, B.; Kwak, S.; Byun, J.; Shin, J.M.; Kim, T.H. Therapeutic Applications of Extracellular Vesicles in Inflammatory Bowel Disease. *Int. J. Mol. Sci.* **2024**, *25*, 745. [CrossRef] [PubMed]
96. Olovo, C.V.; Wiredu Ocansey, D.K.; Ji, Y.; Huang, X.; Xu, M. Bacterial Membrane Vesicles in the Pathogenesis and Treatment of Inflammatory Bowel Disease. *Gut Microbes* **2024**, *16*, 2341670. [CrossRef]
97. Gul, L.; Modos, D.; Fonseca, S.; Madgwick, M.; Thomas, J.P.; Sudhakar, P.; Booth, C.; Stentz, R.; Carding, S.R.; Korcsmaros, T. Extracellular Vesicles Produced by the Human Commensal Gut Bacterium *Bacteroides Thetaiotaomicron* Affect Host Immune Pathways in a Cell-type Specific Manner That Are Altered in Inflammatory Bowel Disease. *J. Extracell. Vesicles* **2022**, *11*, e12189. [CrossRef]
98. Wei, Z.; Hang, S.; Wiredu Ocansey, D.K.; Zhang, Z.; Wang, B.; Zhang, X.; Mao, F. Human Umbilical Cord Mesenchymal Stem Cells Derived Exosome Shuttling Mir-129-5p Attenuates Inflammatory Bowel Disease by Inhibiting Ferroptosis. *J. Nanobiotechnol.* **2023**, *21*, 188. [CrossRef] [PubMed]
99. Liu, C.; Yan, X.; Zhang, Y.; Yang, M.; Ma, Y.; Zhang, Y.; Xu, Q.; Tu, K.; Zhang, M. Oral Administration of Turmeric-Derived Exosome-like Nanovesicles with Anti-Inflammatory and pro-Resolving Bioactions for Murine Colitis Therapy. *J. Nanobiotechnol.* **2022**, *20*, 206. [CrossRef]
100. Sriwastva, M.K.; Deng, Z.; Wang, B.; Teng, Y.; Kumar, A.; Sundaram, K.; Mu, J.; Lei, C.; Dryden, G.W.; Xu, F.; et al. Exosome-like Nanoparticles from Mulberry Bark Prevent DSS-induced Colitis via the AhR/COPS8 Pathway. *EMBO Rep.* **2022**, *23*, e53365. [CrossRef]
101. Zhang, Y.; Belaid, M.; Luo, X.; Daci, A.; Limani, R.; Mantaj, J.; Zilbauer, M.; Nayak, K.; Vllasaliu, D. Probing Milk Extracellular Vesicles for Intestinal Delivery of RNA Therapies. *J. Nanobiotechnol.* **2023**, *21*, 406. [CrossRef]
102. Garbati, P.; Picco, C.; Magrassi, R.; Signorello, P.; Cacopardo, L.; Dalla Serra, M.; Faticato, M.G.; De Luca, M.; Balestra, F.; Scavo, M.P.; et al. Targeting the Gut: A Systematic Review of Specific Drug Nanocarriers. *Pharmaceutics* **2024**, *16*, 431. [CrossRef]
103. Kim, H.I.; Park, J.; Zhu, Y.; Wang, X.; Han, Y.; Zhang, D. Recent Advances in Extracellular Vesicles for Therapeutic Cargo Delivery. *Exp. Mol. Med.* **2024**, *56*, 836–849. [CrossRef]
104. Guo, J.; Wang, F.; Hu, Y.; Luo, Y.; Wei, Y.; Xu, K.; Zhang, H.; Liu, H.; Bo, L.; Lv, S.; et al. Exosome-Based Bone-Targeting Drug Delivery Alleviates Impaired Osteoblastic Bone Formation and Bone Loss in Inflammatory Bowel Diseases. *Cell Rep. Med.* **2023**, *4*, 100881. [CrossRef]
105. Xu, Y.; Zhu, B.W.; Sun, R.; Li, X.; Wu, D.; Hu, J.N. Colon-Targeting *Angelica Sinensis* Polysaccharide Nanoparticles with Dual Responsiveness for Alleviation of Ulcerative Colitis. *ACS Appl. Mater. Interfaces* **2023**, *15*, 26298–26315. [CrossRef] [PubMed]
106. Liu, Y.; Wang, C.; Liu, R.; Zhao, M.; Ding, X.; Zhang, T.; He, R.; Zhu, S.; Dong, X.; Xie, J.; et al. Adhesive Ergothioneine Hyaluronate Gel Protects against Radiation Gastroenteritis by Alleviating Apoptosis, Inflammation, and Gut Microbiota Dysbiosis. *ACS Appl. Mater. Interfaces* **2023**, *15*, 19833–19846. [CrossRef]

107. Deng, L.; Zeng, H.; Hu, X.; Xiao, M.; He, D.; Zhang, Y.; Jin, Y.; Hu, Y.; Zhu, Y.; Gong, L.; et al. Se@Albumin Nanoparticles Ameliorate Intestinal Mucositis Caused by Cisplatin *via* Gut Microbiota-Targeted Regulation. *Nanoscale* **2021**, *13*, 11250–11261. [CrossRef]
108. Sepich-Poore, G.D.; Zitvogel, L.; Straussman, R.; Hasty, J.; Wargo, J.A.; Knight, R. The Microbiome and Human Cancer. *Science* **2021**, *371*, eabc4552. [CrossRef] [PubMed]
109. Matson, V.; Chervin, C.S.; Gajewski, T.F. Cancer and the Microbiome—Influence of the Commensal Microbiota on Cancer, Immune Responses, and Immunotherapy. *Gastroenterology* **2021**, *160*, 600–613. [CrossRef] [PubMed]
110. Chen, F.; Dai, X.; Zhou, C.C.; Li, K.; Zhang, Y.; Lou, X.Y.; Zhu, Y.M.; Sun, Y.L.; Peng, B.X.; Cui, W. Integrated Analysis of the Faecal Metagenome and Serum Metabolome Reveals the Role of Gut Microbiome-Associated Metabolites in the Detection of Colorectal Cancer and Adenoma. *Gut* **2022**, *71*, 1315–1325. [CrossRef]
111. Fernandes, M.R.; Aggarwal, P.; Costa, R.G.F.; Cole, A.M.; Trinchieri, G. Targeting the Gut Microbiota for Cancer Therapy. *Nat. Rev. Cancer* **2022**, *22*, 703–722. [CrossRef] [PubMed]
112. Gubernatorova, E.O.; Gorshkova, E.A.; Bondareva, M.A.; Podosokorskaya, O.A.; Sheynova, A.D.; Yakovleva, A.S.; Bonch-Osmolovskaya, E.A.; Nedospasov, S.A.; Kruglov, A.A.; Drutskaya, M.S. *Akkermansia Muciniphila*-Friend or Foe in Colorectal Cancer? *Front. Immunol.* **2023**, *14*, 1303795. [CrossRef] [PubMed]
113. Sugimura, N.; Li, Q.; Chu, E.S.H.; Lau, H.C.H.; Fong, W.; Liu, W.; Liang, C.; Nakatsu, G.; Su, A.C.Y.; Coker, O.O.; et al. *Lactobacillus Gallinarum* Modulates the Gut Microbiota and Produces Anti-Cancer Metabolites to Protect against Colorectal Tumourigenesis. *Gut* **2022**, *71*, 2011–2021. [CrossRef] [PubMed]
114. Gou, H.; Su, H.; Liu, D.; Wong, C.C.; Shang, H.; Fang, Y.; Zeng, X.; Chen, H.; Li, Y.; Huang, Z.; et al. Traditional Medicine Pien Tze Huang Suppresses Colorectal Tumorigenesis Through Restoring Gut Microbiota and Metabolites. *Gastroenterology* **2023**, *165*, 1404–1419. [CrossRef] [PubMed]
115. Huang, J.; Liu, D.; Wang, Y.; Liu, L.; Li, J.; Yuan, J.; Jiang, Z.; Jiang, Z.; Hsiao, W.W.; Liu, H.; et al. Ginseng Polysaccharides Alter the Gut Microbiota and Kynurenine/Tryptophan Ratio, Potentiating the Antitumour Effect of Antiprogrammed Cell Death 1/Programmed Cell Death Ligand 1 (Anti-PD-1/PD-L1) Immunotherapy. *Gut* **2022**, *71*, 734–745. [CrossRef] [PubMed]
116. Li, X.; Wei, H.; Qi, J.; Ma, K.; Luo, Y.; Weng, L. Interactions of Nanomaterials with Gut Microbiota and Their Applications in Cancer Therapy. *Sensors* **2023**, *23*, 4428. [CrossRef] [PubMed]
117. Lang, T.; Zhu, R.; Zhu, X.; Yan, W.; Li, Y.; Zhai, Y.; Wu, T.; Huang, X.; Yin, Q.; Li, Y. Combining Gut Microbiota Modulation and Chemotherapy by Capecitabine-Loaded Prebiotic Nanoparticle Improves Colorectal Cancer Therapy. *Nat. Commun.* **2023**, *14*, 4746. [CrossRef] [PubMed]
118. Dong, X.; Pan, P.; Zheng, D.W.; Bao, P.; Zeng, X.; Zhang, X.Z. Bioinorganic Hybrid Bacteriophage for Modulation of Intestinal Microbiota to Remodel Tumor-Immune Microenvironment against Colorectal Cancer. *Sci. Adv.* **2020**, *6*, eaba1590. [CrossRef] [PubMed]
119. Wang, M.; Cha, R.; Hao, W.; Du, R.; Zhang, P.; Hu, Y.; Jiang, X. Nanocrystalline Cellulose Cures Constipation *via* Gut Microbiota Metabolism. *ACS Nano* **2022**, *16*, 16481–16496. [CrossRef]
120. Duan, T.; Wang, X.; Dong, X.; Wang, C.; Wang, L.; Yang, X.; Li, T. Broccoli-Derived Exosome-like Nanoparticles Alleviate Loperamide-Induced Constipation, in Correlation with Regulation on Gut Microbiota and Tryptophan Metabolism. *J. Agric. Food Chem.* **2023**, *71*, 16568–16580. [CrossRef]
121. Zhi, X.; Liu, Y.; Lin, L.; Yang, M.; Zhang, L.; Zhang, L.; Liu, Y.; Alfranca, G.; Ma, L.; Zhang, Q.; et al. Oral pH Sensitive GNS@ab Nanoprobes for Targeted Therapy of *Helicobacter Pylori* without Disturbance Gut Microbiome. *Nanomed. Nanotechnol. Biol. Med.* **2019**, *20*, 102019. [CrossRef] [PubMed]
122. Arifa, R.D.N.; De Paula, T.P.; Lima, R.L.; Brito, C.B.; Andrade, M.E.R.; Cardoso, V.N.; Pinheiro, M.V.B.; Ladeira, L.O.; Krambrock, K.; Teixeira, M.M.; et al. Anti-Inflammatory and Antioxidant Effects of the Nanocomposite Fullerol Decrease the Severity of Intestinal Inflammation Induced by Gut Ischemia and Reperfusion. *Eur. J. Pharmacol.* **2021**, *898*, 173984. [CrossRef] [PubMed]
123. Liu, H.; Bai, M.; Xu, K.; Zhou, J.; Zhang, X.; Yu, R.; Huang, R.; Yin, Y. Effects of Different Concentrations of Coated Nano Zinc Oxide Material on Fecal Bacterial Composition and Intestinal Barrier in Weaned Piglets. *J. Sci. Food Agric.* **2021**, *101*, 735–745. [CrossRef] [PubMed]
124. Yu, H.; Zhang, J.; Sun, M.; Chen, H.; Shi, X.; You, F.; Qiao, S. Polymeric Nanohybrids Engineered by Chitosan Nanoparticles and Antimicrobial Peptides as Novel Antimicrobials in Food Biopreservatives: Risk Assessment and Anti-Foodborne Pathogen *Escherichia Coli* O157:H7 Infection by Immune Regulation. *J. Agric. Food Chem.* **2022**, *70*, 12535–12549. [CrossRef] [PubMed]
125. Zhai, C.; Lu, F.; Du, X.; Zhang, M.; Zhang, Y.; Ma, Y.; Zhao, Y.; Huang, H.; Kang, Z. Green Carbon Dots Derived from Atractylodes Macrocephala: A Potential Nanodrug for Treating Alcoholic Gastric Ulcer. *Colloids Surf. B Biointerfaces* **2023**, *230*, 113492. [CrossRef]
126. Li, Y.; Liu, X.; Zheng, Y.; Zhang, Y.; Li, Z.; Cui, Z.; Jiang, H.; Zhu, S.; Wu, S. Ultrasmall *Cortex Moutan* Nanoclusters for the Therapy of Pneumonia and Colitis. *Adv. Healthc. Mater.* **2023**, *12*, 2300402. [CrossRef]
127. Su, X.; Jing, X.; Jiang, W.; Li, M.; Liu, K.; Teng, M.; Wang, D.; Meng, L.; Zhang, Y.; Ji, W. Curcumin-Containing Polyphosphazene Nanodrug for Anti-Inflammation and Nerve Regeneration to Improve Functional Recovery after Spinal Cord Injury. *Int. J. Pharm.* **2023**, *642*, 123197. [CrossRef]

128. Liao, W.; Ni, C.; Ge, R.; Li, Y.; Jiang, S.; Yang, W.; Yan, F. Nel-like Molecule Type 1 Combined with Gold Nanoparticles Modulates Macrophage Polarization, Osteoclastogenesis, and Oral Microbiota in Periodontitis. *ACS Appl. Mater. Interfaces* **2024**, *16*, 8442–8458. [CrossRef]
129. Xu, Y.; Mao, H.; Yang, C.; Du, H.; Wang, H.; Tu, J. Effects of Chitosan Nanoparticle Supplementation on Growth Performance, Humoral Immunity, Gut Microbiota and Immune Responses after Lipopolysaccharide Challenge in Weaned Pigs. *J. Anim. Physiol. Anim. Nutr.* **2020**, *104*, 597–605. [CrossRef]
130. Yang, L.; Cui, Y.; Liang, H.; Li, Z.; Wang, N.; Wang, Y.; Zheng, G. Multifunctional Selenium Nanoparticles with Different Surface Modifications Ameliorate Neuroinflammation through the Gut Microbiota-NLRP3 Inflammasome-Brain Axis in APP/PS1 Mice. *ACS Appl. Mater. Interfaces* **2022**, *14*, 30557–30570. [CrossRef]
131. Al-Okbi, S.Y.; Amin, M.A.; Mohamed, A.E.A.; Edris, A.E.; Sharaf, O.M.; Mabrok, H.B.; Ramadan, A.A. Basil Essential Oil and Its Nanoemulsion Mitigate Non-Alcoholic Steatohepatitis in Rat Model with Special Reference to Gut Microbiota. *J. Oleo Sci.* **2020**, *69*, 913–927. [CrossRef]
132. Sundaram, K.; Mu, J.; Kumar, A.; Behera, J.; Lei, C.; Sriwastva, M.K.; Xu, F.; Dryden, G.W.; Zhang, L.; Chen, S.; et al. Garlic Exosome-like Nanoparticles Reverse High-Fat Diet Induced Obesity via the Gut/Brain Axis. *Theranostics* **2022**, *12*, 1220–1246. [CrossRef] [PubMed]
133. Guo, X.; Li, C.; Zhang, J.; Sun, M.; Xu, J.; Xu, C.; Kuang, H.; Xu, L. Chiral Nanoparticle-Remodeled Gut Microbiota Alleviates Neurodegeneration via the Gut–Brain Axis. *Nat. Aging* **2023**, *3*, 1415–1429. [CrossRef]
134. Liu, N.; Yang, C.; Liang, X.; Cao, K.; Xie, J.; Luo, Q.; Luo, H. Mesoporous Silica Nanoparticle-Encapsulated *Bifidobacterium* Attenuates Brain Aβ Burden and Improves Olfactory Dysfunction of APP/PS1 Mice by Nasal Delivery. *J. Nanobiotechnol.* **2022**, *20*, 439. [CrossRef]
135. Yang, L.; Wang, Y.; Li, Z.; Wu, X.; Mei, J.; Zheng, G. Brain Targeted Peptide-Functionalized Chitosan Nanoparticles for Resveratrol Delivery: Impact on Insulin Resistance and Gut Microbiota in Obesity-Related Alzheimer's Disease. *Carbohydr. Polym.* **2023**, *310*, 120714. [CrossRef] [PubMed]
136. Chen, Y.; Yang, C.; Dai, Q.; Tan, J.; Dou, C.; Luo, F. Gold-Nanosphere Mitigates Osteoporosis through Regulating TMAO Metabolism in a Gut Microbiota-Dependent Manner. *J. Nanobiotechnol.* **2023**, *21*, 125. [CrossRef]
137. Gątarek, P.; Kałużna-Czaplińska, J. Trimethylamine N-Oxide (TMAO) in Human Health. *EXCLI J.* **2021**, *20*, excli2020–excli3239. [CrossRef]
138. Kumar, A.; Sundaram, K.; Teng, Y.; Mu, J.; Sriwastva, M.K.; Zhang, L.; Hood, J.L.; Yan, J.; Zhang, X.; Park, J.W.; et al. Ginger Nanoparticles Mediated Induction of Foxa2 Prevents High-Fat Diet-Induced Insulin Resistance. *Theranostics* **2022**, *12*, 1388–1403. [CrossRef]
139. Li, J.; Wang, L.; Li, S.; Liang, X.; Zhang, Y.; Wang, Y.; Liu, Y. Sustained Oral Intake of Nano-Iron Oxide Perturbs the Gut-Liver Axis. *NanoImpact* **2023**, *30*, 100464. [CrossRef]

pharmaceutics

MDPI

Review

Oromucosal Administration of Oxytocin: The Development of 'Oxipops'

Dan Xu [1], Chunmei Lan [1], Juan Kou [2], Shuxia Yao [1], Weihua Zhao [1,*] and Keith M. Kendrick [1,*]

[1] The Clinical Hospital of Chengdu Brain Science Institute, MOE Key Laboratory for Neuroinformation, Center for Information in Medicine, University of Electronic Science and Technology of China, Chengdu 611731, China; xudan040901@gmail.com (D.X.); chunmeilan.uestc@outlook.com (C.L.); yaoshuxia@uestc.edu.cn (S.Y.)

[2] Institute of Brain and Psychological Sciences, Sichuan Normal University, Chengdu 610066, China; koujuan@sicnu.edu.cn

* Correspondence: zarazhao@uestc.edu.cn (W.Z.); kkendrick@uestc.edu.cn (K.M.K.)

Abstract: The role of the hypothalamic neuropeptide oxytocin in influencing the brain and behavior has been the subject of widespread research over the last few decades due, most notably, to its reported involvement in promoting social cognition and motivation, reducing anxiety, and relieving pain. It is also increasingly being considered as an important therapeutic intervention in a variety of disorders with social dysfunction as a symptom. While, in recent years, studies in humans have administered oxytocin primarily via an intranasal route, since it may partly enter the brain directly this way via the olfactory and trigeminal nerves, there is increasing evidence that many of its functional effects can be peripherally mediated via increasing its concentration in the blood. This has opened up an oromucosal administration route as an alternative, which is beneficial since the oral consumption of peptides is problematic due to their rapid breakdown in the acidic environment of the gastrointestinal system. In this review we will discuss both the methodologies we have developed for administering oxytocin via lingual application and medicated lollipops, 'oxipops', in terms of increasing blood concentrations and the bioavailability of the peptide, and also their validation in terms of functional effects on the brain and behavior. While areas under the curve are significantly greater in terms of plasma oxytocin concentrations following intranasally relative to oromucosally administered oxytocin, with the estimated absolute bioavailability of the latter being around 4.4% compared with 11.1% for intranasal administration, the time to peak concentrations (around 30 min) and functional effects on the brain and behavior are broadly similar. We will also discuss potential therapeutic advantages of the oromucosal administration of oxytocin in different clinical contexts and its wider application for other peptides which are increasingly being developed for therapeutic use.

Keywords: oromucosal administration; oxytocin; medicated lollipops; lingual spray; neuropeptides

1. Introduction

The neuropeptide oxytocin is synthesized by cells in the hypothalamic paraventricular and supraoptic nuclei and transported to the posterior pituitary for release into the blood, where it is most well-known for acting on smooth muscle to stimulate uterine contractions during labor and milk-ejection from the breast [1]. However, there are also extensive projections from hypothalamic oxytocin neurons to many parts of the brain which are important for the control of social cognition, motivation, and a number of other behavioral and physiological functions [2–4]. In recent years, there has therefore been considerable interest in the therapeutic use of oxytocin administration, particularly for social dysfunction in disorders such as autism [5–8]. There is currently no approved medication-based treatment for autism and, while clinical trials have reported some positive effects for improving social symptoms, factors such as the dose magnitude and frequency as well as the route of administration may all be important [5–8]. Furthermore, oxytocin-based treatments may also have beneficial effects for reducing anxiety and depression [9] and for relieving pain [10]. To date, all randomized clinical trials have chosen to use an intranasal route for the chronic administration of oxytocin and have not considered the possibility of using some form of oral administration as an alternative. For pediatric and geriatric patient populations, oral administration would represent a considerable advantage in terms of tolerability and compliance for long periods of treatment. This review firstly details the likely mechanisms whereby oxytocin administration can produce functional effects on the brain and behavior, which demonstrate the potential to use an oral instead of an intranasal route, and, secondly, this review details how an effective oromucosal administration strategy has been developed, which opens up the possibility for orally administered oxytocin to be used in future clinical trials.

2. Mechanisms Whereby Oxytocin Administration May Produce Functional Effects

Oxytocin is a small nine-amino acid peptide with a molecular weight of 1007.2 Daltons and which binds to a single seven-transmembrane domain G protein-coupled receptor. Oxytocin is hydrophilic (logP < 1 for lipophilicity), non-polar, non-charged, and both heat- and UV light-sensitive [2,11]. Its primary clinical use to date has been in the induction of labor and control of post-partum hemorrhage by its intravenous infusion or intramuscular injection through its actions on receptors in uterine smooth muscle [1]. However, there has been increasing interest in administering oxytocin to influence brain and behavioral functions. Small hydrophilic peptides, such as oxytocin, have difficulty crossing the blood–brain barrier, and this has led to its administration by intranasal spray in humans as a method for allowing it to penetrate into the brain to produce its functional effects [3–10]. Using animal models, studies have primarily identified the olfactory and trigeminal nerves as the routes whereby intranasally administered oxytocin can enter the brain, although, additionally, a large amount of the peptide is absorbed by the nasal vasculature and enters the peripheral circulation (see [4]). Oxytocin has receptors in numerous peripheral organs including the cardiovascular and gastrointestinal systems as well as the dorsal root [12] and trigeminal ganglia [13]. Thus, it is possible that peripheral increases in oxytocin may have profound effects on vagal projections to the brain to influence behavior directly without entering the brain, but it could also potentially act via this route to promote endogenous oxytocin release within the brain. However, the potential for oxytocin to produce functional effects on the brain and behavior via these peripheral receptors has been largely overlooked. Additionally, it is possible that increased concentrations of oxytocin in the peripheral circulation may cross the blood–brain barrier to enter the brain after binding to receptors for advanced glycation end-products (RAGE) [14]. This recent discovery has added a further level of complexity to the field, and although experiments using genetically modified animals lacking an expression of RAGE have suggested that this can influence the ability of peripherally administered oxytocin to produce effects on the brain and behavior, it is still unclear whether RAGE might play a similar role in humans.

While the question of the precise mechanism whereby intranasally administered oxytocin might enter the brain, or otherwise influence its function, is still not completely established, what has become increasingly clear is that many of its observed functional effects do indeed appear to depend on increased peripheral concentrations rather than following direct entry into the brain. Three lines of evidence support this conclusion. The first is from a number of intranasal administration studies reporting that functional changes in the brain are associated with peripheral concentration changes [15], the second is from animal model and some human studies demonstrating that behavioral and brain effects can occur via routes of administration where direct entry of the peptide into the brain cannot occur (i.e., intravenous, subcutaneous, and intraperitoneal) (see [4]), and the third, and most recent, line of evidence, is from a study showing that neural effects following intranasal administration can be prevented using pre-treatment with a vasoconstrictor (otrivine), which considerably reduces increased peripheral blood concentrations but should not have any effect on preventing direct entry into the brain. This electroencephalography study found that the effects of a 24 IU intranasal oxytocin dose on increasing cross-frequency coupling in the brain between beta and delta frequencies (which may reflect neural effects of oxytocin on attention) could be almost completely eliminated by pre-treatment with the vasoconstrictor. Additionally, the neural effects of intranasal oxytocin in this study, in the absence of vasoconstrictor treatment, were also associated with increased concentrations of the peptide in the blood [16]. This latter finding effectively demonstrates that, while there may be some functional effects of intranasal oxytocin mediated via direct entry to the brain via the olfactory and trigeminal nerves, it is its increased concentrations in the peripheral circulation which may be of most importance [4].

Taken together, the above lines of evidence demonstrate that functional and potentially therapeutic effects of exogenously administered oxytocin can be achieved via routes which only increase peripheral vascular concentrations without directly entering the brain. For repeated dosing regimens in humans, particularly in pediatric or geriatric populations, intravenous, intramuscular, or subcutaneous injections may not be the best tolerated and this raises the question of whether an oral administration route of some kind might be optimal. While pills or capsules containing oxytocin may have some potential for allowing its absorption into the blood via the gastrointestinal tract, its acidic environment and the presence of peptidases render this method suboptimal [17]. Furthermore, swallowing pills can be problematic for both young children and geriatric patients. For example, for a related neuropeptide, vasopressin, its synthetic analogue desmopressin has been estimated to only achieve a bioavailability from 0.08 to 0.16% when given orally as a pill to be swallowed [18]. One animal study has reported that the absorption of oxytocin into the blood via the gastrointestinal tract can be enhanced following pre-treatment with proton pump inhibitors to reduce the acidic environment [19], but this is not a particularly viable option for long-term treatment in humans, especially in pediatric populations. On the other hand, oromucosal administration where oxytocin can be absorbed by blood vessels in the mouth is far more promising, provided that the method used can permit the peptide to remain in the mouth for a sufficient duration to allow maximum absorption into the blood and be well-tolerated by patients. The main challenge has, therefore, been to develop viable methods for the oromucosal administration of oxytocin which could overcome potential drawbacks of its physicochemical properties and be potentially used in clinical practice, particularly for pediatric and geriatric populations.

3. Oromucosal Administration of Peptides

The oral cavity is easily accessible for the administration of peptides and the main issue is to ensure that they remain in the mouth for a sufficient time to be absorbed into the blood via the mucosae. The two main pathways by which molecules diffuse passively across mucosal membranes are paracellular (passage between adjacent cells, i.e., intercellular) and transcellular (passage through cells) routes [11,20]. The paracellular diffusion route predominates for most lipophilic and hydrophilic molecules when they cross mucosal membranes with two types of pathways within the intercellular space; a hydrophobic pathway through the lipid bilayers and a parallel hydrophilic one along the narrow aqueous regions associated with lipid polar head groups. As the lipophilicity of a molecule increases, the propensity for its diffusion across the epithelial barrier also increases, although the main influence on diffusion is molecular weight, and other factors such as charge can also be important for non-polar molecules to cross the epithelial layer more effectively [11] (see Figure 1). A key advantage of the oromucosal administration of substances, as opposed to oral administation using pills, is that they can enter the blood directly and thereby reduce first-pass metabolism depletion by the liver and gut [20].

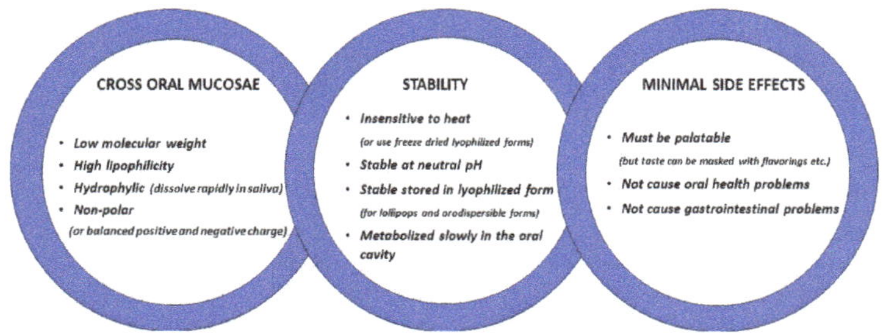

Figure 1. Ideal features for potential peptide-based drugs suitable for oromucosal administration.

The complex structure of peptides represents a challenge for their delivery via a mucosal route, as they have poor physicochemical stability, high molecular weight, and, often, low lipophilicity resulting in problems permeating mucosae and entering the blood [21]. The buccal and sublingual regions of the oral cavity are the main targets for oromucosal administration since they are non-keratinized and highly vascularized, and sub-lingual tissue has a limited number of epithelial cell layers [22]. Currently, there are three main approaches to the oromucosal delivery of drugs: orodispersal using fast-dissolving tablets, films, or gels; intra-oral sprays; and drugs incorporated into lollipops, gum, or chocolate. Of these three approaches, the most often clinically used to date has been the orodispersal method using tablets, films, or gels which dissolve in saliva in the oral cavity and do not require water for swallowing (see [23] for review). Originally, for example, an oromocosal tablet containing oxytocin was used to help induce labor [24,25], although intravenous administration is more effective and now preferred. Currently, only a single therapeutic peptide, desmopressin, a synthetic analogue of arginine vasopressin, is approved and used for oromucosal administration in the treatment of enuresis nocturna [26]. Desmopressin is approximately 10 times more potent as an anti-diuretic agent than vasopressin itself [27], although it has a similar molecular weight (1069 vs. 1084 Daltons). When administered sublingually as a lyophilized tablet, its bioavailability is reportedly only 0.25% [28] in contrast to 5–10% when administered via an intranasal route [29]. Desmopressin's effects on life-threatening hyponatremia are particularly associated with intranasal administration, which has led to the initial approval for its use intranasally being withdrawn by the FDA [30]. Therefore, desmopressin containing minitablets with a mucoadhesive film have been developed for buccal delivery which do not require swallowing, can improve compliance [31], and have a very low incidence of hyponatremia [28]. More recently, orodispersible films and gels have been developed which, when placed on the tongue or cheek, dissolve rapidly to release drugs into the oral cavity [23,32]. However, the substances incorporated into orodispersal mediums may be limited in terms of their concentration, released too fast, and/or swallowed before maximum absorption into the blood occurs, and compliance and tolerance in pediatric and geriatric populations in particular may be more problematic. Thus, the two other main methods for the oromucosal delivery of peptides and other substances, using intraoral sprays and medicated candies, may offer some advantages.

Development of Oromucosal Oxytocin Administration Using Lingual Spray and Medicated Lollipop 'Oxipop' Methodologies

Given that oxytocin is commercially available as an intranasal spray and licensed for use as a lactation enhancer in post-partum women (e.g., Sichuan Defeng, Pharmaceutical Co., Ltd., Chengdu, China), a first step into assessing its efficacy when given orally was to utilize a spray for administration by lingual application. The spray contains oxytocin acetate at a concentration of 4 IUs per 0.1 mL puff and is dissolved in 0.9% saline and stabilized using glycerol. Placebo sprays are identical in composition with the exception that the peptide is excluded. The same protocol was therefore adopted as for intranasal administration with 6 × 4 IU doses being self-administered under and on top of the tongue and with each spray being given at 30 s intervals to match the intranasal protocol (i.e., a total administration duration of 3 min). To maximize absorption, subjects were required to keep the spray in their mouth without swallowing until they self-administered the next dose [33–35]. Initially, in these studies, a pharmacokinetic assessment was carried out in 10 male adult male subjects with blood samples being taken at 15 min intervals before and for 105 min after the lingual administration. The profile of the altered blood concentrations, area under the curve (AUC), Tmax, and bioavailability measures are shown in Figure 2A–D and contrasted with those for 24 IU intranasal oxytocin. The absolute bioavailability was calculated using data for measurements of oxytocin concentrations in the patients' blood following a 10 min intravenous infusion of 10 IU taken from [15], with repeated samples being taken over a similar time course. For lingual administration following a 24 IU dose, the AUC for the altered plasma oxytocin concentrations was significantly less than that for the intranasal administration (mean ± SD 4.79 ± 3.38 (n = 10) vs. 11.93 ± 7.68 pg/mL/h (n = 27), p = 0.008), as was the absolute bioavailability (4.45 ± 3.51% vs. 11.07 ± 7.12%, p = 0.008). The calculated bioavailability for the intranasal administration was very similar to that using data from a previous published paper where a 40 IU dose of oxytocin was used (10.59 ± 7.95%—from [15]). For the time to reach maximum concentrations in blood (Tmax), the lingual administration was 34.5 ± 17.4 min compared with 26.61 ± 14.34 min for the intranasal administration and did not differ significantly (p = 0.159). This obviously contrasts with profiles following intravenous infusions, where blood concentrations rise immediately and sharply [15].

However, lingual sprays where subjects are required to deliberately retain the liquid in their mouth for a period of time to maximize absorption are also clearly not optimal in terms of patient compliance, particularly in pediatric subjects. In recent years, medicated chocolate and candy lollipops have also been increasingly used to administer a variety of substances ranging from vitamin and mineral supplements to antibiotics and pain killers (see [36–38]). Typical lollipop formulations tend to be either hard or soft forms of sugar-free candy, with the substance for medication being incorporated into the candy during the heating stage of its formation. The candy lollipops in particular have a number of advantages for drug administration via oromucosal absorption since, during sucking, they are in constant close contact with the roof of the mouth and tongue and are pleasant to eat, especially for children. The two main disadvantages of such medicated lollipops are that, firstly, since a heating process is used in their conventional manufacture, this precludes using them for heat-sensitive drugs and, secondly, if the drug used has a strong bitter or unpalatable taste, this can also be a problem. Thus, the conventional strategy of incorporating drugs into the whole of a lollipop using a heating process is not suitable for peptides, which are typically heat-sensitive and would therefore degrade using such a strategy. To overcome this problem, the novel step was taken of freeze-drying oxytocin onto the surface of the lollipop to create 'oxipops' rather than trying to incorporate it into the whole lollipop. This had the dual advantage that current commercial sugar-free lollipops could be utilized and that it maximized the peptide being dissolved by the saliva as the child or adult sucked the lollipop with the whole dose being released slowly without the requirement that all of the lollipop needed to be consumed, since the oxytocin dose was only on the surface. These commercial lollipops typically use xylitol as a sweetener, which is widely accepted to be a safe form of low-calorie sweetener that does not cause insulin spikes and can actually promote oral hygiene and even immunocompetence [39]. Clearly, both children and adults may exhibit distinct taste preferences which could potentially influence compliance, although this can be overcome through the use of different flavor alternatives (current options have included orange, grape, pineapple, and pear). Oxytocin does not have a distinctive taste per se, so there is no problem in this respect.

The 'oxipop' protocol involves firstly dissolving different peptide concentrations in volumes from 0.1 to 0.2 mL of 0.9% saline (with glycerol added as a preservative) and then freeze-drying the lollipops using two standard cycles lasting around a total of 48 h in a commercial freeze-dryer [40]. The resultant 'oxipops' are then sealed and placed in a fridge (2–8 deg C) until required (see Figure 3). The 'oxipops' can be stored stably for 3–6 months although possibly for longer periods. The freeze-drying process causes the formation of a white residue on the surface of the lollipop and so it is important for the purposes of blinding in placebo-controlled experiments to also produce placebo lollipops using application of the saline and glycerol solution without the peptide and using the same freeze-drying process. Sucking the 'oxipops' for a total of 3 min can achieve similar increases in plasma concentrations of oxytocin as does direct administration of the same concentration over the same time period using lingual sprays (see Figure 1). The AUC is 4.74 ± 2.41 pg/mL/h ($n = 11$, $p = 0.004$ vs. intranasal and $p = 0.97$ vs. lingual), with an estimated bioavailability of $4.4 \pm 2.23\%$ ($p = 0.008$ vs. intranasal and $p = 0.97$ vs. lingual), thereby confirming in vivo that a similar concentration of oxytocin is being released into the oral cavity and absorbed into the blood as with a direct lingual spray using the same dose. The Tmax was 39.5 ± 21.5, which is not significantly different than that for lingual or intranasal administration (Kruskall–Wallis ANOVA, $p = 0.095$).

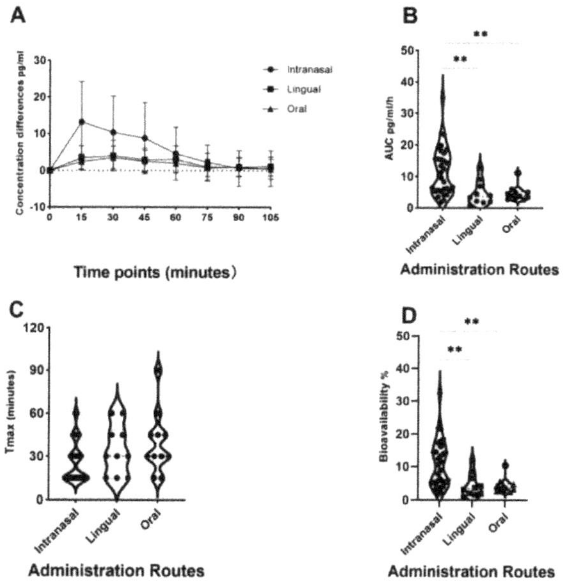

Figure 2. Comparison of pharmacodynamic profiles of oxytocin concentrations in blood following intranasal, lingual, and oral (medicated lollipops, 'oxipops') administration of 24 IU oxytocin. (**A**) Changes in plasma oxytocin concentrations following 24 IU dose administration, means ± SD. Violin plots and individual data points (black dots) showing (**B**) areas under the curve (AUC) (**C**), Tmax, and (**D**) absolute bioavailability. ** $p < 0.01$, for post-hoc tests following significant ($p < 0.001$ for both AUC and bioavailability) one-way ANOVAs (Kruskall–Wallis). Data are taken from [16,33,39]. For bioavailability calculations, plasma concentrations of oxytocin following intravenous infusions are taken from a publication by another group who have made their data publically available [15].

As expected, the saliva concentrations of oxytocin increased considerably after sucking the 'oxipop' for 3 min (from a baseline mean ± SD of 8.70 ± 4.58 pg/mL to = 231.8 ± 116.9 pg/mL, $p < 0.001$ 30 min after sucking the 'oxipop') and remained significantly elevated even 2 h afterwards (30.54 ± 19.12 pg/mL $p < 0.001$) (see Figure 4 and [39]). Interestingly, the pharmacodynamic profiles were similar to those reported for saliva oxytocin concentrations following intranasal administration, reinforcing suggestions that, with the use of nasal sprays, a large proportion of the peptide leaks down into the oral cavity, resulting in prolonged increases in saliva for 2–7 h [41–44]. While there was not a good relationship between the saliva and plasma concentrations of oxytocin at baseline (Spearman r = −0.212, p = 0.5563), in agreement with previous studies [5,45], following oral oxytocin administration using 'oxipops', this became positive by 30 min (r = 0.467, p = 0.174) and by 2 h was significant (r = 0.709, p = 0.0216 = see Figure 3), indicating that alterations in the saliva concentrations post administration were a reasonably accurate guide to likely increases in blood. At this stage it is not known if these peripheral changes following the oromucosal administration of oxytocin also result in increases in cerebrospinal fluid concentrations similar to those reported following intranasal oxytocin [46].

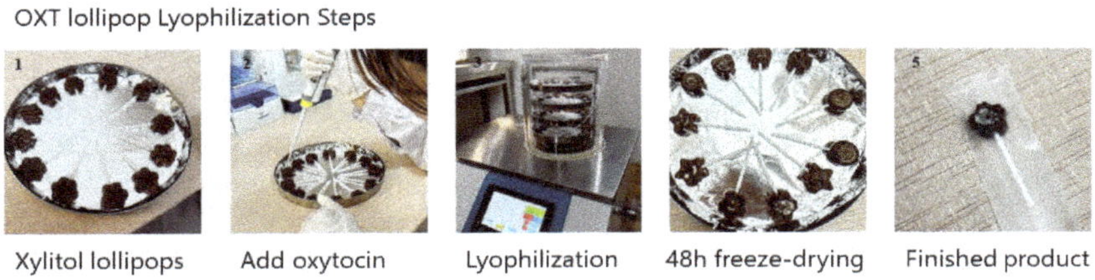
OXT lollipop Lyophilization Steps
1
2
3
5
Xylitol lollipops
Add oxytocin
Lyophilization
48h freeze-drying
Finished product

Figure 3. Method (left to right) for producing sugar-free (xylitol) lollipop candies with oxytocin acetate (OXT) freeze-dried on one surface of the lollipop ('oxipops').

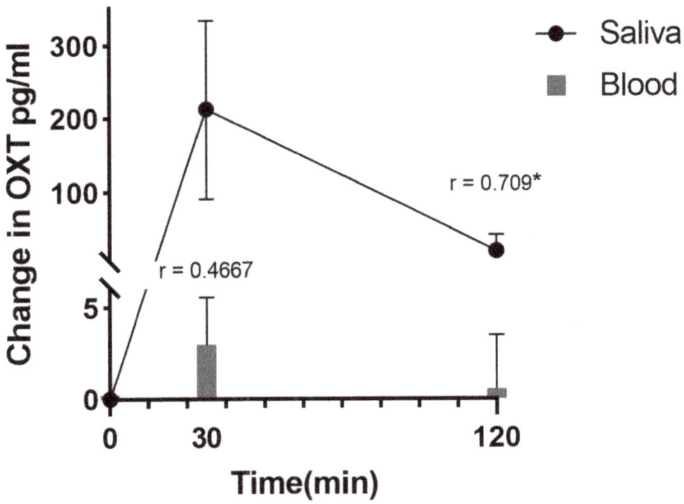

Figure 4. Changes in saliva (line) relative to plasma (histograms) concentrations of oxytocin (OXT) 30 min and 2 h following administration of 24 IU oral oxytocin by medicated lollipop, 'oxipops'. Means ± SDs are plotted. Correlations (Spearman) between changes in saliva and plasma concentrations are also indicated. * $p < 0.05$.

4. Neural and Behavioral Effects of Oromucosal Administration of Oxytocin

A number of proof-of-concept studies have been conducted in human participants where the efficacy of single doses of oxytocin given by intranasal, lingual, and oral 'oxipop' routes was compared using both brain and behavioral measures. The first of these studies used a neural biomarker for the effects of intranasal oxytocin in adult male subjects, where it has been shown to decrease the responses of the amygdala to emotional faces [47,48], although it has been shown to increase them in females [49]. Findings demonstrated that the lingual administration of oxytocin increased rather than decreased amygdala responses in males and also tended to increase them in females. Additionally, lingual oxytocin increased the responses of the putamen (a brain reward region) in both males [34] and females [50], whereas intranasal oxytocin only did so in females. However, overall, lingual and intranasal oxytocin both appeared to influence neural responses to emotional faces, although with some route-dependent differences which might possibly have been due to the fact that increased oxytocin concentrations were greater after intranasal, compared to lingual, administration. Additionally, 24 IU of both intranasal and lingual oxytocin produce a similar facilitation of the perceived pleasantness of soft, caress-like touch, but not of medium pressure touch, as well as increased responses in brain reward (orbitofrontal cortex) and social cognition (superior temporal gyrus) processing regions [33]. Finally, a series of studies investigating the effects of oxytocin on top-down compared with bottom-up attention control found equivalent effects of 24 IU doses administered intranasally, lingually, and via 'oxipops' on top-down attention control, particularly in relation to social stimuli but also to some extent for non-social ones, using an anti-saccade task [35,40]. In this task, subjects were instructed to direct their eye movement (saccade) from a central point either towards (prosaccade) or away (anti-saccade) from a social or non-social stimulus. In general, subjects found it hard to look away from the social stimulus (anti-saccade), made more errors, and were slower to respond relative to when asked to look towards stimuli (pro-saccade). All three routes of oxytocin administration equivalently increased the number of errors subjects made when instructed to look away from stimuli and increased the time taken to look away from social stimuli. As such, this is a very sensitive task for measuring the facilitatory effects of oxytocin on the top-down control of attention and particularly social attention, which has important therapeutic potential in disorders where individuals exhibit impaired attention to social cues.

5. Discussion and Future Potential Developments and Applications

The overall conclusion from the current review is that the oromucosal administration of oxytocin either using lingual spray or medicated lollipops ('oxipops') can produce reliably increased concentrations of the peptide in the peripheral vasculature, and similar functional effects were observed as for the same dose administered intranasally. The timing of peak concentrations of oxytocin were similar for intranasal, lingual spray, and oral 'oxipop' administration routes at around 30 min. On the other hand, the estimated bioavailability of the peptide delivered via the oromucosal routes was around 4.5% compared with around 11% after intranasal administration. The difference in bioavailability between the intranasal and oromucosal routes could reflect greater absorption of the peptide into blood across the nasal mucosa, but since concentrations were additionally greatly increased in saliva for a long duration after intranasal administration, it might also reflect combined absorption across both nasal and oral mucosae.

While there is still the possibility that some functional effects of the intranasal administration of oxytocin might be mediated via its direct entry into the brain via the olfactory and trigeminal nerves, which could not be achieved by an oromucosal route, evidence to date supports the conclusion that many functional effects are mediated by increased blood concentrations [4,16,33–35,40,50]. Most notably, in a recent study where the ability of intranasally administered oxytocin to enter the peripheral circulation was greatly reduced by the pre-administration of a vasoconstrictor (otrivine), the functional effects of a 24 IU intranasal oxytocin dose were almost completely eliminated. This latter finding effectively demonstrated that, while some functional effects of intranasal oxytocin might still be mediated following direct entry to the brain via the olfactory and trigeminal nerves, the increased concentrations in the peripheral circulation are likely to be of the most importance functionally. As such, this renders the potential therapeutic efficacy of the oromucosal administration of oxytocin to be at least equivalent to that of intranasal administration, although possibly actually improved since the oromucosal route offers considerable practical advantages (see [26]). The small size of nasal passages in young children and problems due to nasal blockages during colds or allergic conditions, coupled with the necessity for administration being given by caregivers or medical staff rather than by the individual themselves, makes the intranasal administration of oxytocin, or any other substance, potentially problematic, particularly in pediatric and geriatric populations. Using the novel freeze-drying protocol for oxytocin on the surface of sugar-free lollipops to create 'oxipops' also makes dissolving it into the mouth both rapid and prolonged (the 'oxipop' only needs to be sucked for around 3 min) and has the advantage of being perceived as extremely pleasant by the recipient. A potential drawback of the oral administration of oxytocin, similar to intranasal administration, is that a large amount of the peptide is swallowed and enters the gastrointestinal system. No studies to date using either acute or chronic doses of intranasal oxytocin have reported any significant gastrointestinal side effects and similarly acute doses of oromucosally administered peptide have not been reported to cause problems. Possibly, this reflects the rapid metabolism of oxytocin in the acidic conditions present in the gastrointestinal system.

To date, only the most soluble form of oxytocin, oxytocin acetate, which is soluble up to 5 mg/mL, has been used for oromucosal administration. Evidence suggests that, following administration via an 'oxipop', saliva concentrations remain elevated for at least 2 h and probably much longer given observations from intranasal administration studies. Thus, at this stage, using more stable forms of the peptide may not be that advantageous, although recent studies using the intranasal administration of a more stable analog suggest that the optimum dose required might be considerably reduced (TTA-121 [7]). Therefore, there may be some advantages to using formulations designed to enhance the stability of the peptide. Given that the mucosal barriers in the mouth do reduce the effective absorption of native oxytocin into the peripheral blood stream [11], there may be advantages in producing formulations with an improved ability to permeate the oral mucosae and thereby more efficiently increase blood concentrations. For example, penetrant enhancers such as fatty acids, surfactants, cholates, lauric acid, and alcohols or emulsions in the form of deformable liposomes and nanoparticles have been used as well as materials such as polyacrylic acid, chitosan, cellulose derivatives, alginate, and hyaluronic acid (see reviews [51–53]). However, the main issues limiting the passage of oxytocin across mucosal barriers would appear to be its high molecular weight and low lipophilicity [11], and so the development of peptidomimetic drugs which can circumvent these issues may be a more promising future approach.

Another possibility is that 'oxipops' could additionally contain beneficial concentrations of essential vitamins and minerals. Lollipops containing vitamin C or D and zinc are, for example, currently commercially available for the potential facilitation of immunocompetance. Zinc concentrations are often low in autistic children [53–55] and are associated with symptom severity [56]. There has also been research indicating that oxytocin may become more stable after binding to zinc and that low levels of zinc may actually impair the ability of oxytocin to bind to its receptor [57,58].

At this stage, only the effects of single doses of oromucosally administered oxytocin have been assessed on increased concentrations in blood and saliva and on neural and behavioral effects. Potential therapeutic effects of oxytocin in relation to autism or other disorders are likely to require chronic periods of administration over periods of weeks or months and, to date, this has only been investigated using intranasal administration [5–8, 47]. Clearly, establishing potential therapeutic effects of chronic oxytocin using oromucosal administration is a priority for future research.

The precise mechanism whereby increased peripheral concentrations of oxytocin following oromucosal administration might influence the brain and behavior is also unclear, just as it is for intranasal administration. At this point, the most likely mechanism is via acting on receptors in the vagal system to both influence neural circuitry controlling behavioral functions and possibly additionally an increased release of endogenous peptide within the brain. However, there still remains the possibility that some oxytocin could be transported from the blood into the brain after binding to RAGE and crossing the blood–brain barrier [14]. It will also be important to establish whether there are similar inverted-U dose-dependency issues for oromucosal administration similar to intranasal oxytocin [7,48]. Additionally, for chronic dosing protocols, studies will need to determine whether an infrequent every-other-day dosing strategy produces improved functional effects compared to a more frequent one where doses are given once or twice a day in line with recent findings for repeated doses of intranasal oxytocin [5,47]. However, given increasing evidence for potential therapeutic effects of oxytocin in a range of disorders, including autism, anxiety, depression, schizophrenia, and chronic pain [5–10], the potential for using oromucosal administration as an intervention will be important to establish in future clinical trials.

While the current review has specifically focused on the development of the oromucosal administration of oxytocin to influence brain and behavioral functions, particularly through the use of a freeze-drying protocol where the peptide is simply present on the surface of a lollipop, this strategy has a wider potential application for the administration of oxytocin in other contexts. While intravenous oxytocin infusions and intramuscular injections are used routinely in developed countries for the management of labor and post-partum haemorrhage, in under-resourced, third-world countries, administration via these routes requires skilled medical staff and can be less available and affordable. Post-partum haemorrhage occurs after around 10% of births and is a major contributor to maternal mortality (35–50% of cases) [59,60]. Additionally, given that oxytocin is more stable in its dry form than in solution, there may be advantages for longer-term storage in hot climates with a limited availability of refrigeration. Indeed, one study has reported that lyophilized oxytocin is stable for 12 months when stored at 40 deg. C whereas, in solution, it degrades significantly after a month [60]. Freeze-dried oxytocin for oromucosal administration may therefore offer both practical and cost advantages.

While oromucosal administration using medicated candies is still a relatively novel strategy and has yet to be fully established for other suitable candidate peptide or non-peptide drugs, it may open up future possible avenues for administering either acute or long-term medication to individuals where other routes are less well-tolerated. In recent years for example, there has been a considerable growth in the number of peptide-based therapeutic drugs, with currently > 80 having been approved for use [61]. Peptide drugs offer several advantages over small molecules, including a heightened target specificity and potency and reduced side effects, although few have been developed for oromucosal administration. A full consideration of the current numerous peptide-based drugs, other than oxytocin, is beyond the scope of the current review and has been covered in another publication (see [61]). As outlined in Figure 1, the two obvious potential limitations for the oromucosal administration of peptide-based drugs as opposed to small molecules are that high molecular weights may result in poor penetration through the oral mucosae and that they are often metabolized too rapidly. It is therefore likely that, in a number of cases, more stable peptidomimetic drugs with a smaller molecular weight would have to be developed in order for them to be used with oromucosal administration. There is also the potential issue of peptide-based drugs being unpalatable or causing gastrointestinal problems following their ingestion. A further important issue will be to ensure the long-term stability of drugs for storage prior to use although refrigeration, storage in the dark, and vacuum-sealing should be effective in most cases. Where the refrigerated storage of heat-sensitive compounds is not readily available, they may still be more stable in a dry lyophilized form than in solution, although the addition of chemical stabilizers is another option.

Future developments in technology for the intraoral delivery of drugs may additionally provide alternatives to medicated lollipops. For example, advances in pharmaceutical technology and polymer science are increasingly allowing the manufacture of new types of intraoral administration using sprays, films, tablets, wafers, chewing gums, buccal patches, and bioadhesive tablets to deliver a wide variety of both non-peptide and peptide drugs (see [23,62]). For example, in terms of the oral delivery of peptides, an aerosol droplet application for an insulin delivery system based on a colloidal liquid formulation has recently been developed (Oralin®, Generex Biotechnology Corp., Toronto, ON, Canada) which utilizes a mixture of surfactants as stabilizers and permeation enhancers. This was found to be effective for the rapid oral absorption of insulin and control of glucose levels, and diabetic patients were more compliant than when using the traditional subcutaneous injection method [63]. It is therefore likely that the oromucosal administration of medications will become more widely established in future.

6. Conclusions

In conclusion, since many therapeutic effects of oxytocin appear to be due increasing its peripheral concentrations, oromucosal delivery, particularly using a novel medicated lollipop, 'oxipop', approach, may be an effective way of optimally increasing blood concentrations and offers considerable practical advantages over intravenous or intranasal routes, most notably for chronic use in pediatric and geriatric populations but possibly also for the management of labor and post-partum haemorrhage in some contexts. While the resultant absolute bioavailability using the native peptide is relatively low, concentrations remain significantly elevated for at least 2 h or more. Importantly, robust functional effects on the brain and behavior using acute doses have been observed using a number of different paradigms, although future research is needed to assess dose-dependency and dose-frequency effects. Additionally, using techniques to increase the stability of the peptide and penetrant enhancers to aid its absorption into circulation may be able to improve functional effects, particularly in the context of chronic administration regimes.

Author Contributions: Conceptualization: K.M.K., W.Z. and D.X.; Writing—original draft preparation, K.M.K.; writing—review and editing: D.X., C.L., J.K., S.Y., W.Z. and K.M.K.; visualization: D.X. and K.M.K. All authors have read and agreed to the published version of the manuscript.

Funding: This research was supported by Key Technological Projects of Guangdong Province "Development of New Tools for Diagnosis and Treatment of Autism" grant number 2018B030335001 (K.M.K.) and UESTC High-End Expert Project Development grant number Y0301902610100201 (K.M.K.). Natural Science Foundation of Sichuan Province grant number 2022NSFC1375 (W.Z.).

Institutional Review Board Statement: Not applicable.

Informed Consent Statement: Not applicable.

Data Availability Statement: No new data in this paper.

Conflicts of Interest: The authors declare no conflicts of interest.

References

1. Hermesch, A.C.; Kernberg, A.S.; Layoun, V.R.; Caughey, A.B. Oxytocin: Physiology, pharmacology, and clinical application for labor management. *Am. J. Obstet. Gynecol.* 2023, *in press*. [CrossRef]
2. Gimpl, G.; Fahrenholz, F. The oxytocin receptor system: Structure, function, and regulation. *Physiol. Rev.* **2001**, *81*, 629–683. [CrossRef]
3. Kendrick, K.M.; Guastella, A.J.; Becker, B. Overview of human oxytocin research. *Curr. Top. Behav. Neurosci.* **2017**, *35*, 321–348.
4. Yao, S.; Kendrick, K.M. Effects of Intranasal Administration of Oxytocin and Vasopressin on Social Cognition and Potential Routes and Mechanisms of Action. *Pharmaceutics* **2022**, *14*, 323. [CrossRef]
5. Le, J.; Zhang, L.; Zhao, W.; Zhu, S.; Lan, C.; Kou, J.; Zhang, Q.; Zhang, Y.; Li, Q.; Chen, Z.; et al. Infrequent Intranasal Oxytocin Followed by Positive Social Interaction Improves Symptoms in Autistic Children: A Pilot Randomized Clinical Trial. *Psychother. Psychosom.* **2022**, *91*, 335–347. [CrossRef]
6. Parker, K.J.; Oztan, O.; Libove, R.A.; Sumiyoshi, R.D.; Jackson, L.P.; Karhson, D.S.; Summers, J.E.; Hinman, K.E.; Motonaga, K.S.; Phillips, J.M.; et al. Intranasal oxytocin treatment for social deficits and biomarkers of response in children with autism. *Proc. Natl. Acad. Sci. USA* **2017**, *114*, 8119–8124. [CrossRef]
7. Yamasue, H.; Kojima, M.; Kuwabara, H.; Kuroda, M.; Matsumoto, K.; Kanai, C.; Inada, N.; Owada, K.; Ochi, K.; Ono, N.; et al. Effect of a novel nasal oxytocin spray with enhanced bioavailability on autism: A randomized trial. *Brain* **2022**, *145*, 490–499. [CrossRef]
8. Yatawara, C.J.; Einfeld, S.L.; Hickie, I.B.; Davenport, T.A.; Guastella, A.J. The effect of oxytocin nasal spray on social interaction deficits observed in young children with autism: A randomized clinical crossover trial. *Mol. Psychiatry* **2016**, *21*, 1225–1231. [CrossRef]

9. De Cagna, F.; Fusar-Poli, L.; Damiani, S.; Rocchetti, M.; Giovanna, G.; Mori, A.; Politi, P.; Brondino, N. The Role of Intranasal Oxytocin in Anxiety and Depressive Disorders: A Systematic Review of Randomized Controlled Trials. *Clin. Psychopharmacol. Neurosci.* **2019**, *17*, 1–11. [CrossRef]
10. Bharadwaj, V.N.; Tzabazis, A.Z.; Klukinov, M.; Manering, N.A.; Yeomans, D.C. Intranasal Administration for Pain: Oxytocin and Other Polypeptides. *Pharmaceutics* **2021**, *13*, 1088. [CrossRef] [PubMed]
11. Van Eyk, A.D.; Vand der Bijl, P.; Moll, L.M. Physicochemical characteristics of molecules and their diffusion across human vaginal mucosa. *Eur. J. Inflamm.* **2008**, *2*, 65–71. [CrossRef]
12. Moreno-López, Y.; Martínez-Lorenzana, G.; Condés-Lara, M.; Rojas-Piloni, G. Identification of oxytocin receptor in the dorsal horn and nociceptive dorsal root ganglion neurons. *Neuropeptides* **2013**, *47*, 117–123. [CrossRef]
13. Warfvinge, K.; Krause, D.N.; Maddahi, A.; Grell, A.S.; Edvinsson, J.C.; Haanes, K.A.; Edvinsson, L. Oxytocin as a regulatory neuropeptide in the trigeminovascular system: Localization, expression and function of oxytocin and oxytocin receptors. *Cephalalgia* **2020**, *40*, 1283–1295. [CrossRef]
14. Yamamoto, Y.; Higashida, H. RAGE regulates oxytocin transport into the brain. *Commun. Biol.* **2020**, *3*, 70. [CrossRef]
15. Martins, D.A.; Mazibuko, N.; Zelaya, F.; Vasilakopoulou, S.; Loveridge, J.; Oates, A.; Maltezos, S.; Mehta, M.; Wastling, S.; Howard, M.; et al. Effects of route of administration on oxytocin-induced changes in regional cerebral blood flow in humans. *Nat. Commun.* **2020**, *11*, 1160. [CrossRef]
16. Yao, S.; Chen, Y.; Zhuang, Q.; Zhang, Y.; Lan, C.; Zhu, S.; Becker, B.; Kendrick, K.M. Sniffing oxytocin: Nose to brain or nose to blood? *Mol. Psychiatry* **2023**, *28*, 3083–3091. [CrossRef]
17. Maher, S.; Mrsny, R.J.; Brayden, D.J. Intestinal permeation enhancers for oral peptide delivery. *Adv. Drug Deliv. Rev.* **2016**, *106*, 277–319. [CrossRef]
18. Hashim, H.; Abrams, P. Desmopressin for the treatment of adult nocturia. *Future Med. LTD* **2008**, *5*, 667–683. [CrossRef]
19. Maejima, Y.; Horita, S.; Otsuka, A.; Hidema, S.; Nishimori, K.; Shimomura, K. Oral oxytocin delivery with proton pump inhibitor pretreatment decreases food intake. *Peptides* **2020**, *128*, 170312. [CrossRef]
20. Prego, C.; Garcia, M.; Torres, D.; Alonso, M.J. Transmucosal macromolecular drug delivery. *J. Control. Release* **2005**, *101*, 151–162. [CrossRef]
21. Frokjaer, S.; Otzen, D.E. Protein drug stability: A formulation challenge. *Nat. Rev. Drug Discov.* **2005**, *4*, 298–306. [CrossRef]
22. Rathbone, M.J.; Drummond, B.K.; Tucker, I.G. The oral cavity as a site for systemic drug delivery. *Adv. Drug Deliv. Rev.* **1994**, *13*, 1–22. [CrossRef]
23. Bastos, F.; Pinto, A.C.; Nunes, A.; Simões, S. Oromucosal products—Market landscape and innovative technologies: A review. *J. Control. Release* **2022**, *348*, 305–320. [CrossRef]
24. Mehta, A.C. Buccal and oral drugs: Induction of labour. *Acta. Chir. Hung.* **1986**, *27*, 157–163.
25. Westergaard, J.G.; Lange, A.P.; Pedersen, G.T.; Secher, N.J. Oral oxytocics for induction of labor. A randomized study of prostaglandin E2 tablets and demoxytocin resoriblets. *Acta. Obstet. Gynecol. Scand.* **1983**, *62*, 103–110. [CrossRef]
26. Gleeson, J.P.; Fein, K.C.; Whitehead, K.A. Oral delivery of peptide therapeutics in infants: Challenges and opportunities. *Adv. Drug Deliv. Rev.* **2021**, *173*, 112–124. [CrossRef]
27. Sharman, A.; Low, J. Vasopressin and its role in critical care. *Cont. Ed. Anaesth. Crit. Care Pain* **2008**, *8*, 134–137.26. [CrossRef]
28. van Kerrebroeck, P.; Nørgaard, J.P. Desmopressin for the treatment of primary nocturnal enuresis. *Pediatr. Health* **2009**, *3*, 311–327. [CrossRef]
29. Schiele, J.T.; Quinzler, R.; Klimm, H.-D.; Pruszydlo, M.G.; Haefeli, W.E. Difficulties swallowing solid oral dosage forms in a general practice population: Prevalence, causes, and relationship to dosage forms. *Eur. J. Clin. Pharmacol.* **2013**, *69*, 937–948. [CrossRef]
30. FDA. 2020. Available online: https://www.fda.gov/safety/recalls-market-withdrawals-safety-alerts/ferring-us-issues-voluntary-nationwide-recall-ddavpr-nasal-spray-10-mcg01ml-desmopressin-acetate (accessed on 8 May 2020).
31. Kottke, D.; Burckhardt, B.B.; Knaab, T.C.; Breitkreutz, J.; Fischer, B. Development and evaluation of a composite dosage form containing desmopressin acetate for buccal administration. *Int. J. Pharm. X* **2021**, *9*, 100082. [CrossRef]
32. Hoffmann, E.M.; Breitenbach, A.; Breitkreutz, J. Advances in orodispersible films for drug delivery. *Exp. Op. Drug Deliv.* **2011**, *8*, 299–316. [CrossRef]
33. Chen, Y.; Zou, H.; Hou, X.; Lan, C.; Wang, J.; Qing, Y.; Chen, W.; Yao, S.; Kendrick, K.M. Oxytocin administration enhances pleasantness and neural responses to gentle stroking but not moderate pressure social touch by increasing peripheral concentrations. *Elife* **2023**, *12*, e85847. [CrossRef]
34. Kou, J.; Lan, C.; Zhang, Y.; Wang, Q.; Zhou, F.; Zhao, Z.; Montag, C.; Yao, S.; Becker, B.; Kendrick, K.M. In the nose or on the tongue? Contrasting motivational effects of oral and intranasal oxytocin on arousal and reward during social processing. *Transl. Psychiatry* **2021**, *11*, 94. [CrossRef]
35. Zhuang, Q.; Zheng, X.; Yao, S.; Zhao, W.; Becker, B.; Xu, X.; Kendrick, K.M. Oral Administration of Oxytocin, Like Intranasal Administration, Decreases Top-Down Social Attention. *Int. J. Neuropsychopharmacol.* **2022**, *25*, 912–923. [CrossRef]
36. Pawar, P.G.; Darekar, A.B.; Saudagar, R.B. Medicated chocolate and lollipops: A novel drug delivery system for pediatric patients. *Pharma. Sci. Monitor.* **2018**, *9*, 677–696.
37. Shetty, S.; Kamath, K.; Shabaraya, R.; Miranda, F.C. Design and development of medicated lollipop containing albendazole. *Am. J. Pharmatech. Res.* **2019**, *9*, 275–285. [CrossRef]
38. Tangso, K.J.; Ho, Q.P.; Boyd, B.J. Confectionery-based dose forms. *Curr. Drug Deliv.* **2015**, *12*, 56–62. [CrossRef]

39. Gasmi Benahmed, A.; Gasmi, A.; Arshad, M.; Shanaida, M.; Lysiuk, R.; Peana, M.; Pshyk-Titko, I.; Adamiv, S.; Shanaida, Y.; Bjørklund, G. Health benefits of xylitol. *Appl. Microbiol. Biotechnol.* **2020**, *104*, 7225–7237. [CrossRef]
40. Xu, D.; Li, Q.; Zhuang, Q.; Zhang, Y.; Yao, S.; Zhao, W.; Kendrick, K.M. Oro-mucosal administration of oxytocin using medicated lollipops alters social attention, similar to intranasal and lingual routes: Implications for therapeutic use. *Front. Neurosci.* **2022**, *16*, 1022101. [CrossRef]
41. Daughters, K.; Manstead, A.S.R.; Hubble, K.; Rees, A.; Thapar, A.; van Goozen, S.H.M. Salivary Oxytocin Concentrations in Males following Intranasal Administration of Oxytocin: A Double-Blind, CrossOver Study. *PLoS ONE* **2015**, *10*, e0145104. [CrossRef]
42. van Ijzendoorn, M.H.; Bhandari, R.; van der Veen, R.; Grewen, K.M.; Bakermans-Kranenburg, M.J. Elevated Salivary Levels of Oxytocin Persist More than 7 h after Intranasal Administration. *Front. Neurosci.* **2012**, *6*, 174. [CrossRef]
43. Weisman, O.; Zagoory-Sharon, O.; Feldman, R. Intranasal oxytocin administration is reflected in human saliva. *Psychoneuroendocrinology* **2012**, *37*, 1582–1586. [CrossRef]
44. Weisman, O.; Schneiderman, I.; Zagoory-Sharon, O.; Feldman, R. Salivary vasopressin increases following intranasal oxytocin administration. *Peptides* **2013**, *40*, 99–103. [CrossRef]
45. Martins, D.; Gabay, A.S.; Mehta, M.; Paloyelis, Y. Salivary and plasmatic oxytocin are not reliable trait markers of the physiology of the oxytocin system in humans. *Elife* **2020**, *9*, e62456. [CrossRef]
46. Striepens, N.; Kendrick, K.M.; Hanking, V.; Landgraf, R.; Wüllner, U.; Maier, W.; Hurlemann, R. Elevated cerebrospinal fluid and blood concentrations of oxytocin following its intranasal administration in humans. *Sci. Rep.* **2013**, *3*, 3440. [CrossRef]
47. Kou, J.; Zhang, Y.; Zhou, F.; Sindermann, C.; Montag, C.; Becker, B.; Kendrick, K.M. A randomized trial shows dose-frequency and genotype may determine the therapeutic efficacy of intranasal oxytocin. *Psychol. Med.* **2022**, *52*, 1959–1968. [CrossRef]
48. Spengler, F.B.; Schultz, J.; Scheele, D.; Essel, M.; Maier, W.; Heinrichs, M.; Hurlemann, R. Kinetics and Dose Dependency of Intranasal Oxytocin Effects on Amygdala Reactivity. *Biol. Psychiatry* **2017**, *82*, 885–894. [CrossRef]
49. Lieberz, J.; Scheele, D.; Spengler, F.B.; Matheisen, T.; Schneider, L.; Stoffel-Wagner, B.; Kinfe, T.M.; Hurlemann, R. Kinetics of oxytocin effects on amygdala and striatal reactivity vary between women and men. *Neuropsychopharmacology* **2020**, *45*, 1134–1140. [CrossRef]
50. Lan, C.; Chen, Y.; Zhang, Y.; Kou, J.; Huang, L.; Xu, T.; Yang, X.; Xu, D.; Yang, W.; Kendrick, K.M.; et al. Oral Oxytocin Facilitates Responses to Emotional Faces in Reward and Emotional-Processing Networks in Females. *Neuroendocrinology* **2023**, *113*, 957–970. [CrossRef]
51. Guo, Y.; Singh, A.P. Emerging strategies for enhancing buccal and sublingual administration of nutraceuticals and pharmaceuticals. *J. Drug Deliv. Sci. Tech.* **2019**, *52*, 440–451. [CrossRef]
52. Mazzinelli, E.; Favuzzi, I.; Arcovito, A.; Castagnola, R.; Fratocchi, G.; Mordente, A.; Nocca, G. Oral Mucosa Models to Evaluate Drug Permeability. *Pharmaceutics* **2023**, *15*, 1559. [CrossRef]
53. Nugrahadi, P.P.; Hinrichs, W.L.J.; Frijlink, H.W.; Schöneich, C. Designing formulation strategies for enhanced stability of therapeutic peptides in aqueous solutions: A review. *Pharmaceutics* **2023**, *15*, 935. [CrossRef]
54. Goyal, D.K.; Neil, J.R.; Simmons, S.D.; Mansab, F.; Benjamin, S.; Pitfield, V.; Boulet, S.; Miyan, J. Zinc Deficiency in Autism: A Controlled Study. *Insights Biomed.* **2019**, *4*. [CrossRef]
55. Alsufiani, H.M.; Alkhanbashi, A.S.; Laswad, N.A.B.; Bakhadher, K.K.; Alghamdi, S.A.; Tayeb, H.O.; Tarazi, F.I. Zinc deficiency and supplementation in autism spectrum disorder and Phelan-McDermid syndrome. *J. Neurosci. Res.* **2022**, *100*, 970–978. [CrossRef]
56. Wu, J.; Wang, D.; Yan, L.; Jia, M.; Zhang, J.; Han, S.; Han, J.; Wang, J.; Chen, X.; Zhang, R. Associations of essential element serum concentrations with autism spectrum disorder. *Environ. Sci. Pollut. Res. Int.* **2022**, *29*, 88962–88971. [CrossRef]
57. Liu, D.; Seuthe, A.B.; Ehrler, O.T.; Zhang, X.; Wyttenbach, T.; Hsu, J.F.; Bowers, M.T. Oxytocin-receptor binding: Why divalent metals are essential. *J. Am. Chem. Soc.* **2005**, *127*, 2024–2025. [CrossRef]
58. Avanti, C.; Hinrichs, W.L.; Casini, A.; Eissens, A.C.; Van Dam, A.; Kedrov, A.; Driessen, A.J.M.; Frijlink, H.W.; Permentier, H.P. The formation of oxytocin dimers is suppressed by the zinc-aspartate-oxytocin complex. *J. Pharm. Sci.* **2013**, *102*, 1734–1741. [CrossRef]
59. Khan, K.S.; Wojdyla, D.; Say, L.; Gülmezoglu, A.M.; Van Look, P.F.A. WHO analysis of causes of maternal death: A systematic review. *Lancet* **2006**, *367*, 1066–1074. [CrossRef]
60. Zhu, C.; Estrada, M.; White, J.; Lal, M. Heat-stable sublingual oxytocin tablets as a potential needle-free approach for preventing postpartum hemorrhage in low-resource settings. *Drug. Deliv. Transl. Res.* **2018**, *8*, 853–856. [CrossRef]
61. Rossino, G.; Marchese, E.; Galli, G.; Verde, F.; Finizio, M.; Serra, M.; Linciano, P.; Collina, S. Peptides as Therapeutic Agents: Challenges and Opportunities in the Green Transition Era. *Molecules* **2023**, *28*, 7165. [CrossRef]
62. Alghanem, S.; Dziurkowska, E.; Ordyniec-Kwaśnica, I.; Sznitowska, M. Intraoral medical devices for sustained drug delivery. *Clin. Oral. Investig.* **2023**, *27*, 7157–7169. [CrossRef] [PubMed]
63. Bernstein, G. Delivery of insulin to the buccal mucosa utilizing the rapidmist™ system. *Expert. Opin. Drug. Deliv.* **2008**, *5*, 1047–1055. [CrossRef] [PubMed]

pharmaceutics

MDPI

Review

Delivery Strategies of Probiotics from Nano- and Microparticles: Trends in the Treatment of Inflammatory Bowel Disease—An Overview

Sílvio André Lopes [1], Cesar Augusto Roque-Borda [2,*], Jonatas Lobato Duarte [1], Leonardo Delello Di Filippo [1], Vinícius Martinho Borges Cardoso [1], Fernando Rogério Pavan [1], Marlus Chorilli [1] and Andréia Bagliotti Meneguin [1,*]

[1] Department of Drugs and Medicines, School of Pharmaceutical Sciences, Sao Paulo State University (UNESP), Araraquara 14800-903, Brazil; silvio.lopes@unesp.br (S.A.L.); jl.duarte@unesp.br (J.L.D.); leonardo.filippo@unesp.br (L.D.D.F.); vinicius.mb.cardoso@unesp.br (V.M.B.C.); fernando.pavan@unesp.br (F.R.P.); marlus.chorilli@unesp.br (M.C.)

[2] Vicerrectorado de Investigación, Universidad Católica de Santa María, Arequipa 04000, Peru

* Correspondence: roqueb.cesar@gmail.com (C.A.R.-B.); andreia.meneguin@unesp.br (A.B.M.); Tel.: +55-14-99654-0369 (C.A.R.-B.); +55-16-3301-6976 (A.B.M.)

Abstract: Inflammatory bowel disease (IBD) is a chronic inflammatory disorder, most known as ulcerative colitis (UC) and Crohn's disease (CD), that affects the gastrointestinal tract (GIT), causing considerable symptoms to millions of people around the world. Conventional therapeutic strategies have limitations and side effects, prompting the exploration of innovative approaches. Probiotics, known for their potential to restore gut homeostasis, have emerged as promising candidates for IBD management. Probiotics have been shown to minimize disease symptoms, particularly in patients affected by UC, opening important opportunities to better treat this disease. However, they exhibit limitations in terms of stability and targeted delivery. As several studies demonstrate, the encapsulation of the probiotics, as well as the synthetic drug, into micro- and nanoparticles of organic materials offers great potential to solve this problem. They resist the harsh conditions of the upper GIT portions and, thus, protect the probiotic and drug inside, allowing for the delivery of adequate amounts directly into the colon. An overview of UC and CD, the benefits of the use of probiotics, and the potential of micro- and nanoencapsulation technologies to improve IBD treatment are presented. This review sheds light on the remarkable potential of nano- and microparticles loaded with probiotics as a novel and efficient strategy for managing IBD. Nonetheless, further investigations and clinical trials are warranted to validate their long-term safety and efficacy, paving the way for a new era in IBD therapeutics.

Keywords: inflammatory bowel disease; gastrointestinal tract; probiotics; drug delivery systems; microparticles; nanoparticles

1. Introduction

Inflammatory bowel disease (IBD) is a chronic inflammatory disorder of the gastrointestinal tract (GIT) characterized by unusual immune responses associated with the microbiota of the digestive system in genetically susceptible patients [1,2]. With an estimated 3.1 million individuals affected in the United States alone and an increasing global incidence, IBD presents a substantial public health challenge. Ulcerative colitis (UC) and Crohn's disease (CD) are the two main forms of IBD, which affect various regions of the intestine, particularly the ileum and the large intestine [3,4]. Environmental, genetic, and behavioral factors (lifestyle) may also be related to the onset of these diseases [4]. The course of IBD can be marked by alternating periods of occurrence and remission of the symptoms [4].

The conventional therapeutic options for IBD involve oral administrations of anti-inflammatory drugs, with mesalazine as the first choice, which aim to maintain remission time as long as possible and prevent episodes of inflammation. If left untreated, IBD can exacerbate with more intense symptoms such as rectal bleeding, anemia, gastrointestinal spasm, nausea, fever, fatigue, and loss of weight and appetite [5]. In more advanced cases, IBD patients may show epithelial erosions, ulcerations, and fibrosis [6] that may progress to colorectal cancer [7].

In the current therapy for IBD approved by the US Food and Drug Administration, mesalazine is incorporated into dosage forms based on specific polymers that present several release mechanisms. For example, it includes Asacol (pH-responsive), Colazal (a prodrug with enzymatic reduction), Mezavant (both pH-responsive and prolonged-release), and Pentasa (prolonged-release) (6, 18). The effectiveness of these systems is limited [8]; as many as two-thirds of patients do not respond satisfactorily and require surgery [9]. Also, in this therapy, the anti-inflammatory is administered in high doses and for prolonged periods of time, which leads to systemic adverse side effects [9]. The low efficacy of the treatment and the severe adverse effects occur due to a rapid absorption of most parts of the drug in the jejunum portion, with the remaining portion being released continuously throughout the GIT, before the inflamed site of the intestine. Therefore, only about 20% of the administered drug is effectively released into the colon [10].

This review article aims to provide an in-depth exploration of the potential of nano- and microparticles loaded with probiotics as a cutting-edge approach to IBD treatment. Several studies have shown the important benefits of using probiotics as adjuvants to the traditional treatment of IBD [11]. The use of probiotics was associated with symptom remission or attenuation, angiogenesis blockage, inflammation reduction, intestinal barrier reinforcement, and a reduction in the time to recover from the disease [12–19]. However, their therapeutic potential has been hindered by challenges such as limited stability, viability, and targeted delivery. The strategy of drug delivery directly into the colon, through micro- and nanoparticles, has been studied in the treatment of IBD [20]. The use of these structures is potentially promising due to the ability of these particles to penetrate the mucosal layer and the intestinal epithelium affected by the disease [21]. These particles protect the drug from degradation and allow it to reach the affected colon in high concentrations, conferring prolonged and maximized pharmacological effects and minimizing the adverse side effects [8]. Thus, there is a growing demand for the development of new systems based on micro- and nanotechnologies [9]. Not only anti-inflammatory drugs but also probiotics could benefit from these new delivery systems.

In sum, this review seeks to shed light on the innovative potential of probiotic-loaded particles as a promising avenue for the management of IBD, providing a comprehensive overview of the current research and future prospects in the field.

2. Inflammatory Bowel Disease (IBD)

The main diseases classified as IBD are ulcerative colitis (UC) and Crohn's disease (CD) [1,2], both characterized by the chronic relapse and remission of inflammation in the GIT [22]. These two subtypes differ in the extension of affected regions and the most common symptoms.

2.1. Ulcerative Colitis

Ulcerative colitis (UC) was recognized as a disease for the first time in 1859 by Samuel Wilks [23]. It is characterized by diffuse inflammation of the large intestine, restricted to the mucosa and submucosa and limited to the colon and rectum. The mucosal involvement is continuous and ascending, and the transition between affected and normal tissues is well demarcated [24]. The classification of UC varies according to the symptomatology, as shown in Figure 1. Depending on the extent of the affected colon, colitis is classified as proctitis or left colitis, with both conditions affecting parts of the colon, or pancolitis, affecting the entire colon. Proctitis affects around 30 to 60% of patients with UC and left colitis is observed in range between 16 and 45% of the affected people. Proctitis is the situation in which colitis affects the rectum, associated or not with rectal bleeding and tenesmus. Left-side colitis can affect the rectum and the sigmoid and descending colon, and is associated with bloody diarrhea and severe abdominal cramps. Finally, extensive colitis (or pancolitis) is the condition in which colitis affects the whole organ and is present in 15 to 35% of patients. It includes all the above characteristics plus fatigue and fever [25].

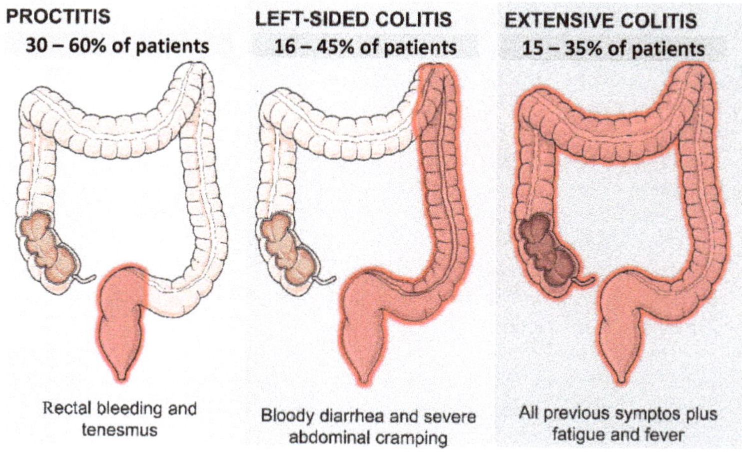

Figure 1. Ulcerative colitis classification with incidence and main symptoms.

The main feature of extensive colitis is diarrhea with the rapid flow of intestinal contents through the inflamed colon causing ulcerative lesions on the inner wall of this organ. Diarrhea crises can be postprandial or even nocturnal, accompanied by rectal bleeding, abdominal pain, fever, weight loss, fatigue, tenesmus (incomplete sensation of evacuation), and general malaise; these are symptoms that may progress to an even more serious clinical picture [24]. The greater the severity of the inflammation, the greater the amount of diarrhea, a mixture of blood and feces. More severe cases of UC, involving severe bleeding, occur in about 10% of patients with urgent colectomies, and about 1% of all affected people have at least one occurrence of massive bleeding, which may require surgical intervention [26]. The main complications of UC comprise symptoms such as toxic megacolon, enterorrhagia, and severe acute colitis [24]. Higher risks of developing colorectal cancer are also associated with UC [7], which may increase by 2.2% in general cases of IBD and 7.0% in cases of long-term UC [27].

2.2. Crohn's Disease

Crohn's disease was first reported in 1932 by Burrill B. Crohn, Leon Ginzburg, and Gordon D. Oppenheimer [28]. CD can discontinuously reach any region of the GI tract, from the mouth to the anus, most frequently the ileum and colon [3]. The most common symptoms are recurrent bouts of diarrhea, fever, severe abdominal pain, and weight loss, impairing the life quality of the patients.

At the beginning of CD, there is hypertrophy of the intestinal mucosa and submucosa, which modifies the normal transverse folds, changing the appearance of hemorrhagic ulcers, which evolve into fissures. In the chronic phase, there are edemas in the submucosa and fissured ulcers. Thus, CD causes histological alterations, the formation of edemas, a reduction in mucus-producing cells, hyperplasia of intestinal crypts, erosions, deep ulcerations, and lymphoid aggregates. In cases of complications, intestinal granulomas, fistulas, stenoses, abscesses [27], and intestinal perforation may occur, a pattern that is not seen in UC. In CD, an increased activity of T helper cells 1 (Th1) and 7 (Th17) leads to dysfunctional inflammation and alters the response of the intestinal immune system, resulting in the excessive release of cytokines such as TNF-alpha, interferon-gamma, IL-12, IL-3, and IL-17 [29]. Therefore, an environmental stimulus in a person who has a genetic predisposition to CD can induce an immune imbalance of Th1 or 17 in relation to regulatory T cells (Treg cells), a situation that may favor the onset of the disease [30].

2.3. Immunopathogenesis

Impairments in the integrity of the intestinal epithelial barrier may be the first step towards the onset of IBD. In immunologically healthy individuals, communication between the epithelial cells of the innate and adaptive immune system ensures intestinal homeostasis [31]. The epithelium, composed of the epidermis and the intestinal mucosa, is the first barrier to defend the body against the invasion of pathogens [32]. Through signaling processes, the epithelium remains in contact with the intestinal microbiota in a state of immunological tolerance, which is maintained by constant sampling through antigen-presenting cells (APCs) [33] of luminal material from the intestine, such as antigens, which triggers the immune response, regulated by the T lymphocytes (T reg cells) [27]. Studies in animal models indicate that the balance between Th17 and Treg cells, which are responsible for the production of pro-inflammatory and anti-inflammatory cytokines, is essential for intestinal homeostasis and is directly affected by the content of the normal microbiota [34].

In a healthy individual, the epithelial layer is renewed every two to three days. Renewal includes apoptosis and enterocyte desquamation of the crypt regions of the colon and the villi structures of the small intestine. If this renewal process is interrupted, the epithelial barrier can be impaired and chronic inflammation can occur [35]. Genetic, immunological, but also microbiological variations affect renewal balance, with disturbances in this process contributing to the onset of gastrointestinal disorders, such as IBD [31]. Thus, defects in the colonic epithelial layer may promote the pathogenesis of IBD through the free passage of microorganisms and triggering the onset of an immune response [35].

In addition to the enterocytes, the microbiota signals the innate immune cells in the lamina propria through the pattern recognition molecule signal receptors [35]. The lamina propria can be understood as a constituent region of the mucosa, present just below the intestinal epithelium, which is reinforced by loose connective tissue and occupied by resident immune cells, such as macrophages and dendritic cells [36]. To enable this mechanism, the recognition of microbial antigens through the action of Toll-like receptors (TLRs) is fundamental. In addition to these receptors, the presence of NOD-like cytoplasmic receptors is essential to initiate the phagocytosis of these microorganisms [37]. Failures in this mechanism result in deficiencies in eliminating bacteria and their products, leading to pathogenic microbial invasions and the progression of IBD [38]. These signals have been shown to be necessary for normal homeostasis and resistance to injury. Cytokines, such as interferon-gamma (IFN-γ), interleukins IL-17 and IL-22, and pathogenic organisms, disturb the epithelium by adjusting the function of the barrier [35]. Thus, UC evolution is associated with changes in the immune homeostasis of the intestine resulting from defects in the mucosal barrier in the affected region, which increases tissue permeability, leading to endotoxin secretion and bacterial translocation, contributing to the establishment of chronic inflammation [31,32].

The colonic epithelial barriers can also be damaged by a decrease in epithelial resistance and of paracellular junction proteins such as claudins and occludins. Consequently, the permeability to ions and water at the injured sites increases. The appearance of lesions, apoptosis, and mucosal necrosis is related to an increase in the release of reactive oxygen species (ROS), tumor necrosis factor (TNF-α), IL-1B, and IFN-γ. The process of apoptosis can allow erosions, ulcers, local leaks, increased transcytosis, and the increased uptake of antigens and bacteria [6]. In the exacerbation phase of IBD, there is an increase in the production of pro-inflammatory cytokines such as IL-1, IL-6, IL-8, and TNF-α [39]. In addition, disturbances in intestinal epithelial cells, such as Paneth cells [40], which produce antimicrobial substances and growth factors [35], are related to important genetic risk factors for IBD and can lead to intestinal inflammation [40].

There are many factors explaining the worsening of IBD. The TLR4 signaling pathway, a subtype of Toll-like receptors, influences this process. Lu et al., reported that TLR4 causes destructive effects on intestinal epithelial tissues and ulceration in patients with UC due to the release of pro-inflammatory cytokines which aggravate intestinal inflammation [41]. Through the activation of TLR4, the inflammation process can favor the development of pathogenic bacteria in addition to changes in the composition of the colonic microbiota. Therefore, the immune system can induce an intense reaction, stimulating the expression of cytokines and favoring the progression of the disease [42].

Because IBD presents disordered immunological responses, a striking characteristic is the chronicity of inflammatory processes. Therefore, immunopathogenesis is one of the most important therapeutic targets in IBD. The identification of new genes reinforces the central roles of innate and adaptive immune cells, as well as autophagic processes in the pathogenesis of IBD. Therefore, autophagy is a crucial point in its pathogenesis, demonstrating the link between changes in immunity and pathogenic factors [43]. In addition, autophagy modulates the balance of pro-inflammatory and anti-inflammatory cytokines through different pathways, different cells in the innate immune system, and non-immune cells, so many immunological changes are linked to this process. Defective autophagy can incite inflammation in the gut region, altering cytokines and innate and adaptive immune cells in IBD. It is believed that effective autophagy can ensure the balance between intestinal tolerance and immune tolerance homeostasis. Thus, autophagy is a potential target for the treatment of IBD, especially when current treatment methods are mainly immune-related therapies [43].

Although the lymphatic system is involved in the initiation and progression of IBD, more studies are needed to better understand this mechanism of action in relation to IBD. In this sense, studies with animal models have investigated the lymphatic system in IBD, showing ascending evidence of the involvement of lymphoid tissues in the pathogenesis of IBD. Lymphadenopathy, a condition described by an increase in the number and size of mesenteric lymph nodes (MLNs), is commonly seen in patients with IBD. The appearance of IBD, stimulated by lymphocyte–dendritic cell interaction, is related to the presence of B and T lymphocytes between the gut-associated lymphoid tissue (GALT) and the intestinal mucosa, induced by lymphocyte–dendritic cell interaction. Furthermore, the luminal microbiota also colonizes lymphoid tissues and can stimulate new local immune responses [44].

2.4. Predisposing Factors

Several environmental and physiological factors, patients' habits, and psychological factors are associated with the occurrence of IBD, as described in Figure 2.

Studies suggest that Caucasian people and inhabitants of urban and industrialized regions are more likely to be affected by autoimmune diseases in general, including IBD [45]. In the highly industrialized countries of North America and Western Europe, IBD is considered a serious public health problem [46]. From 2012 to 2017, the annual incidence ranged from 15.7 cases per 100,000 people in North America to 24.3 in Europe [1,47]. It has been observed that even in areas traditionally of low prevalence, like Brazil, South Korea, and China [34], there has been an increase in the incidence of IBD after processes of urbanization and development. In Brazil, there has been a marked increase in the incidence of CD over the last 40 years. The incidence, which was 0.08 in 1988, increased to 5.48 in 2015 per 100,000 people [48]. Newly industrialized countries in Asia, Africa, South America, and the Middle East have also documented a progressive increase in IBD in recent decades [25,49], at rates higher than 14.9% [36], far above the rates of Europe and North America, which is further evidence that the occurrence of IBD is associated with industrialization and urbanization activities [1,50], and probably as a result of the exposition of a usually increased rate of air pollution [38].

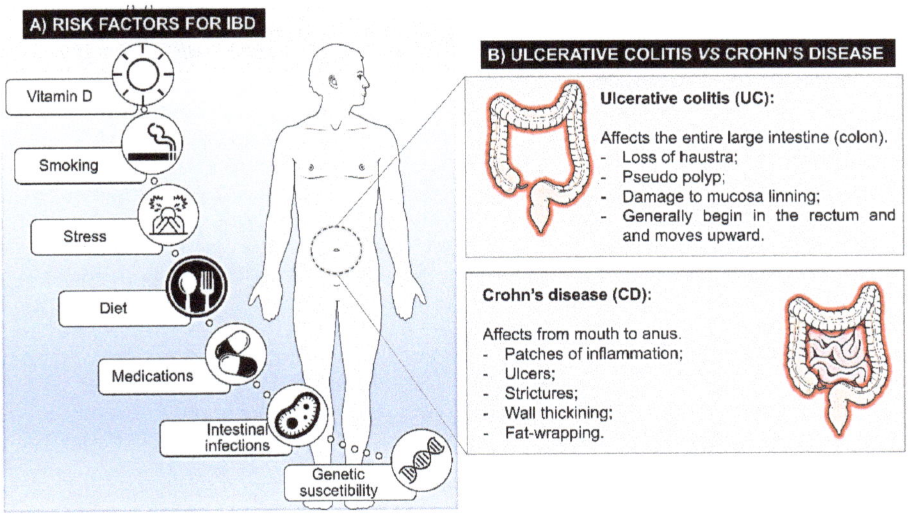

Figure 2. (**A**) Factors of risk for IBD and (**B**) main differences between ulcerative colitis and Crohn's disease.

A deficit in vitamin D, important in calcium metabolism, may favor the onset of IBD [51], and sudden changes in diet; the use of medications such as oral contraceptives; hormone replacement therapy; nonsteroidal anti-inflammatory drugs; physical and mental stress [25]; tobacco consumption [38,51]; and drugs such as Aspirin, Clozapine, Entocapone, Lansoprazole, Omeprazole, Ranitidine, and Sertraline, among others, are cited as predisposing and risk factors. Physical activity, opposite to sedentarism, was associated with a decreased risk of CD occurrence by 44%, and sleep disorders could be a determinant in the development of the active phase of the disease [51]. In addition, between 5 and 15% of adult IBD patients can develop chronic kidney disease over time [52].

As factors that can trigger IBD, alcoholism has a significant effect on in-hospital mortality in IBD patients. Although uncommon in people with IBD, abstaining from alcohol use is highly suggested given the significant risk of mortality associated with alcohol abuse. Furthermore, like IBD, it causes chronic pain and consequent damage to quality of life, which can be a predisposing factor to alcohol abuse [52].

Historically, the 1930s was the time that gastroenterologists and psychiatrists first suggested that emotional life events and experiences could be related to the exacerbation of intestinal symptoms [53], as well as in relapses [54]. Stress processes can stimulate alterations to the motor, secretory, and sensorial functions of the GIT, as well as the thresholds for pain perception, favoring intestinal permeability and inflammatory exacerbation. It is believed that in almost 75% of patients with IBD, events of stress or the own personality of the patients are main contributors to symptom development [55].

It is understood that the consequences of psychological stress to intestinal health are mediated by neuroendocrine-immune pathways related to the brain–gut axis, specifically the hypothalamic–pituitary–adrenal axis (HPA) and the sympathetic nervous system, which can interact directly with the immune system [55], leading to the production of pro-inflammatory cytokines, the activation of macrophages, and changes in permeability and intestinal microbiota [38,51]. Not only are the profiles of cytokines IL-1β, IL6, IL10, IL4, and TNFα altered by stress, but that of the hormone cortisol is too [56,57]. The mucosal mast cells can be activated by stress, thanks to their communication with neurons in the GI tract, through the release of eicosanoids, serotonin, and IL6, situations that may favor the onset of IBD [55].

Psychological stress stimulates corticotropin-releasing factor (CRF) secretion from both central and peripheral parts of the CNS (hypothalamus and adrenal cortex, respectively). Central CRF regulates the ACTH-cortisol system, while peripheral CRF directly influences gastrointestinal motility. In general, CRF, through stress as a trigger, inhibits upper GI motility and stimulates colon motility, so that symptoms such as abdominal pain and changes in bowel function can occur in IBD without significant disease activity [55]. In addition, IBD and stress may be associated with structural and functional changes in limbic structures that may result in the exacerbation of symptoms due to regulation of the autonomic and endocrine pathways of the brain–gut axis [58,59]. Psychological stress can also increase intestinal permeability, possibly as a result of changes in the cholinergic nervous system and mucosal mast cell function. This altered permeability reduces mucosal barrier function and alters host–bacterial interactions [55].

3. Conventional Treatment of IBD

5-aminosalicylic acid, also known as 5-ASA or mesalazine and belonging to the aminosalicylates class, is the drug of first choice for the treatment of mild to moderate IBD [60]. The structural formula and mechanism of action of 5-ASA is shown in Figure 3.

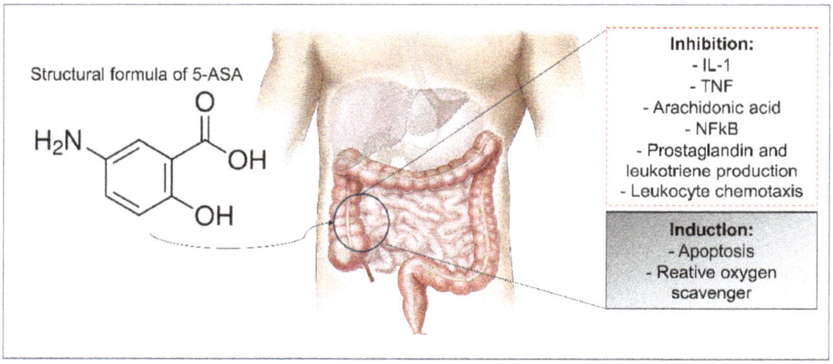

Figure 3. Structural formula and mechanism of action of 5-ASA.

This drug is administered orally, through enteric-coated capsules or tablets; parenterally, through applications of subcutaneous or intravenous injections; or rectally, through suppositories or enemas [6]. It is believed that 5-ASA acts on the intestinal mucosa through a combination of anti-inflammatory effects, involving the inhibition of IL-1 production [61], blocking the production of IL-2 and the inhibition of T cell proliferation and [62], the reduction of TNF-α receptor signaling [63], the inhibition of cyclooxygenase (blocking the production of prostaglandins) and 5-lipoxygenase (blocking the production of leukotrienes) [64,65], and the activation of adhesion molecules in the endothelial cells [66]. It also possesses antioxidant actions that eliminate free radicals [67].

IBD requires long drug therapy, in many cases for indefinite periods. For therapeutic success, total patient compliance with treatment time and correct use of the prescribed drugs are essential, but this is an uncommon situation [45]. Many studies worldwide show a low adherence (40–60%) of patients affected by IBD to 5-ASA treatments [68–72]. Reasons are forgetfulness, bad feeling, the frequency of medication dosage, lack of medication effect, medication unavailability, side or adverse effects, lifelong treatment, and treatment cost [73].

There are situations in which patients do not respond to the use of aminosalicylates [74]. In moderate or severe cases, the administration of corticosteroids, such as dexamethasone, thiopurines (azathioprine), or calcineurin inhibitors (cyclosporine) is common [6,75]. Prednisone [74,76] and budesonide also are employed [74,77,78]. Weight gain, edema, insomnia, emotional lability, psychosis, acne, osteoporosis, cataracts, glaucoma, stretch marks, myopathy, susceptibility to infections, hepatic steatosis, systemic arterial hypertension, *Diabetes mellitus*, and acute pancreatitis are reported as side effects [79]. There are patients resistant to steroids, requiring the administration of immunosuppressive drugs such as azathioprine, tacrolimus, or methotrexate [74,76]. The use of azathioprine may, in turn, cause fever, nausea, vomiting, abdominal pain, medullary depression, changes in liver enzymes and an increased risk of non-Hodgkin's lymphoma, and of methotrexate alopecia, pneumonitis, changes in liver function, liver fibrosis, and teratogenicity [79].

In patients with marked UC activity, parenteral treatment consists of the use, at the hospital-level, of corticosteroids, biological therapy, and cyclosporine. Depending on the situation, infliximab, an anti-TNFα, may be administered [79]. Treatment with azathioprine or anti-TNF-α immunotherapy or vedolizumab is used in cases where the disease is frequently relapsing [27]. If patients do not respond to drug therapy and the disease evolves to extreme cases of intestine perforation and hemorrhagic and toxic megacolon, a surgical intervention (colectomy) may be required [79].

The oral route is the most accepted for drug administration and is the way used for approximately 60% of small molecule drugs that are commercially available [80]. It is noninvasive, safe, and cost-effective, factors that contribute to increased patient adherence [5,80]. In the specific case of 5-ASA, the drug is rapidly and extensively absorbed in the upper portions of the GIT, which results, as already mentioned, in several side effects, in addition to reduced concentrations in the colon (the main affected region), decreasing the effectiveness of IBD treatment. In view of this, the incorporation of the drug to specialized carriers that allow its targeting of the inflamed regions is necessary. This is possible only with the development of drug delivery systems that are specific to the colon. In addition to a significant reduction in unwanted distribution of the drug into the body, such a system would allow for dose reduction, a decrease in adverse and toxic effects, and maximum concentration of the drug in the desired target [5].

The main treatment of mild to moderate cases of IBD involves the use of orally administered drugs. However, the effectiveness of conventional drugs is hampered by several factors, including severe adverse effects, lack of targeting of the inflamed tissue, and others, that are associated with the anatomical and physiological structure of the GIT. These difficulties make the knowledge of the distinct portions of the GIT of paramount importance during the search for alternatives to better treat IBD and for effective targets for drug delivery into the colon.

New and emerging treatments for IBD are being studied as new therapeutic approaches, such as the Inhibition of Immune Cell Trafficking, Sphingosine-1-Phosphate Modulators, the Inhibition of Cytokines, JAK Inhibitors, TLI1A Inhibitors, Phosphodiesterase Inhibitors, and IL-36 Inhibitors [81]. In recent years, many new medications have been developed and therapy for IBD patients has changed significantly. However, current therapies still have unresolved problems, which makes their adherence difficult and contributes to the increase in new numbers of IBD cases around the world. Therefore, new therapies are tremendously urgent [81].

4. Gut Microbiota, Dysbiosis, and the Potential Use of Probiotics in IBD Therapy

The colon has been investigated as a target for the release of drugs [82] and probiotics for local and systemic action. However, the colon as a target poses a great challenge since it is the most distant portion of the GIT. Drug delivery systems with high specificity for the colon are, therefore, necessary [83]. Since this region is a place of great enzymatic activity resulting from the extensive colonic microbiota, it has been successfully explored as a trigger to biologically degrade specific polymers, promoting drug delivery [83].

4.1. The Gut Microbiota

The intestinal microbiota, also known as the gut microbiota or gut microbioma (GM), is a complex and diverse community of microorganisms that inhabit the human digestive tract [82]. This community includes bacteria (Eubacteria and Archaea), viruses, and fungi [84]. In healthy individuals, the GM plays important roles in maintaining the health of the digestive system and the body as a whole. In addition to aiding in digestion, the GM is also involved in a variety of other physiological processes, including immune system regulation and activation, metabolism, and even brain function [59,84]. GM disturbances are involved in several neurological disorders such as depression, anxiety, multiple sclerosis, schizophrenia, [59] anorexia nervosa, Alzheimer's disease, and Parkinson's disease [85].

GM metabolites also contribute to beneficial interactions within the gut microorganisms themselves [86]. The healthy GM works as a homeostatic organ participating in the synthesis of short-chain fatty acids (SCFAs), in processes of fermentation of undigested polysaccharides, in the synthesis of vitamins (such as B and K), in the production of energy, and in the prevention of infections caused by pathogenic microorganisms [34,84]. The SCAFs, produced in the colon, are composed of propionate, butyrate, and acetates. Their synthesis occurs through the fermentation of undigested carbohydrates by obligate anaerobes (mainly Firmicutes and Bacteroidetes), contributing to bacteria that ferment oligosaccharides (e.g., Bifidobacterium) [86]. Butyrate is a primary source of energy for colonic epithelial cells, so, when added to propionate, both can regulate intestinal physiology and immune function. In turn, acetate acts as a substrate for lipogenesis and gluconeogenesis [86]. The predominance of obligate anaerobic bacteria in the colon, belonging to the phyla Firmicutes and Bacteroidetes, provides a strict anaerobic environment. Although colonocytes are the main cellular source of oxygen in the colon, the diffusion of oxygen from colonocytes to the lumen is strictly limited. While superficial colonocytes contain less than 1% oxygen, host tissues contain between 3% and 10% oxygen. Intracellular hypoxia of colonocytes occurs due to the consumption of oxygen inside them through the mitochondrial β-oxidation of butyrate, originating from bacteria, and the production of carbon dioxide, which represents their main energy production pathway. The reduction in butyrate-producing bacteria decreases luminal butyrate levels, resulting in a metabolic reorientation of superficial colonocytes toward anaerobic glycolysis and increased oxygen diffusion into the lumen, thus leading to luminal aerobic and/or facultative anaerobic expansion through aerobic breathing [86].

Unlike the stomach and upper part of the small intestine, where few microorganisms are present, the number and diversity of bacterial species progressively increases from the jejunum to the colon [87]. The number of microorganisms that inhabit a healthy human gut can reach 10^{14} CFU/mL [88]. In the case of bacteria, there are more than one thousand species, predominating representatives of the phyla *Bacteroidetes, Firmicutes, Actinobacteria, Proteobacteria, Fusobacteria, Spirochetes, Tenericutes*, and *Verrucomicrobiota*, including the genera *Bacteroides, Peptococcus, Bifidobacterium, Clostridium, Eubacterium, Streptococcus, Enterobacterium, Enterococcus, Lactobacillus*, and *Fusobacteria* [34,84,89]. These bacteria release large amounts of enzymes responsible for deglucuronidation, decarboxylation, the reduction of double bonds, and hydrolysis reactions [83], all important to the body's metabolism.

In recent work, the importance of bacterial tryptophan metabolism in the human intestinal context was demonstrated [86]. Tryptophan is an amino acid that plays crucial roles in the balance between intestinal immune tolerance and the maintenance of the intestinal microbiota. Tryptophan can be converted into indole-containing bioactive metabolites (indole, indolic acid, skatole, and tryptamine) by intestinal bacteria, and indole derivatives affect the host by triggering the aryl hydrocarbon receptor (AhR). AhR signaling enables host immune homeostasis through the secretion of interleukin (IL)-22 from CD4+ T cells and innate lymphoid cells in the intestine. IL-22 can trigger the release of antimicrobial peptides and modulate microbial composition. Furthermore, AhR activation plays an anti-inflammatory function by developing intraepithelial lymphocytes and innate lymphoid cells [86].

4.2. Dysbiosis

Dysbiosis is any change in the composition or function capacity of the intestinal microbiota, commonly associated with several intestinal pathologies [90]. In patients affected by IBD, when compared with non-affected individuals, there are reports that show that this imbalance comes from the reduction in the number of bacteria that have anti-inflammatory activity and the increase in the number of bacteria with inflammatory activity [91]. This unbalance results in function changes, damages in the fermentation process, and changes in biochemical processes leading to immunological disequilibrium and even drug release [6,34]. Diet, age, host genetics, exercise, antibiotic consumption, smoking, and geographical impacts are factors that can modify the composition of the gut microbiota [84].

The dysbiosis profile most commonly related to patients with IBD is a decrease in the Firmicutes phylum (*Faecalibacterium, Blautia, Roseburia*) [92], in commensal bacterial species in the genera *Firmicutes* (*Clostridium* and *Enterococcus*), *Bacteroides*, and bacteria from the genera *Lactobacillus* and *Eubacterium*. On the other hand, an increase is observed in phylum Proteobacteria belonging to the *Enterobacteriaceae* family (for example, bacteria such as *Escherichia* and *Shigella*) [34,92] and there is a considerable increase in bacteria from the phylum *Bacteroidetes* [93]. In addition, inflammation favors the growth of pathogenic bacteria like *Citrobacter rodentium* and *Salmonella* spp. [92].

Although the association of IBD with the presence of pathogenic species is not clear, adherent-invasive *Escherichia coli* (AIEC) was detected in a higher frequency in patients with Crohn's disease (22%) than in healthy patients (6.2%) [94]. As mentioned, bacteria belonging to the genera *Clostridia* and *Bacteroides*, which are capable of causing anti-inflammatory and T-reg cells responses [95], and polysaccharide A from *Bacteroides fragilis* [96], were detected at higher incidences in the colons of IBD-affected people. Conversely, *Faecalibacterium prausnitzii*, which belongs to the *Firmicutes* phylum, was less frequent in patients with IBD than in healthy controls. This bacterium was associated with a lower severity of endoscopic recurrence after resection in humans and, in mice, minimized colitis symptom severity [97,98].

It has also been demonstrated that patients' diet exerts a strong impact on the gut microbiota, which could influence disease incidence. Diets involving a high intake of animal proteins and saturated fat correlated with the presence of pathogenic *Bacteroides* spp., and those involving the consumption of carbohydrates and fiber correlated with the presence of beneficial *Prevotella* spp. [99,100]. In addition to bacteria, IBD may also involve imbalances in virus, Archaea, and fungi populations. Bacteriophages pertaining to the *Caudovirales* family were at higher incidence in patients with CD and UC, and the susceptibility of mice to chemically induced colitis was influenced by an altered immune response to indigenous fungi in the gut [101,102].

It is important to highlight that dysbiosis is intensified with the chronic use of medications designed to treat IBD, such as anti-inflammatory drugs, which includes the widely used drug 5-ASA [92,103], antibiotics, laxatives, and eating habits, which can alter the secretion of enzymes into the colon [6]. Through constant episodes of evacuation, IBD itself can also contribute to dysbiosis [104].

4.3. Potentials of Probiotics

One way to solve the dysbiosis problem is the use of probiotics. Probiotics can be understood as live microorganisms that, when administered in adequate amounts, confer health benefits [34,105]. The first comprehensive study that associated molecules produced and secreted by one microorganism with factors that could induce the growth of another microorganism was published in 1965 [106]. For a microorganism to be classified as a probiotic, it should be non-pathogenic to the host, be isolated from the same species, survive the transit through the GIT, and, finally, keep its viability during long periods of storage [107]. The most-used probiotics belong to the species of *Lactobacillus, Bifidobacterium, Escherichia, Enterococcus, Streptococcus, Saccharomyces*, and *Propionibacterium*. Most consist of lactic acid-producing bacteria such as lactobacilli, streptococci, enterococci, lactococci, and bifidobacteria. *Bacillus* spp., and fungi such as *Saccharomyces* spp. and *Aspergillus* spp. also have been used [107,108].

Probiotics provide important benefits by restoring or maintaining the balance of the normal intestinal microbiota, inhibiting the growth of pathogenic bacteria, improving the barrier function of the intestine, promoting local immunity, and interfering positively in intestinal inflammatory responses [105,109,110]. Regarding pathogenic bacteria, probiotics compete for adhesion sites through the production of bacteriocins and antimicrobial peptides, such as defensins, lysozymes, and phospholipases [109], by providing nutrients to the host body and by inhibiting the process of apoptosis in the intestinal epithelial cells. Overall, probiotics can improve the treatment of IBD and, consequently, the life quality of patients affected by these diseases [105]. Probiotics affect the immune system in several ways. They work by increasing the levels of cytokine and immunoglobulin, macrophage activation, increasing the activities of natural killer cells, autoimmune modulation, and immune stimulation against pathogenic bacteria and protozoa [14].

Lactobacilli was the first probiotic to be discovered. It belongs to the group of acid-lactic bacteria, comprising 183 known species, with various applications in industrial processes such as the manufacture of preservatives, food flavorings, medicines, and the manufacture of cosmetics. This genus is the dominant group in the gastrointestinal system. It produces large amounts of lactic acid and other metabolites using various substances as sources of carbon such as glucose, fructose, lactose, and galactose. They can be classified according to their metabolism as homofermentative and heterofermentative. The homofermentative group only produces lactic acid, and the heterofermentative group, in addition to lactic acid, produces several other metabolites, including ethanol, acetic acid, and carbon dioxide. *Lactobacilli* can also produce secondary metabolites, including bacteriocins, exopolysaccharides, and enzymes, which are used to increase the quality and shelf life of fermented foods [111].

The probiotics *Lactobacillus* spp. and *Bifidobacterium* spp. also produce the short-chain fatty acids (SCFA) acetate and propionate, which are organic acids that result from carbohydrate metabolism. These probiotics do not produce butyrate, obtaining it from commensal bacteria, such as *Faecalibacterium*, leading to increased levels of this compound in the intestine [110]. Butyrate promotes colon motility, reduces inflammation, increases visceral irrigation, inhibits the progression of tumorigenic cells, and induces the process of apoptosis [112]. SCFAs, in addition to acting as sources of energy, also reduce the pH in the intestinal lumen, hinder the development of pathogenic agents, influence intestinal motility, and reduce colon cancer by stimulating the apoptosis of tumorigenic cells [113]. SCFAs also act as signaling molecules by reducing the production of pro-inflammatory cytokines and increasing the population of regulatory T cells (Treg) in the large intestine [114].

Bifidobacteria are the most abundant microorganisms in the GIT. In addition to the benefits mentioned by other bacteria, *Bifidobacterium* spp. reduces intolerance to lactose, prevents GIT disorders, and decreases ammonia concentrations. The presence of an adequate environment and nutrients, known as "bifidogenic factors", contributes to the viability and activity of bifidobacteria [107].

Direct benefits of probiotics in the treatment of IBD have been shown when several species of probiotics were combined (Table 1). The combination of probiotics *Lactobacillus* spp. and *Bifidobacterium* spp., used in commercial products [115], can be beneficial for the immune system, helping healthy and allergenic people by decreasing inflammatory reactions [14]. When *Bifidobacterium* plus *Lactobacillus* are combined with species of *Streptococcus* or with *E. coli* Nissle 1917, a remission of mild to moderately severe symptoms of UC was observed [15]. Another study reported a meta-analysis procedure to evaluate five clinical studies involving a total of 319 patients with UC in which the therapeutic response to a mixture composed of one strain of *Streptococcus thermophilus*, four of *Lactobacillus* spp., and three *Bifidobacterium* spp. strains, known as VSL#3, was compared with placebo. Symptoms of UC were attenuated in about 44.6% of subjects who were administered VSL#3, compared with a 25.1% reduction in the placebo group [16].

Table 1. Benefits of the use of probiotics, alone or combined with 5-ASA, in the treatment of IBD.

Microorganisms	Benefit	Reference
Lactobacillus spp. and *Bifidobacterium* spp.	Inflammation reduction	[14]
Lactobacillus and *Bifidobacterium* plus *Streptococcus* or *E. coli* Nissle 1917	Symptom remission	[15]
Lactobacillus spp., *Bifidobacterium* spp., and *Streptococcus thermophilus*	Symptom attenuation	[16]
Saccharomyces boulardii	Angiogenesis blockage	[13]
Bacillus	Survive in acid conditions	[17]
Saccharomyces boulardii, *Akkermansia muciniphila*, and *Faecalibacterium prausnitzi*	Intestinal barrier reinforcement; colonic inflammation reduction	[19]
Enterococcus faecium CRL 183 and *Bifidobacterium longum* ATCC 15707	Inflammation and ulceration reduction; *Lactobacillus* spp. and *Bifidobacterium* spp. population increase in rat colon	[12]
5-ASA plus L. *salivarius*, L. *acidophilus*, and *B. bifidum* BGN4	Recovery time reduction; symptom attenuation	[18]

Probiotics have also been compared with the traditional use of 5-ASA. In a randomized clinical trial, *E. coli* strain Nissle 1917 was compared with 5-ASA to treat UC. The trial included 327 patients who were given either a daily dose of the probiotic or 500 mg of 5-ASA three times a day. After a period of twelve months, the patients were evaluated clinically, endoscopically, and histologically. *E. coli* strain Nissle 1917 was as effective as the administration of 5-ASA. A recurrence rate of 36.4% was verified in the *E. coli* Nissle 1917 group against a rate of 33.9% in the 5-ASA group [15]. Although the use of probiotics can be as effective as that of the traditional 5-ASA, the benefit of probiotics can be even greater when they are associated with commonly prescribed anti-inflammatories [116]. The association of 5-ASA with a combination of the probiotics *L. salivarius*, *L. acidophilus*, and *B. bifidum* BGN4 resulted in a reduced time of recovery of IBD symptoms and a more attenuated form of the disease. After more than 2 years of study, the results suggest that probiotic supplementation to conventional drugs should be performed without interruption and administered for a long time, allowing a viable treatment [18].

There is increasing evidence from experimental mouse models and from clinical observations that angiogenesis is an important component of the pathogenesis of IBD [117,118], and the yeast *Saccharomyces boulardii* was found to be associated with this process [13]. Chronically inflamed intestinal tissues exhibit changes in physiology and microvascular functions compared with intestine tissues not affected by IBD. Vascular endothelial growth factor (VEGF) and the VEGF receptor tyrosine kinase family (VEGFR) are proteins that modulate the process of angiogenesis. Transmembrane receptor VEGFR types 1 and 2 are present in endothelial cells and have a high affinity for VEGF. The binding of VEGF to these receptors leads to intracellular receptor phosphorylation which activates various intracellular signaling pathways, leading to endothelial cell proliferation and blood vessel formation [13]. VEGF was shown to be more concentrated in distal colon tissue in the colitis model [119], as well as in tissues and sera from patients with CD and UC [120–122]. Studies conducted in an experimental colitis model suggest that VEGF is an important mediator of IBD by promoting intestinal angiogenesis and inflammation [123]. Therefore, agents that inhibit VEGF/VEGFR signaling may be useful in reducing intestinal inflammation in patients with IBD, and *Saccharomyces boulardii* was found to block angiogenesis of VEGFR signaling and regulate the acute and chronic inflammation of the intestinal mucosa associated with the progression of IBD [13].

Several other reports on the benefits of probiotics to treat IBD exist. For instance, probiotics from the genera *Bacillus* are capable of surviving the hostile environment and low-pH in the upper GIT to reach the small intestine and secrete antimicrobial substances [17]. The yeast *Saccharomyces boulardii* and the bacteria *Akkermansia muciniphila* and *Faecalibacterium prausnitzii* induced reinforcement of the intestinal barrier and reduced colonic inflammation [19]. The population of the species *Akkermansia muciniphila,* although classified as a "next-generation" [115] microorganism, declined in IBD-affected individuals [89] and appeared to not resist storage and GIT conditions [115]. The bacteria *Enterococcus faecium* CRL 183 and *Bifidobacterium longum* ATCC 15707, when administered in the form of soy-based beverages, showed excellent results in the treatment of intestinal colitis. There was a lower degree of inflammation and ulceration in the colons of rats submitted to induced colitis in relation to the control groups, as well as an increase in the population of *Lactobacillus* spp. and *Bifidobacterium* spp. [12].

5. Probiotic Delivery Systems

To treat IBD, the delivery of probiotics directly into the affected sites would offer enormous benefits since it offers a restoration of the normal intestinal microbiota, attenuating the impacts of dysbiosis. However, delivering probiotics into the gut can be challenging, as they must maintain stability and viability, which can be affected by the harsh acidic environment of the stomach, and reach the intestines to be effective. To overcome this challenge, researchers have developed a variety of drug delivery ways such as micro- and nanostructured systems. Examples of works conducted to investigate drug and probiotic delivery systems are provided in the following sections.

5.1. Microparticle-Based Drug Delivery Systems

Microencapsulation covers protective conditions for bioactive compounds, cells, or bacteria. Although they are larger than nanoparticles, there is still no exact definition of the dimensions of each one, which can reach up to 1000 μm [124]. For its part, microencapsulation favors protection and release systems during its passage through the GIT [125]. There are several microencapsulation techniques, but in matters of scaling-up one of them would be spraying via atomization [126]. In food technology, ionic gelation has been widely used for temperature-sensitive compounds [127]. Several reported microparticles with potential GIT protective activity were reported including polymeric systems based on alginate, gelatin, chitosan, hyaluronic acid, pectin, cellulose, and fibrin, among others [128].

Recently, Zhu et al., 2022 [129] reported that during IBD a key target for the release of probiotics would be in specific regions of high production of reactive oxygen species (ROS, up to 0.1 mM). The authors designed a system of ROS-sensitive microbeads with alginate/polyvinyl alcohol (PVA)-based 1,4-phenyleneboronic acid (Pa) embedded in a gelatin-based gel (Figure 4A). The results showed an encapsulation efficiency above 95%, nontoxicity, and the ROS-triggered release of highly active *Lactobacillus plantarum* in intestinal inflammatory sites (Figure 4B). This effect occurred due to reversible reactions formed between PVA (1,2 diol free groups) and Pa (compounds derived from boronic acid and boronate esters) which, in turn, when they come into contact with hydrogen peroxide, are capable of breaking down and effectively releasing the active compound (Figure 4C) [130]. Similarly, polydopamine and catalase, considered powerful antioxidants against free radicals, were used to fabricate ROS scavenging microparticles via coprecipitation and self-polymerization. Dextran sulfate was further applied to modify the microparticles' surface considering its targeting ability toward activated macrophages. Results showed the preparation of 1.1 μm microparticles with excellent ROS scavenging ability in cell experiments and a 40% reduction in disease activity index scores in animal experiments (Figure 4D) [131].

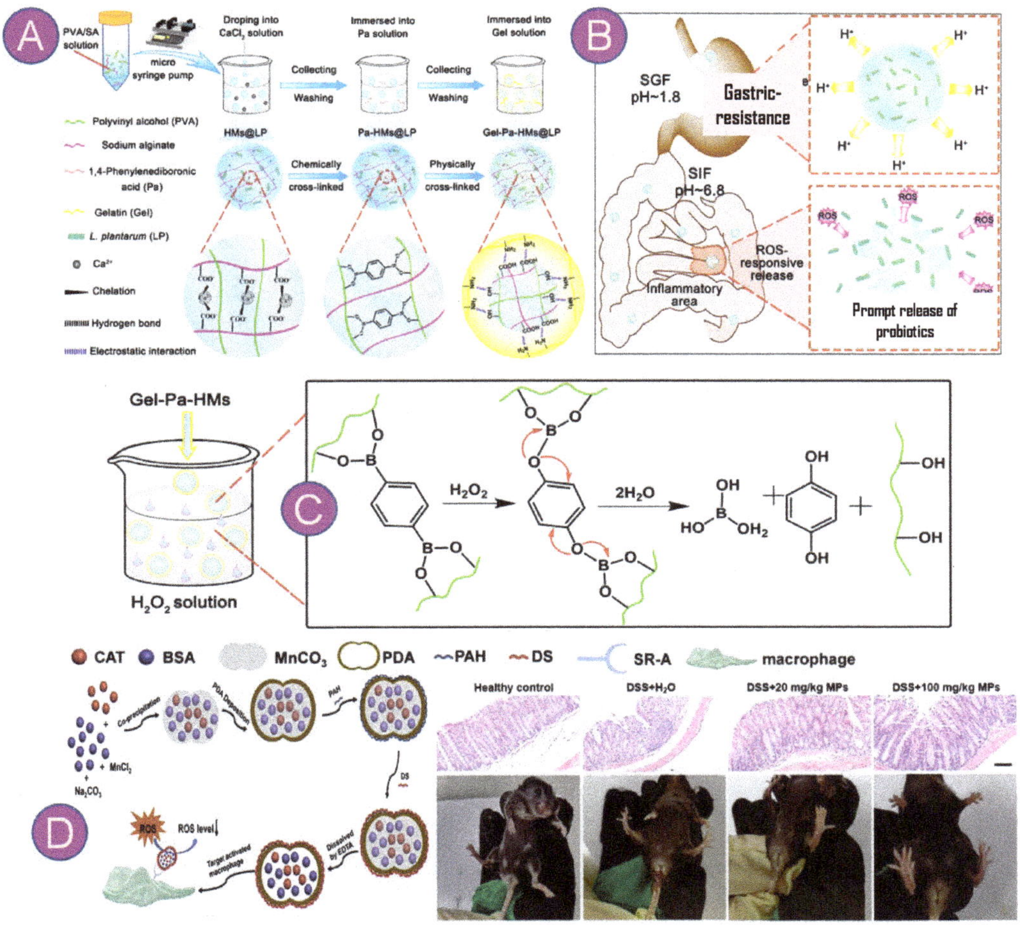

Figure 4. (**A**) Schematic illustration of the fabrication and mechanism of the Gel-Pa-HMs@LP. (**B**) Schematic illustration of the encapsulated *Lactobacillus plantarum* precisely delivered to the inflammatory area and released in response to ROS. (**C**). Schematic illustration of the ROS scavenging mechanism of the Gel-Pa-HMs. Reprinted (adapted) with permission from Zhu et al. [129]. Copyright 2023 American Chemical Society. (**D**) H&E-stained pathological sections of colons of mice with different treatments on day 6, scale bar = 100 µm, and representative photographs of rectal areas of a healthy mouse and IBD mice after treatment with H_2O and 20 and 100 mg/kg microparticles. Reprinted (adapted) with permission from Li et al. [131]. Copyright 2021 American Chemical Society.

In fact, multicomponent microencapsulation could generate better results, as reported by Gąsiorowska et al. The authors showed a clinical study using sodium butyrate microparticles, probiotics, and short-chain fructooligosaccharides in patients with Irritable Bowel Syndrome (IBS), a functional gastrointestinal disorder that can cause symptoms similar to IBD but without damaging the gastrointestinal tract [132]. Probiotics used were two Lactobacillus strains (*L. rhamnosus* and *L. acidophilus*) and three *Bifidobacterium* strains (*B. longum*, *B. bifidum*, and *B. lactis*), and results showed that this combination could be beneficial for an alternative treatment of IBD, as it restores the disturbed functionality of the intestinal microbiota [115].

Microparticles in general present a high rate of protection of bioactive compounds; however, a small premature release of the drug was observed in the stomach, compromising the release in the colon for local treatment. Therefore, a complementary coating alternative was applied to overcome this challenge and optimize the system's effectiveness [133]. Enteric coatings are widely used in the pharmaceutical industry to protect drugs from being broken down by stomach acid before they can be absorbed in the small intestine. Commonly used for active agents that are sensitive to the acidic environment of the stomach, such as probiotics and some antibiotics, enteric coatings can help improve their effectiveness and reduce the risk of side effects. Among the main polymers explored for such applications are cellulose acetate phthalate, polyvinyl acetate phthalate, and methacrylic acid copolymers [134]. Cellulose derivatives are widely used for this purpose, since their structure allows one to obtain rigid, plasticized, and pH-responsible structures [135,136].

Several polymers have been approved by the FDA for this technological process, but some are still under investigation. Park et al. (2016) coated microparticles containing the probiotics *Lactobacillus acidophilus* and *Bifidobacteria animalis* ssp. *Lactis* with hydroxypropyl methylcellulose acetate succinate (HPMCAS) using a dry powder coating technique. The preparation process did not affect the growth of the probiotics, which was improved in acidic conditions compared with encapsulated and uncoated bacteria. As a result, coated probiotics were able to colonize the small and large intestinal membrane, providing pharmacological advantages in relation to the free probiotics [137].

The probiotic *Lactobacillus acidophilus* and prebiotic Reishi medicinal mushroom (*Ganoderma lingzhi*) extract were co-encapsulated in calcium-alginate microparticles aiming to prolong their stability in gastric conditions. Microparticles were prepared with an ionotropic gelation technique using calcium lactate as a crosslinker agent. As a strategy to increase the stability of encapsulated agents, microparticles were double-coated with the same polyelectrolyte layer and a second crosslinking solution (6% calcium lactate + 0.4% chitosan). Single-layered and double-layered microparticles were 1.5 mm and 2.3 mm in diameter and showed 83% and 74% of encapsulation efficiency, respectively. The number of viable bacteria was higher for double-layer coating microparticles in relation to single-layer-ones, demonstrating the influence of coatings on reducing the release rate of the active molecules in harsh conditions of the upper GIT [138].

Another designed microsystem was using double-layer gelatin-mucin-alginate and chitosan-mucin-alginate to protect *Lactobacillus plantarum* B2, responsible for riboflavin production. The authors showed that the inclusion of mucin in the formulation made it possible to maintain the structural characteristics of the microcapsules even after lyophilization, in addition to increasing the rate of adherence in the intestinal tract and stimulating greater production of vitamin B2 [139]. Curiously, the application of mucin in other biomaterials has been shown to generate a positive immunological response for the patient since they would have been related to the expression of cytokines [140]. Likewise, Eudragit® S100 (anionic polymer) is used as an enteric coating which, in the majority of its formulations, allows for the blocking of the release of biomolecules in acidic pH; as such, after the microencapsulation of *L. acidophilus* and the coating (chitosan nanoparticles and Eu S100) were incorporated into Iranian Doogh drinks, they showed that the storage time would be up to 42 days without changes in their morphology, preserving their organoleptic properties and their bacterial viability [141].

The structural modification of polymers can improve their biophysical properties of both release and adherence to the intestinal mucosa since there are some reports indicating the use of thiol groups as potential mucoadhesive agents [142,143]. Zhang et al. developed a multinucleated bilayer microsystem of thiolated carboxymethyl cellulose, allowing for greater adherence between probiotics (*Bifidobacterium adolescence* FS2-3 and *Bacillus subtilis* SN15-2) and the mucosa; significant repairs were observed in the microbiota and the site of inflammation induced by *Escherichia coli* O157:H7 [144]. On the other hand, some lipid supplements can be added to these microsystems to improve their versatility. A double emulsion of *L. rhamnosus* and krill oil based on protein showed a high content of monounsaturated and polyunsaturated fatty acids capable of avoiding the appearance of neurodegenerative diseases, obesity, and cancer, which lead to a multi-objective application of prevention [145]. Various emulsions were generated during recent years where probiotics were incorporated, but, curiously, the use of Okara oil allowed for the modulation and regulation of the size of the microcapsule structure since the size would be related to the concentration of the oily phase [146]. However, it is necessary to be careful at the time of formulation as there may be an induced stress which would allow some bacteria, such as *Lactobacillus plantarum*, when combined with Omega 3, to lose the anticancer activity that each component possessed individually [147].

A recent study indicated that the incorporation of *Akkermansia muciniphila* would be beneficial to prevent some diseases, including IBD, since a study in mice indicated that the counts of these bacteria in high-fat diets were significantly lower than those in healthy mice. Thus, Marcial-Coba et al., reported a study where *A. muciniphila* and *Lactobacillus* cases were included in xanthan/gellan gum microcapsules and incorporated into dark chocolate; they achieved gastric protection, a long storage period, high bacterial viability, and no significant difference in its organoleptic properties [148]. *Akkermansia* spp. is a bacterial family that is difficult to isolate and manipulate, and there is little information about its role in the microbiota as well as its role in the appearance of gastrointestinal diseases reported to date.

5.2. Nanoparticle-Based Drug Delivery Systems

With the advent of nanotechnology, it was possible to explore new delivery platforms that were able to solve problems related to the low stability and bioavailability of probiotics given orally. The encapsulation of probiotics in nanosystems can protect them against degradation, improving their stability during product processing and digestion, which improves their bioavailability in the large intestine by delivering a higher fraction of viable probiotics to the colon. In this session, the biological properties of nanosystems containing probiotics will be discussed as a therapeutic alternative for the management of IBD [149,150].

To ensure the therapeutic efficacy of probiotics, they must remain viable and intact within their formulation and resist various pH fluctuations during transit through different regions of the GIT, including the oral cavity, stomach, and intestines. Additionally, these probiotics must be able to withstand the effects of digestive enzymes, such as amylase, pepsin, and trypsin. This is crucial, as oral administration requires that the probiotics survive the harsh environment of the stomach and be released in the colon. Polymeric nanoparticles have proven to be particularly useful in the transport and delivery of probiotics as they can be designed from natural or synthetic polymers having some of the peculiarities of the colon as a trigger mechanism for release. Among them, the characteristics most explored to initiate the release are the distinct pH range (such as sodium-alginate- and Eudragit®-based systems), the specific enzymatic biodegradability (resistant starch-based systems), as well as the longer transit time (ethyl cellulose coating). The latter can be exploited by systems based on polymers that have poor aqueous solubility and that require longer contact time with gastrointestinal fluids for release [151,152].

Bacillus amyloliquefaciens loaded nanoparticles (BANPs) were designed to achieve a long-lasting effect in the prevention and treatment of IBD. The chitosan nanoparticles were more stable in simulated intestinal and gastric juice than free bacillus. After colitis induction, rats treated with BANPs had a higher survival rate and greater recovery of liver and kidney function. Fecal Lcn-2 levels were significantly decreased in rats treated with BANPs compared with the colitic group. The BANP group also showed reconstructed colon epithelium in some areas with reduced inflammatory cell infiltration and detachment of the epithelial lining. The study suggests that orally administered BANPs have potential therapeutic effects on colitis [153].

In a similar study, *B. amyloliquefacies* was associated with *Lactobacillus acidophilus* and *Bifidobacterium bifidum* in chitosan nanoparticles. Similar to the previous study, the nanoparticle system improved the stability of probiotics in the GIT and reduced the severity of clinical signs in colitic rats, including weight loss, diarrhea, and rectal bleeding. Additionally, the nanoparticle system reduced inflammatory markers and increased the expression of anti-inflammatory cytokines in colon tissues. The study suggests that the nanoparticle system has potential as a treatment for colitis [154].

Ebrahimnejad and coworkers (2017) developed chitosan-based nanoparticles for the encapsulation of *L. acidophilus* (1643 PTCC) as a probiotic agent. The polymeric nanoparticles were obtained using chitosan and tripolyphosphate anions via an ionic gelation technique and presented an average size of 100 to 250 nm with a distinct spherical regular shape, as confirmed with scanning electron microscopy. The optimal bacterial loading was achieved using the lowest chitosan concentration (0.05 mg/mL). The authors assessed the survival of *L. acidophilus* in vitro using simulated gastric fluid (pH 2), and results showed a better protective effect in encapsulated bacteria compared with its free form, corroborating the results described in the literature, where probiotic encapsulation seems to increase bacterial viability after exposure to the acidic conditions of the stomach. In intestinal conditions, the number of free cells remarkably decreased after 120 min, while encapsulated bacteria did not. The results suggest the encapsulation of probiotics using chitosan can improve the stability of probiotics in different pH conditions, improving their delivery to the colon [155].

Biodegradable chitosan-coated PLGA nanoparticles (NPs) for the delivery of probiotic *Lactobacillus plantarum* extract (LPE) to treat colitis were developed by Saadatzadeh et al. The NPs show a particle size of 226.3 nm, positive surface zeta potential, and biphasic controlled drug release. Treatment with LPE and NPs reduced colonic damage, decreased levels of inflammatory cytokines TNF-α and IL-1β, and reduced myeloperoxidase and lipid peroxidation activity in colitic rats. The study concluded that the LPE-loaded NPs can be a promising approach for treating colitis [156]. These studies suggest that chitosan-based nanoparticle systems have potential as a treatment for colitis by improving the stability and delivery of probiotics.

Sahu and coauthors explored agricultural waste as an opportunity to design eggshell nanoparticle-based (ESNP) gel for probiotic delivery. ESNPs were prepared using sterile air-dried eggshells that were processed in a ball mill. The ESNPs presented a size <300 nm. The gel was prepared using a suspension of *L. plantarum* (MTCC2621) and the ESNPs. After incorporation, the gel presented 80% of the initial *L. plantarum* content. This concentration decreased by 40% in the gel after 60 days of storage, while 100% of cells were lost after 60 days in the conventional formulation, suggesting a protective effect of ESNP gel. The stability in simulated gastric fluid was assessed using simulated gastric fluid prepared with pepsin and other salts at pH 2. The gel did not present a reduction in viability even after 120 min, while for free cells a reduction of 50% was observed. These results reinforce the ability of ESNP-based gels to improve probiotic delivery by shielding the bacteria from the acidic pH of the gastric fluid and their potential use in the management of intestinal diseases [157].

Self-assembling hyaluronic acid (HA)-based nanoparticles capable of scavenging reactive oxygen species (ROS) conjugated with probiotic *Escherichia coli* Nissle 1917 (EcN) within a nanogel layer containing hinokitiol (HPN), a natural anti-inflammatory compound for targeted delivery to inflamed colon tissues, were developed by Liu et al. The nanoparticles effectively protect the EcN against environmental assaults, such as simulated gastric fluid and bile salts, and exhibited enhanced survival rates compared with uncoated EcN. The conjugation of HPN onto the surface of EcN has the potential to exhibit synergy for enhanced therapeutic efficacy in IBDs. The treatment was tested on mice with induced colitis and was found to significantly reduce weight loss, increase colon length, and minimize colon damage compared with other treatments. The therapy also modulated the gut microbiota by increasing the relative abundance of beneficial bacteria and decreasing virulent bacteria [158].

Regarding inorganic nanoparticles, their use for food and medical applications is limited due to issues related to their low solubility and intrinsic toxicity resulting from the use of heavy metals in their fabrication. Furthermore, when compared to other nanofabrication techniques, inorganic nanoparticles do not provide significant advantages in protecting probiotics from degradation.

Interestingly, Wei and colleagues explored one possible use of mesoporous silica nanoparticles (MSNPs) to create a multi-purpose nanoprobiotic. The authors encapsulated *B. infantis* (ATCC 15697) with MSNPs, which were further coated with bacterially derived quantum dots (QDs) produced either by *L. acidophilus* or *E. coli*. This multi-purpose nanoprobiotic (MPNPs) was successfully fabricated, as techniques such as infra-red spectroscopy and scanning electron microscopy confirmed the MSNP coating in *B. infantis* and the further attachment of bacterially derived QDs on its surface. In vitro exposure of MPNPs to simulated gastric fluid and antibiotics demonstrated better protection compared with uncoated *B. infantis*, suggesting that an MSNP coating could be useful to protect probiotics from gastric fluid. The MPNPs also showed increased mucoadhesion on an intestinal epithelial layer colonized by *E. coli* when compared with uncoated *B. infantis*, suggesting a possible therapeutic effect against Enterobacteriaceae colonization. Additionally, the QD-coated nanoprobiotics showed an increased killing effect on *E. coli* due to the increased generations of reactive oxygen species. These techniques together could lead to an enhancement of the properties of *B. infantis*, representing a new generation of engineered nanoprobiotics [159].

Probiotic-inspired nanomedicines were developed by coating MSNP with an *Escherichia coli* Nissle 1917-derived membrane. The researchers found that the nanoparticles were effective in treating IBDs by regulating the redox balance and immune responses in a mouse model of colitis. Compared with other nanoformulations and conventional therapeutics, the nanoparticles demonstrated the greatest therapeutic effects, including reduced weight loss, a lower disease activity index (DAI), increased colon length, and decreased colonic histological damage scores. The treatment with the nanoparticles also improved the integrity of the colonic mucosal barrier, as indicated by increased levels of tight junction markers. It is suggested that the adhesion of the membrane shell to the mucus layer and the accumulation of the nanoparticles in inflammatory tissue contributed to its therapeutic efficacy. The NP was found to decrease myeloperoxidase (MPO) activity and pro-inflammatory cytokine secretion while increasing the secretion of the anti-inflammatory factor interleukin-10 (IL-10) in the colon tissue of acute colitis mice [160].

In recent decades, research related to the use of lipid nanoparticles for the delivery of probiotics has gained prominence with the advent of nanocoating techniques that have improved the biopharmaceutical properties of colloidal lipid carriers such as liposomes. Polysaccharides and protein-coated liposomes are capable of protecting probiotics against degradation, significantly increasing the number of viable probiotics after exposure to simulated gastric juice and simulated intestinal juice, reinforcing their potential application in the delivery of probiotics to the intestine [152,161,162].

The use of nanotechnology has provided a promising strategy for the delivery of probiotics in the treatment of IBD. The encapsulation of probiotics in nanosystems protects them from degradation, improves their stability and bioavailability, and enhances their therapeutic efficacy. Polymeric nanoparticles, particularly those designed to withstand the harsh conditions of the GIT, have shown potential in the targeted delivery of probiotics to the colon in addition to providing bioadhesive properties for the formulations. Several studies have demonstrated the benefits of probiotic-loaded nanoparticles in reducing the severity of clinical signs of IBD and restoring the epithelial lining in the colon [163]. These findings indicate that nanotechnology-based approaches have the potential to improve the effectiveness of probiotics in the treatment of intestinal inflammatory diseases.

6. Conclusions

This review underscores the immense promise of probiotics delivered through micro- and nanoparticles as a novel strategy for managing IBD. While substantial progress has been made in understanding the potential benefits and mechanisms of probiotic-loaded particles, numerous avenues for future research and exploration remain. To pave the way for more effective IBD treatments, it is imperative that further investigation and research are undertaken.

Future research in this field should focus on optimizing the formulation of probiotic-loaded particles. This includes developing more advanced and targeted delivery systems, enhancing the stability of probiotics during transit through the GIT, and exploring innovative encapsulation methods to ensure prolonged probiotic viability. Moreover, personalized medicine holds significant potential. Investigating the tailoring of probiotic therapies to individual patient profiles based on their unique gut microbiota composition can provide more personalized and effective treatment regimens. Longitudinal studies and clinical trials are required to assess the sustained safety, efficacy, and potential long-term side effects of probiotic-loaded particles for IBD. Additionally, a deeper understanding of the immunomodulatory mechanisms and the interactions between probiotics and the host's immune system in the context of IBD is essential for refining treatment strategies. This would involve exploring the specific strains of probiotics and their dosages that yield the most favorable outcomes for various IBD subtypes.

The potential future research directions in the field of IBD treatment with probiotics in micro- and nanoparticles are vast. These investigations will not only enhance our comprehension of the therapeutic potential of probiotics but also offer innovative, patient-specific solutions for managing this challenging and prevalent disease. It is with these prospects in mind that we look forward to the continued evolution of IBD therapeutics and the improved quality of life for patients affected by this condition.

Author Contributions: Conceptualization, writing—original draft: S.A.L. and A.B.M.; methodology: J.L.D., L.D.D.F., V.M.B.C., M.C. and F.R.P.; writing—review and editing: C.A.R.-B. and A.B.M.; graphics: S.A.L. and C.A.R.-B.; funding acquisition, A.B.M. All authors have read and agreed to the published version of the manuscript.

Funding: This study was financed in part by the Coordenação de Aperfeiçoamento de Pessoal de Nível Superior—Brasil (CAPES)—Finance Code 001 and EDITAL 01/2023 PROPe-Retificado-Prorrogado—Apoio à publicação científica com autoria de alunos de Iniciação Científica e Tecnológica (ICT), Pós-Doutorandos (PD) e Assistentes de Suporte Acadêmico (ASA) from UNESP. São Paulo Research Foundation (FAPESP) Fellowships: 2020/16573-3 and 2021/14603-5.

Institutional Review Board Statement: Not applicable.

Informed Consent Statement: Not applicable.

Data Availability Statement: The data presented in this study are available in this article.

Conflicts of Interest: The authors declare no conflict of interest.

References

1. Molodecky, N.A.; Soon, I.S.; Rabi, D.M.; Ghali, W.A.; Ferris, M.; Chernoff, G.; Benchimol, E.I.; Panaccione, R.; Ghosh, S.; Barkema, H.W.; et al. Increasing Incidence and Prevalence of the Inflammatory Bowel Diseases with Time, Based on Systematic Review. *Gastroenterology* **2012**, *142*, 46–54.e42. [CrossRef]
2. Oka, A.; Sartor, R.B. Microbial-Based and Microbial-Targeted Therapies for Inflammatory Bowel Diseases. *Dig. Dis. Sci.* **2020**, *65*, 757–788. [CrossRef] [PubMed]
3. Baumgart, D.C.; Sandborn, W.J. Crohn's Disease. *Lancet* **2012**, *380*, 1590–1605. [CrossRef] [PubMed]
4. Brito, R.C.V.; Peres De, C.L.; Silveira, K.A.F.; Arruda, E.L.; de Almeida Júnior, M.P. Doenças Inflamatórias Intestinais No Brasil: Perfil Das Internações, Entre Os Anos de 2009 a 2019. *Rev. Educ. Saúde* **2020**, *8*, 127–135. [CrossRef]
5. Kulkarni, N.; Jain, P.; Shindikar, A.; Suryawanshi, P.; Thorat, N. Advances in the Colon-Targeted Chitosan Based Multiunit Drug Delivery Systems for the Treatment of Inflammatory Bowel Disease. *Carbohydr. Polym.* **2022**, *288*, 119351. [CrossRef]
6. Kotla, N.G.; Rana, S.; Sivaraman, G.; Sunnapu, O.; Vemula, P.K.; Pandit, A.; Rochev, Y. Bioresponsive Drug Delivery Systems in Intestinal Inflammation: State-of-the-Art and Future Perspectives. *Adv. Drug Deliv. Rev.* **2018**, *146*, 248–266. [CrossRef]

7. Lee, J.; Jee, S.R.; Kim, H.W.; Baek, D.H.; Song, G.A.; Moon, W.; Park, S.J.; Kim, H.J.; Lee, J.H.; Park, J.H.; et al. Factors Associated with Low Adherence to Oral 5-Aminosalicylic Acid in Patients with Ulcerative Colitis. *PLoS ONE* **2019**, *14*, e0214129. [CrossRef]
8. Zhang, M.; Merlin, D. Nanoparticle-Based Oral Drug Delivery Systems Targeting the Colon for Treatment of Ulcerative Colitis. *Inflamm. Bowel Dis.* **2018**, *24*, 1401–1415. [CrossRef]
9. Shah, B.M.; Palakurthi, S.S.; Khare, T.; Khare, S.; Palakurthi, S. Natural Proteins and Polysaccharides in the Development of Micro/Nano Delivery Systems for the Treatment of Inflammatory Bowel Disease. *Int. J. Biol. Macromol.* **2020**, *165*, 722–737. [CrossRef]
10. Cottone, M.; Renna, S.; Modesto, I.; Orlando, A. Is 5-ASA Still the Treatment of Choice for Ulcerative Colitis? *Curr. Drug Targets* **2011**, *12*, 1396–1405. [CrossRef]
11. Coqueiro, A.Y.; Raizel, R.; Bonvini, A.; Tirapegui, J.; Rogero, M.M. Probiotics for Inflammatory Bowel Diseases: A Promising Adjuvant Treatment. *Int. J. Food Sci. Nutr.* **2019**, *70*, 20–29. [CrossRef]
12. Celiberto, L.S.; Bedani, R.; Dejani, N.N.; Ivo de Medeiros, A.; Sampaio Zuanon, J.A.; Spolidorio, L.C.; Tallarico Adorno, M.A.; Amâncio Varesche, M.B.; Carrilho Galvão, F.; Valentini, S.R.; et al. Effect of a Probiotic Beverage Consumption (Enterococcus Faecium CRL 183 and Bifidobacterium Longum ATCC 15707) in Rats with Chemically Induced Colitis. *PLoS ONE* **2017**, *12*, e0175935. [CrossRef]
13. Chen, X.; Yang, G.; Song, J.-H.; Xu, H.; Li, D.; Goldsmith, J.; Zeng, H.; Parsons-Wingerter, P.A.; Reinecker, H.-C.; Kelly, C.P. Probiotic Yeast Inhibits VEGFR Signaling and Angiogenesis in Intestinal Inflammation. *PLoS ONE* **2013**, *8*, e64227. [CrossRef]
14. Ghasemian, A.; Eslami, M.; Shafiei, M.; Najafipour, S.; Rajabi, A. Probiotics and Their Increasing Importance in Human Health and Infection Control. *Rev. Med. Microbiol.* **2018**, *29*, 153–158. [CrossRef]
15. Kruis, W.; Fric, P.; Pokrotnieks, J.; Lukaš, M.; Fixa, B.; Kaščák, M.; Kamm, M.A.; Wiesmueller, J.; Beglinger, C.; Stolte, M.; et al. Maintaining Remission of Ulcerative Colitis with the Probiotic Escherichia Coli Nissle 1917 Is as Effective as with Standard Mesalazine. *Gut* **2004**, *53*, 1617–1623. [CrossRef]
16. Mardini, H.E.; Grigorian, A.Y. Probiotic Mix VSL#3 Is Effective Adjunctive Therapy for Mild to Moderately Active Ulcerative Colitis. *Inflamm. Bowel Dis.* **2014**, *20*, 1562–1567. [CrossRef]
17. Mingmongkolchai, S.; Panbangred, W. Bacillus Probiotics: An Alternative to Antibiotics for Livestock Production. *J. Appl. Microbiol.* **2018**, *124*, 1334–1346. [CrossRef]
18. Palumbo, V.D.; Romeo, M.; Gammazza, A.M.; Carini, F.; Damiani, P.; Damiano, G.; Buscemi, S.; Lo Monte, A.I.; Gerges-Geagea, A.; Jurjus, A.; et al. The Long-Term Effects of Probiotics in the Therapy of Ulcerative Colitis: A Clinical Study. *Biomed. Pap.* **2016**, *160*, 372–377. [CrossRef] [PubMed]
19. Wieërs, G.; Belkhir, L.; Enaud, R.; Leclercq, S.; Philippart de Foy, J.-M.; Dequenne, I.; de Timary, P.; Cani, P.D. How Probiotics Affect the Microbiota. *Front. Cell. Infect. Microbiol.* **2020**, *9*, 454. [CrossRef] [PubMed]
20. Li, S.; Zhang, Y.-X. Sensitive Delivery Systems and Novel Encapsulation Technologies for Live Biotherapeutic Products and Probiotics. *Crit. Rev. Microbiol.* **2023**, 1–14. [CrossRef] [PubMed]
21. Collnot, E.-M.; Ali, H.; Lehr, C.-M. Nano- and Microparticulate Drug Carriers for Targeting of the Inflamed Intestinal Mucosa. *J. Control. Release* **2012**, *161*, 235–246. [CrossRef]
22. Haneishi, Y.; Furuya, Y.; Hasegawa, M.; Picarelli, A.; Rossi, M.; Miyamoto, J. Inflammatory Bowel Diseases and Gut Microbiota. *Int. J. Mol. Sci.* **2023**, *24*, 3817. [CrossRef] [PubMed]
23. Wilks, S. Morbid Appearances in the Intestine of Miss Bankes. *London Med. Gaz.* **1859**, *2*, 264–265.
24. Fumery, M.; Singh, S.; Dulai, P.S.; Gower-Rousseau, C.; Peyrin-Biroulet, L.; Sandborn, W.J. Natural History of Adult Ulcerative Colitis in Population-Based Cohorts: A Systematic Review. *Clin. Gastroenterol. Hepatol.* **2018**, *16*, 343–356.e3. [CrossRef] [PubMed]
25. Ungaro, R.; Mehandru, S.; Allen, P.B.; Peyrin-Biroulet, L.; Colombel, J.-F. Ulcerative Colitis. *Lancet* **2017**, *389*, 1756–1770. [CrossRef] [PubMed]
26. Becker, J.M. Surgical Therapy for Ulcerative Colitis and Crohn's Disease. *Gastroenterol. Clin. N. Am.* **1999**, *28*, 371–390. [CrossRef]
27. Hartwig, O.; Shetab Boushehri, M.A.; Shalaby, K.S.; Loretz, B.; Lamprecht, A.; Lehr, C.-M. Drug Delivery to the Inflamed Intestinal Mucosa—Targeting Technologies and Human Cell Culture Models for Better Therapies of IBD. *Adv. Drug Deliv. Rev.* **2021**, *175*, 113828. [CrossRef] [PubMed]
28. Crohn, B.B.; Ginzburg, L.; Oppenheimer, G.D. Regional ileitis. *J. Am. Med. Assoc.* **1932**, *99*, 1323. [CrossRef]
29. Pinho, M. A Biologia Molecular Das Doenças Inflamatórias Intestinais. *Rev. Bras. Coloproctol.* **2008**, *28*, 119–123. [CrossRef]
30. Gomes, J.P.; Watad, A.; Shoenfeld, Y. Nicotine and Autoimmunity: The Lotus' Flower in Tobacco. *Pharmacol. Res.* **2018**, *128*, 101–109. [CrossRef]
31. Khor, B.; Gardet, A.; Xavier, R.J. Genetics and Pathogenesis of Inflammatory Bowel Disease. *Nature* **2011**, *474*, 307–317. [CrossRef] [PubMed]
32. Zhang, J.; Zhao, Y.; Hou, T.; Zeng, H.; Kalambhe, D.; Wang, B.; Shen, X.; Huang, Y. Macrophage-Based Nanotherapeutic Strategies in Ulcerative Colitis. *J. Control. Release* **2020**, *320*, 363–380. [CrossRef]
33. Guo, X.Y.; Liu, X.J.; Hao, J.Y. Gut Microbiota in Ulcerative Colitis: Insights on Pathogenesis and Treatment. *J. Dig. Dis.* **2020**, *21*, 147–159. [CrossRef]
34. Khan, I.; Ullah, N.; Zha, L.; Bai, Y.; Khan, A.; Zhao, T.; Che, T.; Zhang, C. Alteration of Gut Microbiota in Inflammatory Bowel Disease (IBD): Cause or Consequence? IBD Treatment Targeting the Gut Microbiome. *Pathogens* **2019**, *8*, 126. [CrossRef]
35. Wallace, K.L.; Zheng, L.-B.; Kanazawa, Y.; Shih, D.Q. Immunopathology of Inflammatory Bowel Disease. *World J. Gastroenterol.* **2014**, *20*, 6. [CrossRef] [PubMed]

36. Porter, R.J.; Kalla, R.; Ho, G.-T. Ulcerative Colitis: Recent Advances in the Understanding of Disease Pathogenesis. *F1000Research* **2020**, *9*, 294. [CrossRef]
37. Rogler, G.; Biedermann, L.; Scharl, M. New Insights into the Pathophysiology of Inflammatory Bowel Disease: Microbiota, Epigenetics and Common Signalling Pathways. *Swiss Med. Wkly.* **2018**, *148*, w14599. [CrossRef]
38. Zhang, Y.-Z.; Li, Y.-Y. Inflammatory Bowel Disease: Pathogenesis. *World J. Gastroenterol.* **2014**, *20*, 91. [CrossRef] [PubMed]
39. Costello, S.P.; Soo, W.; Bryant, R.V.; Jairath, V.; Hart, A.L.; Andrews, J.M. Systematic Review with Meta-Analysis: Faecal Microbiota Transplantation for the Induction of Remission for Active Ulcerative Colitis. *Aliment. Pharmacol. Ther.* **2017**, *46*, 213–224. [CrossRef]
40. Cader, M.Z.; Kaser, A. Recent Advances in Inflammatory Bowel Disease: Mucosal Immune Cells in Intestinal Inflammation. *Gut* **2013**, *62*, 1653–1664. [CrossRef]
41. Lu, Y.; Li, X.; Liu, S.; Zhang, Y.; Zhang, D. Toll-like Receptors and Inflammatory Bowel Disease. *Front. Immunol.* **2018**, *9*, 79. [CrossRef] [PubMed]
42. Dvornikova, K.A.; Bystrova, E.Y.; Churilov, L.P.; Lerner, A. Pathogenesis of the Inflammatory Bowel Disease in Context of SARS-COV-2 Infection. *Mol. Biol. Rep.* **2021**, *48*, 5745–5758. [CrossRef] [PubMed]
43. Li, Y.; Law, H.K.W. Deciphering the Role of Autophagy in the Immunopathogenesis of Inflammatory Bowel Disease. *Front. Pharmacol.* **2022**, *13*, 184. [CrossRef] [PubMed]
44. Nikolakis, D.; de Voogd, F.A.E.; Pruijt, M.J.; Grootjans, J.; van de Sande, M.G.; D'Haens, G.R. The Role of the Lymphatic System in the Pathogenesis and Treatment of Inflammatory Bowel Disease. *Int. J. Mol. Sci.* **2022**, *23*, 1854. [CrossRef]
45. De Souza, F.G.; Lo Prete, A.C.; Ribeiro, C.H.M.A. Adesão Ao Tratamento Farmacológico Em Pacientes Com Doenças Inflamatórias Intestinais: Uma Revisão Integrativa Da Literatura. *Rev. Eletrônica Acervo Saúde* **2021**, *13*, e4601. [CrossRef]
46. Kesharwani, S.S.; Ahmad, R.; Bakkari, M.A.; Rajput, M.K.S.; Dachineni, R.; Valiveti, C.K.; Kapur, S.; Jayarama Bhat, G.; Singh, A.B.; Tummala, H. Site-Directed Non-Covalent Polymer-Drug Complexes for Inflammatory Bowel Disease (IBD): Formulation Development, Characterization and Pharmacological Evaluation. *J. Control. Release* **2018**, *290*, 165–179. [CrossRef]
47. Shivashankar, R.; Tremaine, W.J.; Harmsen, W.S.; Loftus, E.V. Incidence and Prevalence of Crohn's Disease and Ulcerative Colitis in Olmsted County, Minnesota From 1970 Through 2010. *Clin. Gastroenterol. Hepatol.* **2017**, *15*, 857–863. [CrossRef]
48. Windsor, J.W.; Kaplan, G.G. Evolving Epidemiology of IBD. *Curr. Gastroenterol. Rep.* **2019**, *21*, 40. [CrossRef]
49. Kaplan, G.G. The Global Burden of IBD: From 2015 to 2025. *Nat. Rev. Gastroenterol. Hepatol.* **2015**, *12*, 720–727. [CrossRef]
50. Ng, S.C.; Shi, H.Y.; Hamidi, N.; Underwood, F.E.; Tang, W.; Benchimol, E.I.; Panaccione, R.; Ghosh, S.; Wu, J.C.Y.; Chan, F.K.L.; et al. Worldwide Incidence and Prevalence of Inflammatory Bowel Disease in the 21st Century: A Systematic Review of Population-Based Studies. *Lancet* **2017**, *390*, 2769–2778. [CrossRef]
51. Ananthakrishnan, A.N. Epidemiology and Risk Factors for IBD. *Nat. Rev. Gastroenterol. Hepatol.* **2015**, *12*, 205–217. [CrossRef] [PubMed]
52. Chhoun, C.; Blair, B.; Joo, L.; Hashir, M.; Dasu, N.; Khalid, Y.; Chiesa, D.; Walters, R.; Suga, H. S22 Outcomes of Patients With Inflammatory Bowel Disease and Alcohol Use From the National Inpatient Sample. *Am. J. Gastroenterol.* **2022**, *117*, S6. [CrossRef]
53. Keefer, L.; Keshavarzian, A.; Mutlu, E. Reconsidering the Methodology of "Stress" Research in Inflammatory Bowel Disease. *J. Crohn's Colitis* **2008**, *2*, 193–201. [CrossRef] [PubMed]
54. Araki, M.; Shinzaki, S.; Yamada, T.; Arimitsu, S.; Komori, M.; Shibukawa, N.; Mukai, A.; Nakajima, S.; Kinoshita, K.; Kitamura, S.; et al. Psychologic Stress and Disease Activity in Patients with Inflammatory Bowel Disease: A Multicenter Cross-Sectional Study. *PLoS ONE* **2020**, *15*, e0233365. [CrossRef]
55. Sajadinejad, M.S.; Asgari, K.; Molavi, H.; Kalantari, M.; Adibi, P. Psychological Issues in Inflammatory Bowel Disease: An Overview. *Gastroenterol. Res. Pract.* **2012**, *2012*, 106502. [CrossRef]
56. Bernstein, C.N.; Singh, S.; Graff, L.A.; Walker, J.R.; Miller, N.; Cheang, M. A Prospective Population-Based Study of Triggers of Symptomatic Flares in IBD. *Am. J. Gastroenterol.* **2010**, *105*, 1994–2002. [CrossRef]
57. Mawdsley, J.E.; Rampton, D.S. Psychological Stress in IBD: New Insights into Pathogenic and Therapeutic Implications. *Gut* **2005**, *54*, 1481–1491. [CrossRef]
58. Agostini, A.; Filippini, N.; Cevolani, D.; Agati, R.; Leoni, C.; Tambasco, R.; Calabrese, C.; Rizzello, F.; Gionchetti, P.; Ercolani, M.; et al. Brain Functional Changes in Patients with Ulcerative Colitis. *Inflamm. Bowel Dis.* **2011**, *17*, 1769–1777. [CrossRef] [PubMed]
59. Morais, L.H.; Schreiber, H.L.; Mazmanian, S.K. The Gut Microbiota–Brain Axis in Behaviour and Brain Disorders. *Nat. Rev. Microbiol.* **2021**, *19*, 241–255. [CrossRef]
60. Tavares Junior, A.G.; De Araújo, J.T.C.; Duarte, J.L.; Silvestre, A.L.P.; Di Filippo, L.D.; Chorilli, M. Polymeric Systems for Colon-Specific Mesalazine Delivery in the Intestinal Bowel Diseases Management. *Curr. Med. Chem.* **2023**, *30*, 1351–1367. [CrossRef]
61. Rachmilewitz, D.; Karmeli, F.; Schwartz, L.W.; Simon, P.L. Effect of Aminophenols (5-ASA and 4-ASA) on Colonic Interleukin-1 Generation. *Gut* **1992**, *33*, 929–932. [CrossRef] [PubMed]
62. Stevens, C.; Corp, D.; Strom, T.B.; Lipman, M.; Peppercorn, M.A.; Moscovitch-lopatin, M.; Strom, T.B.; Hospital, B.I. 5-Aminosalicylic Acid Abrogates T-CelI Proliferation by Blocking Lnterleukin-2 Production in Peripheral Blood Mononuclear Cells. *J. Pharmacol. Exp. Ther.* **1995**, *272*, 399–406. [PubMed]
63. Kaiser, G.C.; Yan, F.; Polk, D.B. Mesalamine Blocks Tumor Necrosis Factor Growth Inhibition and Nuclear Factor KB Activation in Mouse Colonocytes. *Gastroenterology* **1999**, *116*, 602–609. [CrossRef]

64. Abdu Allah, H.H.; A El Shorbagi, A.N.; Abdel-Moty, S.G.; El-Awady, R.; Abdel-Alim, A.-A.M. 5-Aminosalyclic Acid (5-ASA): A Unique Anti-Inflammatory Salicylate. *Med. Chem.* **2016**, *6*, 306–315. [CrossRef]
65. Bantel, H. Mesalazine Inhibits Activation of Transcription Factor NF-KB in Inflamed Mucosa of Patients with Ulcerative Colitis. *Am. J. Gastroenterol.* **2000**, *95*, 3452–3457. [CrossRef]
66. Pooley, N.; Ghosh, L.; Sharon, P. Up-Regulation of E-Selectin and Intercellular Adhesion Molecule-1 Differs between Crohn's Disease and Ulcerative Colitis. *Dig. Dis. Sci.* **1995**, *40*, 219–225. [CrossRef]
67. Joshi, R.; Kumar, S.; Unnikrishnan, M.; Mukherjee, T. Free Radical Scavenging Reactions of Sulfasalazine, 5-Aminosalicylic Acid and Sulfapyridine: Mechanistic Aspects and Antioxidant Activity. *Free Radic. Res.* **2005**, *39*, 1163–1172. [CrossRef]
68. Bucci, C.; Zingone, F.; Tammaro, S.; Iovino, P.; Santonicola, A.; Ciacci, C. Factors Predicting the Adherence to the Therapy of Italian IBD Patients. *Gastroenterol. Res. Pract.* **2017**, *2017*, 1–6. [CrossRef]
69. Červený, P.; Bortlík, M.; Kuběna, A.; Vlček, J.; Lakatos, P.L.; Lukáš, M. Nonadherence in Inflammatory Bowel Disease: Results of Factor Analysis. *Inflamm. Bowel Dis.* **2007**, *13*, 1244–1249. [CrossRef]
70. Coenen, S.; Weyts, E.; Ballet, V.; Noman, M.; Van Assche, G.; Vermeire, S.; Van Emelen, J.; Ferrante, M. Identifying Predictors of Low Adherence in Patients with Inflammatory Bowel Disease. *Eur. J. Gastroenterol. Hepatol.* **2016**, *28*, 503–507. [CrossRef]
71. Kane, S.; Huo, D.; Aikens, J.; Hanauer, S. Medication Nonadherence and the Outcomes of Patients with Quiescent Ulcerative Colitis. *Am. J. Med.* **2003**, *114*, 39–43. [CrossRef] [PubMed]
72. Shale, M.J.; Riley, S.A. Studies of Compliance with Delayed-Release Mesalazine Therapy in Patients with Inflammatory Bowel Disease. *Aliment. Pharmacol. Ther.* **2003**, *18*, 191–198. [CrossRef]
73. Tomar, S.K.; Kedia, S.; Singh, N.; Upadhyay, A.D.; Kamat, N.; Bopanna, S.; Yadav, D.P.; Goyal, S.; Jain, S.; Makharia, G.; et al. Higher Education, Professional Occupation, and Upper Socioeconomic Status Are Associated with Lower Adherence to Medications in Patients with Inflammatory Bowel Disease. *JGH Open* **2019**, *3*, 302–309. [CrossRef]
74. Su, H.-J.; Chiu, Y.-T.; Chiu, C.-T.; Lin, Y.-C.; Wang, C.-Y.; Hsieh, J.-Y.; Wei, S.-C. Inflammatory Bowel Disease and Its Treatment in 2018: Global and Taiwanese Status Updates. *J. Formos. Med. Assoc.* **2019**, *118*, 1083–1092. [CrossRef] [PubMed]
75. Baumgart, D.C.; Vierziger, K.; Sturm, A.; Wiedenmann, B.; Dignass, A.U. Mesalamine Promotes Intestinal Epithelial Wound Healing in Vitro through a TGF-Beta-Independent Mechanism. *Scand. J. Gastroenterol.* **2005**, *40*, 958–964. [CrossRef]
76. Ho, G.-T.; Lees, C.; Satsangi, J. Ulcerative Colitis. *Medicine* **2011**, *39*, 224–228. [CrossRef]
77. Bernstein, C.N.; Eliakim, A.; Fedail, S.; Fried, M.; Gearry, R.; Goh, K.-L.; Hamid, S.; Khan, A.G.; Khalif, I.; Ng, S.C.; et al. World Gastroenterology Organisation Global Guidelines Inflammatory Bowel Disease. *J. Clin. Gastroenterol.* **2016**, *50*, 803–818. [CrossRef]
78. Feuerstein, J.D.; Cheifetz, A.S. Ulcerative Colitis. *Mayo Clin. Proc.* **2014**, *89*, 1553–1563. [CrossRef]
79. Fróes, R.D.S.B. Tratamento Convencional Na Doença Inflamatória Intestinal. *Rev. Hosp. Univ. Pedro Ernesto* **2012**, *11*, 27–32.
80. Alqahtani, M.S.; Kazi, M.; Alsenaidy, M.A.; Ahmad, M.Z. Advances in Oral Drug Delivery. *Front. Pharmacol.* **2021**, *12*, 618411. [CrossRef] [PubMed]
81. Higashiyama, M.; Hokaria, R. New and Emerging Treatments for Inflammatory Bowel Disease. *Digestion* **2023**, *104*, 74–81. [CrossRef]
82. Hua, S. Advances in Oral Drug Delivery for Regional Targeting in the Gastrointestinal Tract—Influence of Physiological, Pathophysiological and Pharmaceutical Factors. *Front. Pharmacol.* **2020**, *11*, 524. [CrossRef]
83. Arévalo-Pérez, R.; Maderuelo, C.; Lanao, J.M. Recent Advances in Colon Drug Delivery Systems. *J. Control. Release* **2020**, *327*, 703–724. [CrossRef] [PubMed]
84. Gomaa, E.Z. Human Gut Microbiota/Microbiome in Health and Diseases: A Review. *Antonie Van Leeuwenhoek* **2020**, *113*, 2019–2040. [CrossRef] [PubMed]
85. Manos, J. The Human Microbiome in Disease and Pathology. *APMIS* **2022**, *130*, 690–705. [CrossRef]
86. Andoh, A.; Nishida, A. Alteration of the Gut Microbiome in Inflammatory Bowel Disease. *Digestion* **2023**, *104*, 16–23. [CrossRef] [PubMed]
87. Sartor, R.B. Microbial Influences in Inflammatory Bowel Diseases. *Gastroenterology* **2008**, *134*, 577–594. [CrossRef] [PubMed]
88. Sender, R.; Fuchs, S.; Milo, R. Are We Really Vastly Outnumbered? Revisiting the Ratio of Bacterial to Host Cells in Humans. *Cell* **2016**, *164*, 337–340. [CrossRef] [PubMed]
89. Hajela, N.; Ramakrishna, B.S.; Nair, G.B.; Abraham, P.; Gopalan, S.; Ganguly, N.K. Gut Microbiome, Gut Function, and Probiotics: Implications for Health. *Indian J. Gastroenterol.* **2015**, *34*, 93–107. [CrossRef]
90. Buttó, L.F.; Schaubeck, M.; Haller, D. Mechanisms of Microbe–Host Interaction in Crohn's Disease: Dysbiosis vs. Pathobiont Selection. *Front. Immunol.* **2015**, *6*, 555. [CrossRef]
91. Nishida, A.; Inoue, R.; Inatomi, O.; Bamba, S.; Naito, Y.; Andoh, A. Gut Microbiota in the Pathogenesis of Inflammatory Bowel Disease. *Clin. J. Gastroenterol.* **2018**, *11*, 1–10. [CrossRef] [PubMed]
92. Xu, J.; Chen, N.; Wu, Z.; Song, Y.; Zhang, Y.; Wu, N.; Zhang, F.; Ren, X.; Liu, Y. 5-Aminosalicylic Acid Alters the Gut Bacterial Microbiota in Patients With Ulcerative Colitis. *Front. Microbiol.* **2018**, *9*, 1274. [CrossRef]
93. Fuentes, S.; Rossen, N.G.; van der Spek, M.J.; Hartman, J.H.A.; Huuskonen, L.; Korpela, K.; Salojärvi, J.; Aalvink, S.; de Vos, W.M.; D'Haens, G.R.; et al. Microbial Shifts and Signatures of Long-Term Remission in Ulcerative Colitis after Faecal Microbiota Transplantation. *ISME J.* **2017**, *11*, 1877–1889. [CrossRef]

94. Darfeuille-Michaud, A.; Boudeau, J.; Bulois, P.; Neut, C.; Glasser, A.-L.; Barnich, N.; Bringer, M.-A.; Swidsinski, A.; Beaugerie, L.; Colombel, J.-F. High Prevalence of Adherent-Invasive Escherichia Coli Associated with Ileal Mucosa in Crohn's Disease. *Gastroenterology* **2004**, *127*, 412–421. [CrossRef]
95. Mucida, D.; Park, Y.; Kim, G.; Turovskaya, O.; Scott, I.; Kronenberg, M.; Cheroutre, H. Reciprocal T H 17 and Regulatory T Cell Differentiation Mediated by Retinoic Acid. *Science* **2007**, *317*, 256–260. [CrossRef]
96. Round, J.L.; Mazmanian, S.K. Inducible Foxp3+ Regulatory T-Cell Development by a Commensal Bacterium of the Intestinal Microbiota. *Proc. Natl. Acad. Sci. USA* **2010**, *107*, 12204–12209. [CrossRef]
97. Martín, R.; Chain, F.; Miquel, S.; Lu, J.; Gratadoux, J.-J.; Sokol, H.; Verdu, E.F.; Bercik, P.; Bermúdez-Humarán, L.G.; Langella, P. The Commensal Bacterium Faecalibacterium Prausnitzii Is Protective in DNBS-Induced Chronic Moderate and Severe Colitis Models. *Inflamm. Bowel Dis.* **2014**, *20*, 417–430. [CrossRef] [PubMed]
98. Sokol, H.; Seksik, P.; Furet, J.P.; Firmesse, O.; Nion-Larmurier, I.; Beaugerie, L.; Cosnes, J.; Corthier, G.; Marteau, P.; Doré, J. Low Counts of Faecalibacterium Prausnitzii in Colitis Microbiota. *Inflamm. Bowel Dis.* **2009**, *15*, 1183–1189. [CrossRef]
99. David, L.A.; Maurice, C.F.; Carmody, R.N.; Gootenberg, D.B.; Button, J.E.; Wolfe, B.E.; Ling, A.V.; Devlin, A.S.; Varma, Y.; Fischbach, M.A.; et al. Diet Rapidly and Reproducibly Alters the Human Gut Microbiome. *Nature* **2014**, *505*, 559–563. [CrossRef]
100. Wu, G.D.; Chen, J.; Hoffmann, C.; Bittinger, K.; Chen, Y.-Y.; Keilbaugh, S.A.; Bewtra, M.; Knights, D.; Walters, W.A.; Knight, R.; et al. Linking Long-Term Dietary Patterns with Gut Microbial Enterotypes. *Science* **2011**, *334*, 105–108. [CrossRef] [PubMed]
101. Iliev, I.D.; Funari, V.A.; Taylor, K.D.; Nguyen, Q.; Reyes, C.N.; Strom, S.P.; Brown, J.; Becker, C.A.; Fleshner, P.R.; Dubinsky, M.; et al. Interactions Between Commensal Fungi and the C-Type Lectin Receptor Dectin-1 Influence Colitis. *Science* **2012**, *336*, 1314–1317. [CrossRef]
102. Norman, J.M.; Handley, S.A.; Baldridge, M.T.; Droit, L.; Liu, C.Y.; Keller, B.C.; Kambal, A.; Monaco, C.L.; Zhao, G.; Fleshner, P.; et al. Disease-Specific Alterations in the Enteric Virome in Inflammatory Bowel Disease. *Cell* **2015**, *160*, 447–460. [CrossRef]
103. Kaufman, J.; Griffiths, T.A.; Surette, M.G.; Ness, S.; Rioux, K.P. Effects of Mesalamine (5-Aminosalicylic Acid) on Bacterial Gene Expression. *Inflamm. Bowel Dis.* **2009**, *15*, 985–996. [CrossRef]
104. Guarino, M.; Altomare, A.; Emerenziani, S.; Di Rosa, C.; Ribolsi, M.; Balestrieri, P.; Iovino, P.; Rocchi, G.; Cicala, M. Mechanisms of Action of Prebiotics and Their Effects on Gastro-Intestinal Disorders in Adults. *Nutrients* **2020**, *12*, 1037. [CrossRef] [PubMed]
105. Shen, Z.-H.; Zhu, C.-X.; Quan, Y.-S.; Yang, Z.-Y.; Wu, S.; Luo, W.-W.; Tan, B.; Wang, X.-Y. Relationship between Intestinal Microbiota and Ulcerative Colitis: Mechanisms and Clinical Application of Probiotics and Fecal Microbiota Transplantation. *World J. Gastroenterol.* **2018**, *24*, 5–14. [CrossRef]
106. Lilly, D.M.; Stillwell, R.H. Probiotics: Growth-Promoting Factors Produced by Microorganisms. *Science* **1965**, *147*, 747–748. [CrossRef] [PubMed]
107. Sarao, L.K.; Arora, M. Probiotics, Prebiotics, and Microencapsulation: A Review. *Crit. Rev. Food Sci. Nutr.* **2017**, *57*, 344–371. [CrossRef] [PubMed]
108. Cao, F.; Gui, S.-Y.; Gao, X.; Zhang, W.; Fu, Z.-Y.; Tao, L.-M.; Jiang, Z.-X.; Chen, X.; Qian, H.; Wang, X. Research Progress of Natural Product-Based Nanomaterials for the Treatment of Inflammation-Related Diseases. *Mater. Des.* **2022**, *218*, 110686. [CrossRef]
109. Nath, A.; Haktanirlar, G.; Varga, Á.; Molnár, M.A.; Albert, K.; Galambos, I.; Koris, A.; Vatai, G. Biological Activities of Lactose-Derived Prebiotics and Symbiotic with Probiotics on Gastrointestinal System. *Medicina* **2018**, *54*, 18. [CrossRef]
110. Sanders, M.E.; Merenstein, D.J.; Reid, G.; Gibson, G.R.; Rastall, R.A. Probiotics and Prebiotics in Intestinal Health and Disease: From Biology to the Clinic. *Nat. Rev. Gastroenterol. Hepatol.* **2019**, *16*, 605–616. [CrossRef]
111. De Melo Pereira, G.V.; de Oliveira Coelho, B.; Magalhães Júnior, A.I.; Thomaz-Soccol, V.; Soccol, C.R. How to Select a Probiotic? A Review and Update of Methods and Criteria. *Biotechnol. Adv.* **2018**, *36*, 2060–2076. [CrossRef] [PubMed]
112. Ríos-Covián, D.; Ruas-Madiedo, P.; Margolles, A.; Gueimonde, M.; de los Reyes-Gavilán, C.G.; Salazar, N. Intestinal Short Chain Fatty Acids and Their Link with Diet and Human Health. *Front. Microbiol.* **2016**, *7*, 185. [CrossRef]
113. Tsai, Y.-L.; Lin, T.-L.; Chang, C.-J.; Wu, T.-R.; Lai, W.-F.; Lu, C.-C.; Lai, H.-C. Probiotics, Prebiotics and Amelioration of Diseases. *J. Biomed. Sci.* **2019**, *26*, 3. [CrossRef] [PubMed]
114. Corrêa-Oliveira, R.; Fachi, J.L.; Vieira, A.; Sato, F.T.; Vinolo, M.A.R. Regulation of Immune Cell Function by Short-Chain Fatty Acids. *Clin. Transl. Immunol.* **2016**, *5*, e73. [CrossRef]
115. Yao, M.; Xie, J.; Du, H.; McClements, D.J.; Xiao, H.; Li, L. Progress in Microencapsulation of Probiotics: A Review. *Compr. Rev. Food Sci. Food Saf.* **2020**, *19*, 857–874. [CrossRef]
116. Jakubczyk, D.; Leszczyńska, K.; Górska, S. The Effectiveness of Probiotics in the Treatment of Inflammatory Bowel Disease (IBD)—A Critical Review. *Nutrients* **2020**, *12*, 1973. [CrossRef]
117. Danese, S. Negative Regulators of Angiogenesis in Inflammatory Bowel Disease: Thrombospondin in the Spotlight. *Pathobiology* **2008**, *75*, 22–24. [CrossRef]
118. Papa, A.; Scaldaferri, F.; Danese, S.; Guglielmo, S.; Roberto, I.; Bonizzi, M.; Mocci, G.; Felice, C.; Ricci, C.; Andrisani, G.; et al. Vascular Involvement in Inflammatory Bowel Disease: Pathogenesis and Clinical Aspects. *Dig. Dis.* **2008**, *26*, 149–155. [CrossRef] [PubMed]
119. Chidlow, J.H.; Shukla, D.; Grisham, M.B.; Kevil, C.G. Pathogenic Angiogenesis in IBD and Experimental Colitis: New Ideas and Therapeutic Avenues. *Am. J. Physiol. Liver Physiol.* **2007**, *293*, G5–G18. [CrossRef]
120. Kanazawa, S.; Tsunoda, T.; Onuma, E.; Majima, T.; Kagiyama, M.; Kikuchi, K. VEGF, Basic-FGF, and TGF-Beta in Crohn's Disease and Ulcerative Colitis: A Novel Mechanism of Chronic Intestinal Inflammation. *Am. J. Gastroenterol.* **2001**, *96*, 822–828. [CrossRef]

121. Kapsoritakis, A.; Sfiridaki, A.; Maltezos, E.; Simopoulos, K.; Giatromanolaki, A.; Sivridis, E.; Koukourakis, M.I. Vascular Endothelial Growth Factor in Inflammatory Bowel Disease. *Int. J. Colorectal Dis.* **2003**, *18*, 418–422. [CrossRef]
122. Tsiolakidou, G.; Koutroubakis, I.E.; Tzardi, M.; Kouroumalis, E.A. Increased Expression of VEGF and CD146 in Patients with Inflammatory Bowel Disease. *Dig. Liver Dis.* **2008**, *40*, 673–679. [CrossRef]
123. Scaldaferri, F.; Vetrano, S.; Sans, M.; Arena, V.; Straface, G.; Stigliano, E.; Repici, A.; Sturm, A.; Malesci, A.; Panes, J.; et al. VEGF-A Links Angiogenesis and Inflammation in Inflammatory Bowel Disease Pathogenesis. *Gastroenterology* **2009**, *136*, 585–595.e5. [CrossRef] [PubMed]
124. Zulham, Z.Z.; Wilar, G.; Susilawati, Y.; Subarnas, A.; Chaerunisaa, A.Y. Microparticles of Herbal Extracts with Antioxidant Activity. *Pharmacogn. J.* **2021**, *13*, 285–295. [CrossRef]
125. Da Silva, A.B.; Miniter, M.; Thom, W.; Hewitt, R.E.; Wills, J.; Jugdaohsingh, R.; Powell, J.J. Gastrointestinal Absorption and Toxicity of Nanoparticles and Microparticles: Myth, Reality and Pitfalls Explored through Titanium Dioxide. *Curr. Opin. Toxicol.* **2020**, *19*, 112–120. [CrossRef] [PubMed]
126. Kaul, S.; Kaur, K.; Mehta, N.; Dhaliwal, S.S.; Kennedy, J.F. Characterization and Optimization of Spray Dried Iron and Zinc Nanoencapsules Based on Potato Starch and Maltodextrin. *Carbohydr. Polym.* **2022**, *282*, 119107. [CrossRef]
127. Barajas-Álvarez, P.; González-Ávila, M.; Espinosa-Andrews, H. Recent Advances in Probiotic Encapsulation to Improve Viability under Storage and Gastrointestinal Conditions and Their Impact on Functional Food Formulation. *Food Rev. Int.* **2023**, *39*, 992–1013. [CrossRef]
128. How, Y.; Pui, L. Survivability of Microencapsulated Probiotics in Nondairy Beverages: A Review. *J. Food Process. Preserv.* **2021**, *45*, e15641. [CrossRef]
129. Zhu, Y.; Wang, Q.; Chen, Y.; Xie, Y.; Han, G.; Liu, S.; Song, Y.; Lu, W.; Guo, Y. Living Probiotics—Loaded Hydrogel Microspheres with Gastric Acid Resistance and ROS Triggered Release for Potential Therapy of Inflammatory Bowel Disease. *ACS Appl. Polym. Mater.* **2023**, *5*, 957–967. [CrossRef]
130. Williams, G.T.; Sedgwick, A.C.; Sen, S.; Gwynne, L.; Gardiner, J.E.; Brewster, J.T.; Hiscock, J.R.; James, T.D.; Jenkins, A.T.A.; Sessler, J.L. Boronate Ester Cross-Linked PVA Hydrogels for the Capture and H_2O_2-Mediated Release of Active Fluorophores. *Chem. Commun.* **2020**, *56*, 5516–5519. [CrossRef]
131. Li, J.; Qiu, H.; Gong, H.; Tong, W. Broad-Spectrum Reactive Oxygen Species Scavenging and Activated Macrophage-Targeting Microparticles Ameliorate Inflammatory Bowel Disease. *Biomacromolecules* **2021**, *22*, 3107–3118. [CrossRef] [PubMed]
132. Gąsiorowska, A.; Romanowski, M.; Walecka-Kapica, E.; Kaczka, A.; Chojnacki, C.; Padysz, M.; Siedlecka, M.; Bierła, J.B.; Steinert, R.E.; Cukrowska, B. Effects of Microencapsulated Sodium Butyrate, Probiotics and Short Chain Fructooligosaccharides in Patients with Irritable Bowel Syndrome: A Study Protocol of a Randomized Double-Blind Placebo-Controlled Trial. *J. Clin. Med.* **2022**, *11*, 6587. [CrossRef]
133. Pinto, L.A.; Corá, L.A.; Rodrigues, G.S.; Prospero, A.G.; Soares, G.A.; de Andreis, U.; de Arruda Miranda, J.R. Pharmacomagnetography to Evaluate the Performance of Magnetic Enteric-Coated Tablets in the Human Gastrointestinal Tract. *Eur. J. Pharm. Biopharm.* **2021**, *161*, 50–55. [CrossRef] [PubMed]
134. Maderuelo, C.; Lanao, J.M.; Zarzuelo, A. Enteric Coating of Oral Solid Dosage Forms as a Tool to Improve Drug Bioavailability. *Eur. J. Pharm. Sci.* **2019**, *138*, 105019. [CrossRef]
135. Roque-Borda, C.A.; de Mesquita Souza Saraiva, M.; Macedo Junior, W.D.; Márquez Montesinos, J.C.E.; Meneguin, A.B.; Toledo Borges, A.B.; Crusca Junior, E.; Garrido, S.S.; de Almeida, A.M.; Marchetto, R.; et al. Chitosan and HPMCAS Double-Coating as Protective Systems for Alginate Microparticles Loaded with Ctx(Ile21)-Ha Antimicrobial Peptide to Prevent Intestinal Infections. *Biomaterials* **2023**, *293*, 121978. [CrossRef]
136. Roque-Borda, C.A.; de Mesquita Souza Saraiva, M.; Monte, D.F.M.; Rodrigues Alves, L.B.; de Almeida, A.M.; Ferreira, T.S.; de Lima, T.S.; Benevides, V.P.; Cabrera, J.M.; Claire, S.; et al. HPMCAS-Coated Alginate Microparticles Loaded with Ctx(Ile 21)-Ha as a Promising Antimicrobial Agent against Salmonella Enteritidis in a Chicken Infection Model. *ACS Infect. Dis.* **2022**, *8*, 472–481. [CrossRef]
137. Park, H.J.; Lee, G.H.; Jun, J.H.; Son, M.; Choi, Y.S.; Choi, M.K.; Kang, M.J. Formulation and in Vivo Evaluation of Probiotics-Encapsulated Pellets with Hydroxypropyl Methylcellulose Acetate Succinate (HPMCAS). *Carbohydr. Polym.* **2015**, *136*, 692–699. [CrossRef]
138. Mirmazloum, I.; Ladányi, M.; Omran, M.; Papp, V.; Ronkainen, V.-P.; Pónya, Z.; Papp, I.; Némedi, E.; Kiss, A. Co-Encapsulation of Probiotic Lactobacillus Acidophilus and Reishi Medicinal Mushroom (*Ganoderma Lingzhi*) Extract in Moist Calcium Alginate Beads. *Int. J. Biol. Macromol.* **2021**, *192*, 461–470. [CrossRef]
139. Zhu, Y.-Y.; Thakur, K.; Zhang, W.-W.; Feng, J.-Y.; Zhang, J.-G.; Hu, F.; Liao, C.; Wei, Z.-J. Double-Layer Mucin Microencapsulation Enhances the Stress Tolerance and Oral Delivery of Lactobacillus Plantarum B2. *Food Hydrocoll.* **2023**, *141*, 108678. [CrossRef]
140. Yan, H.; Seignez, C.; Hjorth, M.; Winkeljann, B.; Blakeley, M.; Lieleg, O.; Phillipson, M.; Crouzier, T. Immune-Informed Mucin Hydrogels Evade Fibrotic Foreign Body Response In Vivo. *Adv. Funct. Mater.* **2019**, *29*, 1902581. [CrossRef]
141. Pourjafar, H.; Noori, N.; Gandomi, H.; Basti, A.A.; Ansari, F. Viability of Microencapsulated and Non-Microencapsulated Lactobacilli in a Commercial Beverage. *Biotechnol. Rep.* **2020**, *25*, e00432. [CrossRef]
142. Roque-Borda, C.A.; Antunes, B.F.; Toledo Borgues, A.B.; Costa de Pontes, J.T.; Meneguin, A.B.; Chorilli, M.; Trovatti, E.; Teixeira, S.R.; Pavan, F.R.; Vicente, E.F. Conjugation of Ctx(Ile^{21})-Ha Antimicrobial Peptides to Chitosan Ultrathin Films by

N-Acetylcysteine Improves Peptide Physicochemical Properties and Enhances Biological Activity. *ACS Omega* **2022**, *7*, 28238–28247. [CrossRef]
143. Shahzadi, I.; Fürst, A.; Akkus-Dagdeviren, Z.B.; Arshad, S.; Kurpiers, M.; Matuszczak, B.; Bernkop-Schnürch, A. Less Reactive Thiol Ligands: Key towards Highly Mucoadhesive Drug Delivery Systems. *Polymers* **2020**, *12*, 1259. [CrossRef] [PubMed]
144. Zhang, H.; Liu, Z.; Fang, H.; Chang, S.; Ren, G.; Cheng, X.; Pan, Y.; Wu, R.; Liu, H.; Wu, J. Construction of Probiotic Double-Layered Multinucleated Microcapsules Based on Sulfhydryl-Modified Carboxymethyl Cellulose Sodium for Increased Intestinal Adhesion of Probiotics and Therapy for Intestinal Inflammation Induced by Escherichia Coli O157:H7. *ACS Appl. Mater. Interfaces* **2023**, *15*, 18569–18589. [CrossRef]
145. Zavaleta, E.B.; Coavichi, L.I.L.; Rodríguez, L.C.V.; Andrade, E.F.; García, H.S.; Rascón Díaz, M.P. Co-Microencapsulation of Lactobacillus Rhamnosus and Krill Oil by Spray-Drying. *Food Biosci.* **2022**, *50*, 102133. [CrossRef]
146. Quintana, G.; Gerbino, E.; Alves, P.; Simões, P.N.; Rúa, M.L.; Fuciños, C.; Gomez-Zavaglia, A. Microencapsulation of Lactobacillus Plantarum in W/O Emulsions of Okara Oil and Block-Copolymers of Poly(Acrylic Acid) and Pluronic Using Microfluidic Devices. *Food Res. Int.* **2021**, *140*, 110053. [CrossRef]
147. Sharifi, E.; Yazdani, Z.; Najafi, M.; Hosseini-khah, Z.; Jafarpour, A.; Rafiei, A. The Combined Effect of Fish Oil Containing Omega-3 Fatty Acids and Lactobacillus Plantarum on Colorectal Cancer. *Food Sci. Nutr.* **2022**, *10*, 4411–4418. [CrossRef]
148. Marcial-Coba, M.S.; Saaby, L.; Knøchel, S.; Nielsen, D.S. Dark Chocolate as a Stable Carrier of Microencapsulated *Akkermansia muciniphila* and *Lactobacillus casei*. *FEMS Microbiol. Lett.* **2019**, *366*, 74. [CrossRef] [PubMed]
149. Jiang, Z.; Li, M.; McClements, D.J.; Liu, X.; Liu, F. Recent Advances in the Design and Fabrication of Probiotic Delivery Systems to Target Intestinal Inflammation. *Food Hydrocoll.* **2022**, *125*, 107438. [CrossRef]
150. Thakur, V.; Singh, B.; Sharma, A.; Kumari, N.; Kumar, I.; Verma, K.; Kumar, A.; Rana, S. Importance of Nanocarriers and Probiotics in the Treatment of Ulcerative Colitis. *Int. J. Appl. Pharm.* **2021**, *13*, 77–85. [CrossRef]
151. Razavi, S.; Janfaza, S.; Tasnim, N.; Gibson, D.L.; Hoorfar, M. Nanomaterial-Based Encapsulation for Controlled Gastrointestinal Delivery of Viable Probiotic Bacteria. *Nanoscale Adv.* **2021**, *3*, 2699–2709. [CrossRef]
152. Xu, C.; Ban, Q.; Wang, W.; Hou, J.; Jiang, Z. Novel Nano-Encapsulated Probiotic Agents: Encapsulate Materials, Delivery, and Encapsulation Systems. *J. Control. Release* **2022**, *349*, 184–205. [CrossRef] [PubMed]
153. Alkushi, A.G.; Abdelfattah-Hassan, A.; Eldoumani, H.; Elazab, S.T.; Mohamed, S.A.M.; Metwally, A.S.; El-Shetry, S.E.; Saleh, A.A.; ElSawy, N.A.; Ibrahim, D. Probiotics-Loaded Nanoparticles Attenuated Colon Inflammation, Oxidative Stress, and Apoptosis in Colitis. *Sci. Rep.* **2022**, *12*, 5116. [CrossRef]
154. Alkushi, A.G.; Elazab, S.T.; Abdelfattah-Hassan, A.; Mahfouz, H.; Salem, G.A.; Sheraiba, N.I.; Mohamed, E.A.A.; Attia, M.S.; El-Shetry, E.S.; Saleh, A.A.; et al. Multi-Strain-Probiotic-Loaded Nanoparticles Reduced Colon Inflammation and Orchestrated the Expressions of Tight Junction, NLRP3 Inflammasome and Caspase-1 Genes in DSS-Induced Colitis Model. *Pharmaceutics* **2022**, *14*, 1183. [CrossRef]
155. Ebrahimnejad, P.; Khavarpour, M.; Khalili, S. Survival of Lactobacillus Acidophilus as Probiotic Bacteria Using Chitosan Nanoparticles. *Int. J. Eng.* **2017**, *30*, 456–463. [CrossRef]
156. Saadatzadeh, A.; Atyabi, F.; Fazeli, M.R.; Dinarvand, R.; Jamalifar, H.; Abdolghaffari, A.H.; Mahdaviani, P.; Mahbod, M.; Baeeri, M.; Baghaei, A.; et al. Biochemical and Pathological Evidences on the Benefit of a New Biodegradable Nanoparticles of Probiotic Extract in Murine Colitis. *Fundam. Clin. Pharmacol.* **2012**, *26*, 589–598. [CrossRef]
157. Sahu, B.K.; Sharma, S.; Kaur, K.; Chandel, M.; Sood, P.; Singh, M.; Shanmugham, V. Farm Waste-Eggshell Nanoparticles Constitute Gel for Safe Navigation of Probiotic across the Stomach. *Mater. Today Commun.* **2023**, *34*, 104876. [CrossRef]
158. Liu, J.; Wang, Y.; Heelan, W.J.; Chen, Y.; Li, Z.; Hu, Q. Mucoadhesive Probiotic Backpacks with ROS Nanoscavengers Enhance the Bacteriotherapy for Inflammatory Bowel Diseases. *Sci. Adv.* **2022**, *8*, eabp8798. [CrossRef]
159. Wei, H.; Geng, W.; Yang, X.-Y.; Kuipers, J.; van der Mei, H.C.; Busscher, H.J. Activation of a Passive, Mesoporous Silica Nanoparticle Layer through Attachment of Bacterially-Derived Carbon-Quantum-Dots for Protection and Functional Enhancement of Probiotics. *Mater. Today Bio* **2022**, *15*, 100293. [CrossRef] [PubMed]
160. Xu, J.; Xu, J.; Shi, T.; Zhang, Y.; Chen, F.; Yang, C.; Guo, X.; Liu, G.; Shao, D.; Leong, K.W.; et al. Probiotic-Inspired Nanomedicine Restores Intestinal Homeostasis in Colitis by Regulating Redox Balance, Immune Responses, and the Gut Microbiome. *Adv. Mater.* **2023**, *35*, 2207890. [CrossRef]
161. Cao, Z.; Wang, X.; Pang, Y.; Cheng, S.; Liu, J. Biointerfacial Self-Assembly Generates Lipid Membrane Coated Bacteria for Enhanced Oral Delivery and Treatment. *Nat. Commun.* **2019**, *10*, 5783. [CrossRef] [PubMed]
162. Zhou, X.; Guo, Q.; Guo, M.; Li, B.; Peng, W.; Wang, D.; Ming, D.; Zheng, B. Nanoarmour-Shielded Single-Cell Factory for Bacteriotherapy of Parkinson's Disease. *J. Control. Release* **2021**, *338*, 742–753. [CrossRef] [PubMed]
163. Zhang, C.; Li, Q.; Shan, J.; Xing, J.; Liu, X.; Ma, Y.; Qian, H.; Chen, X.; Wang, X.; Wu, L.-M.; et al. Multifunctional Two-Dimensional Bi_2Se_3 Nanodiscs for Anti-Inflammatory Therapy of Inflammatory Bowel Diseases. *Acta Biomater.* **2023**, *160*, 252–264. [CrossRef] [PubMed]

pharmaceutics

Systematic Review

Advances in the Oral Administration of Somatostatin Receptor Ligands in Acromegaly: A Systematic Review Focusing on Biochemical Response

Clémence Reverdiau [1] and Damien Denimal [2,3,*]

[1] Department of Pharmacy, Faculté des Sciences de Santé, Université de Bourgogne, F-21000 Dijon, France
[2] Department of Clinical Biochemistry, Centre Hospitalier Universitaire Dijon-Bourgogne, F-21000 Dijon, France
[3] Center for Translational and Molecular Medicine, Université de Bourgogne, F-21000 Dijon, France
* Correspondence: damien.denimal@u-bourgogne.fr; Tel.: +33-03-80-29-38-23

Abstract: Recent advances in pharmaceutical technology, aimed at overcoming poor drug permeation across the intestinal–epithelial membrane and the challenges posed by the acidic gastrointestinal environment, have led to the development of orally administered somatostatin receptor ligands (SRLs). This development represents a promising step forward in the management of acromegaly, offering an alternative to the limitations associated with injectable SRLs. Several key clinical findings have emerged in the past two years, notably including the results from the extension phase of the MPOWERED trial, which evaluated oral octreotide capsules (OOCs), and the placebo-controlled PATHFNDR-1 trial using paltusotine. This prompted us to conduct a systematic review of the literature focusing on the efficacy of oral SRLs in controlling acromegaly, based on biochemical response. Of the 136 reports identified through our search on Medline and ClinicalTrials.gov, twelve were included, encompassing data from five interventional trials. Both OOCs and paltusotine demonstrated the ability to maintain biochemical control in patients previously controlled with injectable SRLs. While long-term maintenance was confirmed for OOCs, no data are yet available for paltusotine. Several gaps remain, such as the need for head-to-head comparisons between OOCs and paltusotine, and clinical trials in patients who have not received prior injectable SRL treatment.

Keywords: octreotide; paltusotine; acromegaly; oral route

1. Introduction

Acromegaly is characterized by an excessive production of growth hormone (GH) by the anterior pituitary gland. The prevalence of acromegaly is estimated at 5.9 cases per 100,000 individuals, with an incidence rate of approximately 0.38 cases per 100,000 person-years [1]. Medical therapy is recommended for patients with persistent disease despite surgical resection of the adenoma as well as for patients in whom surgery is not appropriate [2]. The long-acting formulations of the somatostatin receptor ligands (SRLs) octreotide and lanreotide are currently recommended as first-line medical therapy, while long-acting pasireotide could be considered as a second-line treatment [2]. SRLs bind to somatostatin receptors and mimic their physiological effects, leading to a reduction in GH secretion and subsequently insulin growth factor (IGF)-1 secretion by the liver.

Octreotide, lanreotide, and pasireotide are SRLs of a peptide nature, initially developed in injectable formulations due to their susceptibility to enzymatic degradation and low epithelial permeability in the intestine. They are administered through monthly intramuscular or subcutaneous injections of long-acting formulations. Injectable SRLs (iSRLs) exhibit numerous disadvantages such as injection site pain, nodules, bruising, inflammation, and scarring [3–5]. A real-world survey showed that 70% of patients reported experiencing pain at the injection site lasting up to a week, with other common adverse effects including nodules (38%), swelling (28%), bruising (16%), scar tissue formation (8%), and inflammation (7%) [3]. In addition, nurses have only a small amount of confidence that the octreotide syringe will not be clogged and will be somewhat easy to use during injection [6].

The development of oral formulations of SRLs has raised hope in mitigating these adverse effects and increasing compliance and quality of life [7]. Significant advances in oral formulations of SRLs have been made in the last decade. In particular, oral octreotide capsules (OOCs) have been developed through the enteric coating of capsules with a pH-dependent methacrylic acid copolymer preventing chemical and enzymatic degradation, but above all through the development of absorption enhancers to overcome low epithelial permeability [8]. In particular, the Transient Permeation Enhancer® technology (TPE®, Chiasma™, Jerusalem, Israel) has been used for the development of OOCs [9]. TPE® consists of an oily suspension of the peptide drug, sodium caprylate (C8), glyceryl monocaprylate and tricaprylate, and polyvinylpyrrolidone. C8 plays the role of a permeation enhancer by causing a transient opening of the intestinal epithelial tight junctions, thus creating a paracellular pathway for peptides with a molecular weight lower than 10 kDa (octreotide: 1.14 kDa) [10].

The pharmacokinetic parameters, such as peak plasma concentration and area under the curve, are similar after oral administration of 20 mg octreotide or subcutaneous administration of 100 µg octreotide in human subjects [11]. The first results of phase III trials for OOCs were published in 2015 through the open-label CH-ACM-01 trial [12], followed by the results of the randomized controlled treatment OPTIMAL trial in 2020 [13]. Subsequently, Mycapssa® (OOC) received regulatory approval from the US Food and Drug Administration (FDA) in June 2020 for the long-term maintenance and treatment of patients with acromegaly who have responded to and tolerated treatment with injectable octreotide or lanreotide. The European Medicines Agency delivered a marketing authorization for Mycapssa® in December 2022.

In addition to OOC, paltusotine, a novel oral SRL, has been recently developed by Crinetics Pharmaceuticals™ [14]. Paltusotine is original among oral SRLs due to its nonpeptide nature (Figure 1) and its high specificity for the somatostatin receptor subtype 2, while octreotide has an affinity for both somatostatin receptor subtype 2 and subtype 5. The placebo-controlled phase II ACROBAT Evolve trial (NCT03792555) was designed to assess the safety and efficacy of paltusotine in patients that are responders to long-acting iSRLs, but the results were not published due to the positive results of the ACROBAT Edge trial (NCT03789656). This open-label, phase II, single-arm study demonstrated satisfactory maintenance of biochemical response, leading the FDA to grant orphan drug designation to paltusotine for the treatment of acromegaly. Very interestingly, the first results of the placebo-controlled phase III PATHFNDR-1 trial (NCT04837040) evaluating oral paltusotine in patients with acromegaly previously controlled with iSRLs were recently published in June 2024 [15].

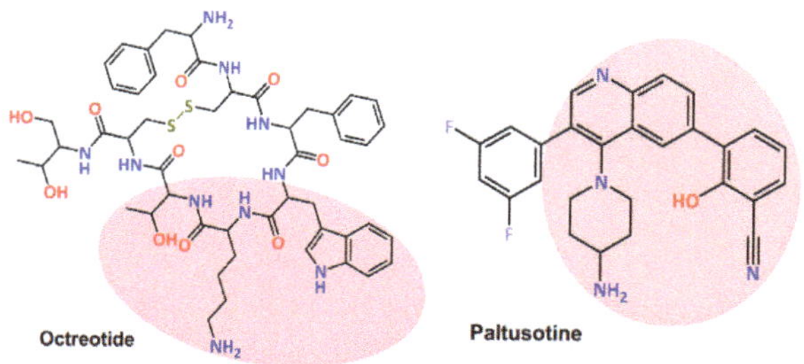

Figure 1. Chemical structures of the somatostatin receptor ligands octreotide and paltusotine. Pink area highlights similar moieties. Reproduced from [16] under a Creative Commons Attribution 4.0 International License (http://creativecommons.org/licenses/by/4.0/).

This prompted us to conduct a systematic review of clinical trials of SRLs administrated via the oral route in patients with acromegaly by focusing on their efficacy based on the biochemical response, which is the strongest predictor of patient outcomes.

2. Materials and Methods

Our systematic review was presented according to the PRISMA 2020 statement [17].

2.1. Eligibility Criteria

Table 1 shows the inclusion and exclusion criteria used to select the clinical trials for the review, according to the Population, Intervention, Comparison, Outcome, Study (PICOS) format.

Table 1. Inclusion and exclusion criteria for the selection of studies.

PICOS Parameter	Inclusion Criteria	Exclusion Criteria
Population	Adult individuals with confirmed acromegaly. Any study population size, gender, disease duration, prior treatment (surgery, radiotherapy, none), and degree of clinical and biochemical control.	Non-human animals. Healthy individuals. Patients with syndromic acromegaly: McCune Albright syndrome (OMIM [1]: #174800), Carney syndrome (#160980), X-linked acrogigantism (#300942).
Intervention	Oral administration of SRLs (octreotide, lanreotide, pasireotide, and paltusotine). Any duration, dose, and administration frequency.	Treatment with a drug other than SRLs in order to treat acromegaly; in particular, dopamine and GH receptor agonists.
Comparison	With or without a comparison group (placebo, iSRLs, other drug, radiotherapy, surgery).	
Outcomes	Proportion of responders at the end of the intervention based on serum IGF-1 and/or GH levels (any threshold).	
Study design	Any design (open-label, double blind) Records published in English. Results published in peer-review journals.	Reviews, meta-analysis, case reports, case series, commentaries.

[1] OMIM: Online Mendelian Inheritance in Man.

2.2. Information Sources and Search Strategy

We conducted a search procedure using the PubMed/MEDLINE and ClinicalTrials.gov databases. The search strategy was based on the following words: "acromegaly", "octreotide", "lanreotide", "pasireotide", "paltusotine", and "oral". In addition, the references cited in the included studies were examined to select additional reports for screening. All reports published up to 15 June 2024 were included for further screening.

2.3. Selection and Data Collection Process

The two authors independently screened the titles and abstracts, excluding reports and studies based on the predefined inclusion and exclusion criteria. The remaining studies were integrally read to definitively judge on their inclusion. Disagreements on the eligibility of studies were resolved through discussion and consensus between the two authors. Data from each report were independently collected in Excel sheets by the two authors. No automation tool was used in the selection process or in data collection.

2.4. Data Items (Outcomes)

The primary outcome was the proportion of responders at the end of the treatment period, as determined by serum IGF-1 and GH levels.

2.5. Study Risk of Bias Assessment

The risk of bias in the included studies was independently evaluated by the two authors using the revised Cochrane risk-of-bias tool for randomized trials (RoB 2) and the ROBINS-I tool for uncontrolled trials [18]. Any discrepancies in judgment between the two authors were resolved through discussion.

2.6. Effect Measures

The effect measure of the primary outcome was the percentage of responders among enrolled participants.

2.7. Synthesis Methods

When the 95% confidence intervals of the proportion of responders were not available in the reports, they were determined using the modified Wald method (GraphPad Prism, version 9.5.0).

3. Results

3.1. Study Selection

The flowchart in Figure 2 illustrates the selection process for the studies included in our systematic review. Initially, 136 reports were identified through our search strategy. The majority (n = 87, 64.0%) were excluded based on the initial screening of their titles and abstracts due to non-adherence to our inclusion criteria. An additional fourteen records (10.3%) were excluded either due to non-retrieval or because the biochemical results were not yet available. The unpublished biochemical results were related to the following trials: ACROBAT Evolve (NCT03792555) [19,20], ACROBAT Advance (NCT04261712) [21], and PATHFNDR-2 (NCT05192382) [22].

Of the nineteen studies assessed for eligibility, five were excluded since they were literature reviews, one which was a preclinical study on animals [23], and another one involving a study population of healthy volunteers [24]. The interim results from the single-arm ACROBAT Advance study presented at the Endocrine Society's annual meeting ENDO 2023 in June 2023 were not included in our review due to the lack of a peer-review process [25]. For the same reason, we did not include the results from the double-blind placebo-controlled PATHFNDR-2 study presented at ENDO 2024 in June 2024 [25].

Ultimately, we included twelve reports from the following five clinical trials: CH-ACM-01 (NCT01412424), OPTIMAL (NCT03252353), MPOWERED (NCT02685709), ACROBAT Edge (NCT03789656), and PATHFNDR-1 (NCT04837040). Tables 2 and 3 summarize the key characteristics of these five interventional trials. Three of these trials assessed the efficacy of OOCs (CH-ACM-01, OPTIMAL, and MPOWERED), while the remaining two evaluated oral paltusotine (ACROBAT Edge and PATHFNDR-1).

All the selected trials were designed to include a core phase followed by a single-arm extension phase. The core phase consisted of open-label single arm trials (CH-ACM-01 and ACROBAT Edge), double-blind placebo-controlled trials (OPTIMAL and PATHFNDR-1), and a double-blind iSRL-controlled trial (MPOWERED). A total of 458 individuals with acromegaly, all of whom had achieved biochemical control on iSRLs, were enrolled in the core phases of these trials. Among them, 234 received OOCs, and 77 received paltusotine. The extension phases of these trials were structured as open-label single-arm studies, with biochemical results available for CH-ACM-01, OPTIMAL, and MPOWERED. The extension phases evaluating paltusotine are currently ongoing.

Biochemical measurements of serum IGF-I and GH levels were conducted using the iSYS analyzer with dedicated reagents (ImmunoDiagnostic Systems™, Boldon, UK) across all five clinical trials.

Table 2. Characteristics of the selected studies.

Ref., Publication Year	Trial Name (ClinicalTrials ID) Sponsor	Study Design	Study Population	Intervention
[12,26], 2015	CH-ACM-01 (NCT01412424) Chiasma™	Phase III trial Single-arm Open-label	151 patients with acromegaly and IGF-1 < 1.3 ULN and 2 h integrated GH < 2.5 ng/mL receiving iSRL for ≥3 months.	Core phase (7 months): Administration of the first OOC dose ≥ 4 weeks after the last SRLs injection. OOC 40 mg, escalation to 60, and then 80 mg/d if there was inadequate IGF-1 suppression (2–5 months) followed by a fixed-dose period up to the end of the core phase. Extension phase (6 months): At the fixed-dose determined during the core phase.
[13,27], 2020	OPTIMAL (NCT03252353) Chiasma™	Phase III trial Placebo-controlled Double-blind	56 patients with acromegaly and IGF-1 ≤ 1.0 × ULN after ≥6 months on long-acting iSRL.	Core phase (9 months): OOC (*n* = 28) or placebo (*n* = 28) twice daily (administration of the first dose ≥4 weeks after the last SRLs injection). OOC 40 mg/d, escalation to 60, and then 80 mg/d if there was inadequate IGF-1 (increase ≥ 30% to >1.0 × ULN or >1.0 × ULN for 2 consecutive visits) and/or symptoms suppression.
[28], 2022		Phase III trial Single-arm Open-label	40 patients with completion of the 9-month placebo-controlled phase (20 from the OOC group and 20 from the placebo group).	Extension phase (11 months): OOC 60 mg/d followed by a subsequent dose escalation (80 mg/d, 67.5%) or de-escalation (40 mg/d, 7.5%) based on biochemical results, safety and disease symptoms.
[29,30], 2021	MPOWERED (NCT02685709) Chiasma™	Phase III trial iSRL-controlled Open-label	146 patients with acromegaly and IGF-1 < 1.3 × ULN and mean integrated GH < 2.5 ng/mL on long-acting iSRL for ≥6 months. 92 patients with IGF-1 < 1.3 × ULN and mean integrated GH < 2.5 ng/mL at the end of the run-in phase.	Run-in phase (6 months): OOC 40 mg/d, escalation to 60 or 80 mg/d based on IGF-1 results and acromegaly symptoms. Randomized treatment phase (8.3 months): OOC at the final dose achieved during the run-in-phase (*n* = 55) or iSRL at the dose and interval before trial enrolment (*n* = 37).
[31], 2023		Phase III trial Single-arm Open-label	60 patients with acromegaly and IGF-1 < 1.3 × ULN after the core trial.	Extension phase (≤3.5 years): OOC at the final dose achieved during the run-in-phase.
[32,33], 2022	ACROBAT Edge (NCT03789656) Crinetics Pharmaceuticals™	Phase II trial Single-arm Open-label	47 patients with acromegaly with stable treatment for ≥3 months (including a group of 25 partial responders previously treated with iSRL with IGF-1 ≤ 2.5 × ULN, and a group of 15 partial responders previously treated with iSRL plus dopamine agonist).	Treatment phase (13 weeks): Paltusotine 10 mg/d, escalation to 20, 30, and 40 mg/d. Washout phase (1 month): No treatment
[15,34], 2024	PATHFNDR-1 (NCT04837040) Crinetics Pharmaceuticals™	Phase III trial Placebo-controlled Double-blind	58 patients with acromegaly and IGF-1 ≤ 1.0 × ULN on iSRL for at least 12 weeks.	Core phase (8.3 months): Paltusotine (*n* = 30) or placebo (*n* = 28). Paltusotine 40 mg 1x/d, escalation to 60 mg/d if IGF-1 > 0.9 ULN.

Table 3. Characteristics of participants within the studies included in the review.

Ref.	Trial	Inclusion and Exclusion Criteria
[12]	CH-ACM-01	Inclusion: Adult subjects between 18 and 75 years; patients with acromegaly and documented evidence of a GH-secreting pituitary tumor that is abnormally responsive to glucose, or documented elevated IGF-1, who are currently receiving a stable dose of iSRL for at least the previous 3 months; a serum IGF-1 level < 1.3 × ULN and a serum-integrated GH response over 2 h < 2.5 ng/mL. Exclusion: GH antagonist (within <3 months) or dopamine agonist (within <2 months); radiotherapy within 10 years; pituitary surgery within 6 months before screening; conditions (e.g., bariatric surgery) significantly affecting gastric acidity or emptying; Current use (within 1 month) of proton pump inhibitors and current chronic use of H2-antagonists; female patients who are pregnant or lactating.
[13]	OPTIMAL	Inclusion: Adult subjects ≥ 18 years; confirmed acromegaly: pituitary tumor on imaging or pathology analysis and IGF-1 ≥ 1.3 ULN; IGF-1 ≤ 1.0 × ULN (based on the average of two assessments); treatment with long-acting iSRLs (octreotide or lanreotide) ≥6 months with a stable dose for ≥3 months. Exclusion: Treatment with iSRLs not as indicated in the label; pituitary surgery within 6 months; pituitary radiotherapy; participation in the CH-ACM-01 or MPOWERED trials; symptomatic cholelithiasis; treatment with pegvisomant within 24 weeks, dopamine agonists within 12 weeks, or pasireotide within 24 weeks.
[29]	MPOWERED	Inclusion: Confirmed diagnosis of acromegaly; biochemical control at screening (IGF-1 < 1.3 × ULN and mean integrated GH < 2.5 ng/mL over 2 h); treatment with long-acting forms of iSRL for ≥6 months. Exclusion: Injections of iSRLs at a dosing interval >8 weeks; pituitary radiotherapy within 5 years; pituitary surgery within 6 months; previous participation in the CH-ACM-01 trial; any clinically significant uncontrolled concomitant disease; symptomatic cholelithiasis; treatment with pegvisomant (within 12 weeks), dopamine agonists (within 6 weeks), or pasireotide (within 12 weeks).
[32]	ACROBAT Edge	Inclusion: Age between 18 and 70 years; confirmed diagnosis of acromegaly with either a partial or complete response with SRLs. Exclusion: Treatment-naïve acromegaly subjects; prior treatment with paltusotine; pituitary surgery within 6 months prior to screening; history or presence of malignancy except adequately treated basal cell and squamous cell carcinomas of the skin within the past 5 years; use of any investigational drug within the past 30 days or 5 half-lives; positive screening for human immunodeficiency virus, hepatitis B surface antigen, or hepatitis C antibody or has a history of a positive result; history of alcohol or substance abuse in the past year; any condition that, in the opinion of the investigator, would jeopardize the subject's appropriate participation in this study; cardiovascular conditions or medications associated with prolonged QT or those which predispose subjects to heart rhythm abnormalities; subjects with symptomatic cholelithiasis; subjects with clinically significant abnormal findings during the screening period, and any other medical condition(s) or laboratory findings that might jeopardize the subject's safety or ability to complete the study; subjects taking injectable octreotide at a dose higher than 40 mg, or lanreotide depot at a dose higher than 120 mg, or pasireotide LAR at a dose higher than 60 mg; patients who usually take injectable octreotide or lanreotide depot less frequently than every 4 weeks.
[15]	PATHFNDR-1	Inclusion: Age ≥ 18 years; confirmed diagnosis of acromegaly; biochemical control as measured by IGF-1 ≤ 1.0 × ULN via stable dose of iSRL therapy; females either surgically sterile, post-menopausal, or using an effective method of birth control. Exclusion: Treatment-naïve or treatment-withdrawn acromegaly subjects; prior treatment with paltusotine; pituitary surgery within 24 weeks prior to screening or history of pituitary radiation therapy; history or presence of malignancy except adequately treated basal cell and squamous cell carcinomas of the skin within the past 5 years; use of any investigational drug within the past 30 days or 5 half-lives, whichever is longer; history of HIV, hepatitis B, or active hepatitis C; pregnancy; history of alcohol or substance abuse in the past 12 months; any condition that, in the opinion of the investigator, would jeopardize the subject's appropriate participation in this study; cardiovascular conditions or medications associated with prolonged QT or those which predispose subjects to heart rhythm abnormalities; subjects with symptomatic cholelithiasis; subjects with clinically significant abnormal findings during the screening period, or any other medical condition(s) or laboratory findings that, in the opinion of the Investigator, might jeopardize the subject's safety or ability to complete the study; subjects currently taking long-acting pasireotide (within 24 weeks prior to screening) or pegvisomant, dopamine agonists (within 12 weeks prior to screening), or short-acting somatostatin analogs (within 12 weeks prior to first dose of study drug).

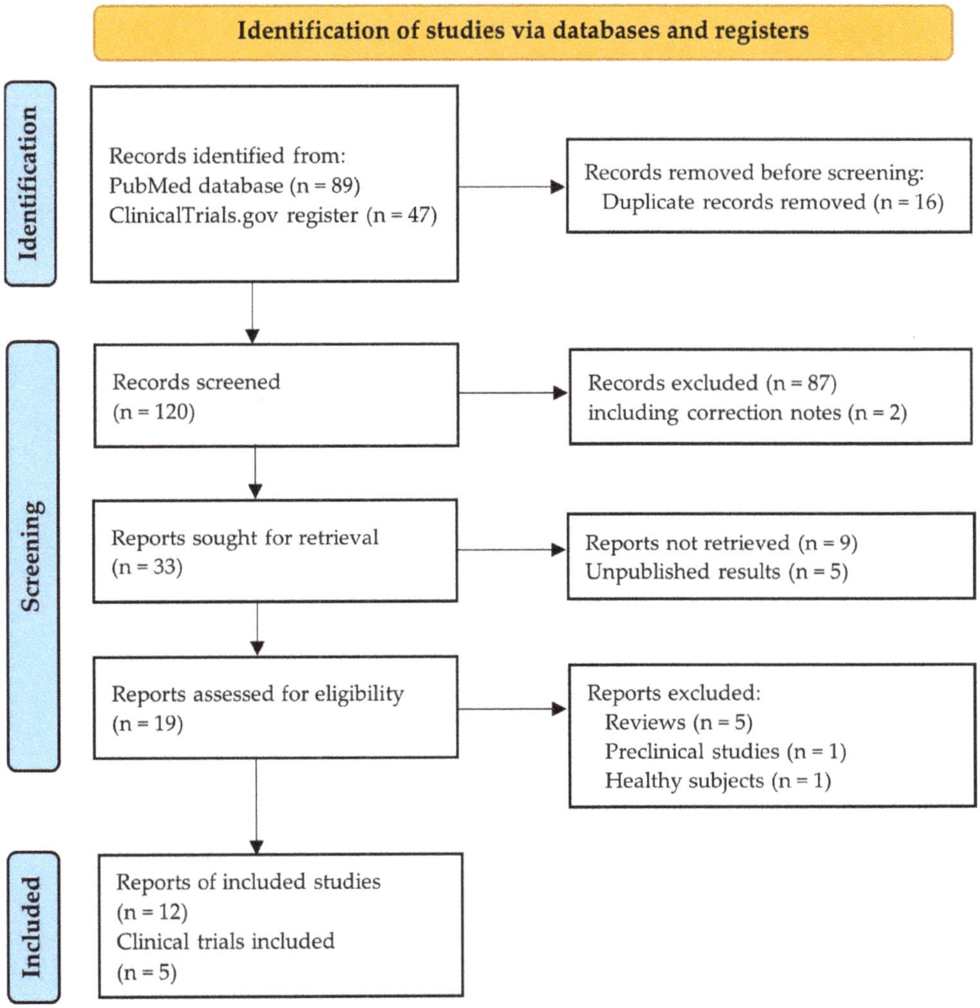

Figure 2. PRISMA flowchart.

3.2. Risk of Bias

Tables 4 and 5 present the assessment of the risk of bias in the randomized and uncontrolled interventional trials, respectively. Several potential biases were identified. In the CH-ACM-01 trial, at baseline in both the core and extension phases, 11% and 17% of participants, respectively, had IGF-1 levels exceeding 1.3 × ULN, despite having IGF-1 levels below this threshold at the time of inclusion. In the open-label MPOWERED trial, six participants were randomly assigned to the OOC group with IGF-I levels greater than 1.3 × ULN, whereas none in the iSRL group had IGF-1 levels above this threshold. Additionally, patients receiving the OOC had higher pre-inclusion doses of iSRLs. Moreover, the proportion of participants in the MPOWERED trial achieving IGF-1 levels below 1.0 times ULN at the end of the OOC treatment was not reported. In the PATHFNDR-1 trial, there were baseline imbalances between the paltusotine and placebo groups in terms of sex ratio, disease duration, and previous injectable octreotide dosage.

Table 4. Assessment of the quality of the randomized interventional trials. Green indicates a low risk of bias, while orange signifies some concerns regarding the risk of bias.

	Randomization Process	Deviations from Intended Interventions	Missing Data	Measurement of the Outcome	Selection of the Results	Overall Judgment
OPTIMAL (core phase)	Green	Green	Orange	Green	Green	Green
MPOWERED (core phase)	Orange	Orange	Green	Orange	Green	Orange
PATHFNDR-1 (core phase)	Green	Orange	Green	Green	Green	Green

Table 5. Assessment of the quality of the uncontrolled interventional trials. Green indicates a low risk of bias, while orange signifies some concerns regarding the risk of bias.

	Confounding	Selection Bias	Missing Data	Measurement of the Outcome	Selection of the Results	Overall Judgment
CH-ACM-01 (core and extension phases)	Orange	Green	Green	Green	Green	Green
ACROBAT Edge (treatment phase)	Green	Green	Orange	Orange	Green	Orange

3.3. Biochemical Response

Table 6 summarizes the rate of responders based on IGF-1 and GH levels in the five selected interventional trials. In the single-arm CH-ACM-01 trial, the rate of responders (i.e., IGF-1 < 1.3 × ULN) reduced from 91.4% at baseline to 64.2% after a 7-month treatment with OOC [12]. The reduction in the proportion of responders was only 6.3% during the extension phase.

Table 6. Efficacy of oral SRLs based on biochemical response.

Ref.	Trial Sponsor	Biochemical Response
[12]	CH-ACM-01	From baseline to the end of the core phase (OOC for 7 months) (n = 151): • IGF-1 < 1.3 × ULN: from 91.4% (85.7–95.3%) to 64.2% (56.0–71.9%). • IGF-1 < 1.3 × ULN + mean GH < 2.5 ng/mL: from 88.7% (82.6–93.3%) to 61.6% (53.3–69.4%). • IGF-1 ≤ 1.0 × ULN: from 63.6% (55.4–71.3%) to 37.8% (30.0–46.0%). • IGF-1 ≤ 1.0 × ULN + mean GH < 1.0 ng/mL: from 43.1% (35.0–51.4%) to 32.5% (25.1–40.5%). From baseline to the end of the extension phase (OOC up to 13 months) (n = 110): • IGF-1 < 1.3 × ULN + mean integrated GH < 2.5 ng/mL: from 82.7% (74.4–89.3%) to 74.6% (65.4–82.4%). • IGF-1 < 1.3 × ULN: from 82.7% (74.4–89.3%) to 76.4% (67.3–83.9%). • IGF-1 ≤ 1.0 × ULN: from 53.6% (43.9–63.2%) to 47.3% (37.7–57.0%).

Table 6. *Cont.*

Ref.	Trial Sponsor	Biochemical Response
[13,28]	OPTIMAL	From baseline to the end of the core phase (9 months) (n = 56): • IGF-1 $\leq$ 1.0 × ULN: - OOC: from 96.4% (81.7–99.9%) to 58.2% (37.4–75.8%). - Placebo: from 82.1% (63.1–93.9%) to 19.4% (7.4–38.2%). - p = 0.008 for the comparison between the two groups at the end of the treatment. • GH < 2.5 ng/mL: - OOC: from 96.4% (81.7–99.9%) to 77.7% (57.6–91.8%). - Placebo: from 89.3% (71.8–97.7%) to 30.4% (15.0–50.5%). - p < 0.001 for the comparison between the two groups at the end of the treatment. • IGF-1 < 1.3 × ULN: - OOC: from 100.0% (87.8–100.0%) to 71.4% (51.3–86.8%). - Placebo: data not available. From baseline to the end of the open-label extension phase (11 months) (n = 40): • IGF-1 $\leq$ 1.0 × ULN: 70.0% (53.5–83.4%) at baseline - From 73.7% (48.8–90.9%) to 52.6% (28.9–75.6%) in patients who received OOC during the core phase, but with a responder rate of 92.6% (78.7–100%) when accounting for missing IGF-1 data.
[29,31]	MPOWERED	From baseline to the end of the randomized treatment phase (n = 92): • IGF-1 < 1.3 × ULN (time-weighted average): - OOC: 89.1% (77.8–95.3%) to 90.9% (80.0–96.5%). - iSRL: 100.0% (90.5–100.0%) to 100.0% (90.5–100.0%). - Statistical non-inferiority of OOC compared to iSRL. Annual evaluation during the extension phase ($\leq$3.5 years) (n = 60): • IGF-1 $\leq$ 1.3 × ULN: - Year 1: from 100% (94.0–100.0%) to 89.7% (78.8–96.1) at the end of year 1 (n = 58). - Year 2: 87.8% (73.8–95.9) at the end of year 2 (n = 41). - Year 3: 93.5% (78.6–99.2) at the end of year 3 (n = 31).
[32]	ACROBAT Edge	From baseline to the end of the treatment phase (13 weeks): • IGF-1 levels: - Patients previously on iSRL monotherapy (n = 25): from 1.34 (1.08–1.47) to 1.34 (1.17–1.45) × ULN (p = 0.63). - Patients previously treated with iSRL plus dopamine agonist (n = 15): from 1.21 × ULN (0.93–1.50) to 1.44 × ULN (1.09–2.08) (p = 0.002). • GH levels: - Patients previously on iSRL monotherapy: from 0.69 ng/mL (0.49–1.55) to 0.72 ng/mL (0.48–1.75) (p = 0.63). - Patients previously treated with iSRL plus dopamine agonist: from 1.04 ng/mL (0.51–1.61) to 1.46 ng/mL (0.62–3.65) (p = 0.0067).
[15]	PATHFNDR-1	From baseline to the end of the core phase (8.3 months) (n = 58): • IGF-1 $\leq$ 1.0 × ULN: - Paltusotine: from 100.0% (88.4–100.0%) to 83.3% (65.3–94.4%). - Placebo: from 100.0% (87.7–100.0%) to 3.6% (0.1–18.4%). - p < 0.0001 between the two groups. • Mean GH < 1.0 ng/mL (n = 41): - Paltusotine (n = 23): from 100.0% (85.2–100.0%) to 87.0% (66.4–97.2%). - Placebo (n = 18): from 100.0% (81.5–100.0%) to 27.8% (9.7–53.5%). - p = 0.0003 between the two groups.

Data are percentage of responders (95% confidence interval) or mean (interquartile range), as appropriate.

In the placebo-controlled OPTIMAL trial, all participants had IGF-1 levels lower than 1.3 × ULN at inclusion but this reduced to 71.4% after 9 months with OOC treatment. The OOC had higher efficacy than placebo in maintaining IGF-1 levels below 1.0 × ULN (+62.7%). The responder rate was 92.6% (78.7–100%) during the 11-month extension phase with OOC.

In the iSRL-controlled MPOWERED trial, the rate of participants with IGF-1 levels inferior to 1.3 × ULN remained stable after 8 months of OOC treatment. The efficacy was not inferior to that of iSRLs. It should be noted that only responders to the OOC during the run-in phase were enrolled in the randomized trial.

In the ACROBAT Edge trial, IGF-1 levels were expressed in concentrations rather than in percentage of responders. Nevertheless, the comparison between the levels at baseline and after paltusotine showed that monotherapy with paltusotine for 13 weeks maintained IGF-1 levels in patients previously on iSRL monotherapy.

Lastly, the core phase of the PATHFNDR-1 trial revealed that oral paltusotine for 8 months maintained IGF-1 levels below 1 × ULN in 83.3% of patients in comparison to 3.6% in the placebo group.

4. Discussion

The oral administration of SRLs, such as OOCs and oral paltusotine, represents an active area of research aiming to provide an efficient alternative to iSRLs in the management of acromegaly. It represents a genuine hope to improve the quality of life of patients with acromegaly. This development represents a promising step forward in the management of acromegaly, offering an alternative to the limitations associated with iSRLs. In particular, iSRLs exhibit disadvantages such as injection-site pain, nodules, swelling, bruising, inflammation, and scarring. Additionally, some patients may experience worsening symptoms of acromegaly and higher IGF-1 levels close to the date of their next injection [5,35]. However, a recent survey revealed that 65% of patients preferred subcutaneous injections administered once every fourth weeks using a pen at home, compared to oral capsules taken twice daily, suggesting that the required three-hour fasting period remains a significant burden [36]. The transition from injectable to oral SRLs should not compromise disease control. Our review indicates that the current data are reassuring in this regard.

The most studied formulation is OOCs, administered twice daily in a fasting state. The pharmacokinetic parameters in human subjects are similar after oral administration of 20 mg octreotide or subcutaneous administration of 100 µg octreotide, particularly regarding the peak plasma concentration and the area under the curve [11]. The mean of the apparent steady state elimination half-life ranged from 3.19 ± 1.07 h on 40 mg of oral octreotide, to 4.47 ± 2.02 h on 80 mg [12]. The first phase III trial, CH-ACM-01, demonstrated a biochemical response after seven months of treatment in approximately two-thirds of patients previously controlled by iSRLs. A similar magnitude of biochemical response was observed after nine months in the OPTIMAL trial, which also showed a clear superiority of the OOC compared to the placebo. Notably, the degree of baseline control on iSRLs was predictive of subsequent biochemical response to the OOC. In CH-ACM-01, the proportion of responders to the OOC reached 84.5% in patients with baseline IGF-1 levels below 1.0 × ULN, compared to 61.6% in the overall study population. The MPOWERED study was the first head-to-head comparison of an OOC with iSRLs in patients previously controlled with iSRLs. It demonstrated the non-inferiority of OOCs to iSRLs after an 8-month treatment period. In addition, it showed that the biochemical response remained satisfactory over three years of maintenance therapy.

In contrast to OOCs, paltusotine offers the advantage of once-daily administration. Paltusotine is associated with increased plasma concentrations to doses up to 40 mg, and is eliminated with a half-life of approximately 30 h [24]. Preclinical studies have demonstrated that paltusotine, an agonist of somatostatin receptor subtype 2, dose-dependently suppresses recombinant GH-releasing hormone-stimulated GH secretion in rats, and dose-dependently reduces IGF-1 levels [37]. In clinical trials conducted in humans, the ACRO-

BAT Edge trial demonstrated that switching from iSRLs to oral paltusotine for thirteen weeks did not compromise biochemical control in patients previously well-managed on iSRL monotherapy. Recently published data from the PATHFNDR-1 trial further confirmed that paltusotine can maintain the biochemical response in over 80% of patients previously controlled with iSRLs, even after eight months of treatment.

Several gaps remain in the clinical validation of oral SRLs, including the need for direct head-to-head comparisons between OOCs and paltusotine. Furthermore, no peer-reviewed data are currently available on the efficacy of oral SRLs in patients who have not received prior treatment with injectable SRLs. However, the ongoing double-blind, placebo-controlled PATHFNDR-2 trial (NCT05192382) is assessing paltusotine in patients who were either treatment-naïve or previously treated but had discontinued medications for at least four months. Preliminary findings from PATHFNDR-2, presented at the ENDO 2024 meeting, reported that, after 24 weeks of treatment, 42.5% of patients in the paltusotine group achieved serum IGF-1 levels below 1.0 × ULN, compared to only 2.4% in the placebo group [22]. Finally, data on the long-term efficacy of paltusotine are still pending. The open-label phase II ACROBAT Advance trial (NCT04261712) is currently ongoing and is designed to evaluate the safety and efficacy of paltusotine over one year of treatment.

One limitation of our study is that the search strategy was restricted to the PubMed/MEDLINE and ClinicalTrials.gov databases. As a result, we may have missed some eligible studies. However, PubMed is one of the largest biomedical bibliographic databases, and ClinicalTrials.gov is a key reference database for interventional trials.

5. Conclusions

Recent advances in pharmaceutical technology have enabled the development of orally administered SRLs, providing a promising alternative to iSRLs in the management of acromegaly. OOCs have demonstrated efficacy in maintaining long-term biochemical control in patients previously stabilized on iSRLs. paltusotine has shown the ability to sustain biochemical control, but its long-term efficacy has yet to be conclusively established.

Author Contributions: Conceptualization, D.D.; methodology, D.D.; formal analysis, C.R. and D.D.; data curation, C.R. and D.D.; writing—original draft preparation, D.D.; writing—review and editing, C.R. and D.D.; supervision, D.D. All authors have read and agreed to the published version of the manuscript.

Funding: This research received no external funding.

Data Availability Statement: The raw data supporting the conclusions of this article will be made available by the authors on request.

Conflicts of Interest: The authors declare no conflicts of interest.

References

1. Crisafulli, S.; Luxi, N.; Sultana, J.; Fontana, A.; Spagnolo, F.; Giuffrida, G.; Ferraù, F.; Gianfrilli, D.; Cozzolino, A.; Cristina De Martino, M.; et al. Global Epidemiology of Acromegaly: A Systematic Review and Meta-Analysis. *Eur. J. Endocrinol.* **2021**, *185*, 251–263. [CrossRef] [PubMed]
2. Melmed, S.; Bronstein, M.D.; Chanson, P.; Klibanski, A.; Casanueva, F.F.; Wass, J.A.H.; Strasburger, C.J.; Luger, A.; Clemmons, D.R.; Giustina, A. A Consensus Statement on Acromegaly Therapeutic Outcomes. *Nat. Rev. Endocrinol.* **2018**, *14*, 552–561. [CrossRef]
3. Strasburger, C.J.; Karavitaki, N.; Störmann, S.; Trainer, P.J.; Kreitschmann-Andermahr, I.; Droste, M.; Korbonits, M.; Feldmann, B.; Zopf, K.; Sanderson, V.F.; et al. Patient-Reported Outcomes of Parenteral Somatostatin Analogue Injections in 195 Patients with Acromegaly. *Eur. J. Endocrinol.* **2016**, *174*, 355–362. [CrossRef] [PubMed]
4. O'Toole, D.; Kunz, P.L.; Webb, S.M.; Goldstein, G.; Khawaja, S.; McDonnell, M.; Boiziau, S.; Gueguen, D.; Houchard, A.; Ribeiro-Oliveira, A.; et al. PRESTO 2: An International Survey to Evaluate Patients' Injection Experiences with the Latest Devices/Formulations of Long-Acting Somatostatin Analog Therapies for Neuroendocrine Tumors or Acromegaly. *Adv. Ther.* **2023**, *40*, 671–690. [CrossRef]
5. Geer, E.B.; Sisco, J.; Adelman, D.T.; Ludlam, W.H.; Haviv, A.; Liu, S.; Mathias, S.D.; Gelbaum, D.; Shi, L. Patient Reported Outcome Data from Acromegaly Patients Treated with Injectable Somatostatin Receptor Ligands (SRLs) in Routine Clinical Practice. *BMC Endocr. Disord.* **2020**, *20*, 117. [CrossRef]

6. Adelman, D.; Truong Thanh, X.-M.; Feuilly, M.; Houchard, A.; Cella, D. Evaluation of Nurse Preferences between the Lanreotide Autogel New Syringe and the Octreotide Long-Acting Release Syringe: An International Simulated-Use Study (PRESTO). *Adv. Ther.* **2020**, *37*, 1608–1619. [CrossRef]
7. Chen, G.; Kang, W.; Li, W.; Chen, S.; Gao, Y. Oral Delivery of Protein and Peptide Drugs: From Non-Specific Formulation Approaches to Intestinal Cell Targeting Strategies. *Theranostics* **2022**, *12*, 1419–1439. [CrossRef]
8. Kim, J.C.; Park, E.J.; Na, D.H. Gastrointestinal Permeation Enhancers for the Development of Oral Peptide Pharmaceuticals. *Pharmaceuticals* **2022**, *15*, 1585. [CrossRef]
9. Brayden, D.J.; Maher, S. Transient Permeation Enhancer® (TPE®) Technology for Oral Delivery of Octreotide: A Technological Evaluation. *Expert Opin. Drug Deliv.* **2021**, *18*, 1501–1512. [CrossRef]
10. Tuvia, S.; Pelled, D.; Marom, K.; Salama, P.; Levin-Arama, M.; Karmeli, I.; Idelson, G.H.; Landau, I.; Mamluk, R. A Novel Suspension Formulation Enhances Intestinal Absorption of Macromolecules via Transient and Reversible Transport Mechanisms. *Pharm. Res.* **2014**, *31*, 2010–2021. [CrossRef]
11. Tuvia, S.; Atsmon, J.; Teichman, S.L.; Katz, S.; Salama, P.; Pelled, D.; Landau, I.; Karmeli, I.; Bidlingmaier, M.; Strasburger, C.J.; et al. Oral Octreotide Absorption in Human Subjects: Comparable Pharmacokinetics to Parenteral Octreotide and Effective Growth Hormone Suppression. *J. Clin. Endocrinol. Metab.* **2012**, *97*, 2362–2369. [CrossRef] [PubMed]
12. Melmed, S.; Popovic, V.; Bidlingmaier, M.; Mercado, M.; van der Lely, A.J.; Biermasz, N.; Bolanowski, M.; Coculescu, M.; Schopohl, J.; Racz, K.; et al. Safety and Efficacy of Oral Octreotide in Acromegaly: Results of a Multicenter Phase III Trial. *J. Clin. Endocrinol. Metab.* **2015**, *100*, 1699–1708. [CrossRef] [PubMed]
13. Samson, S.L.; Nachtigall, L.B.; Fleseriu, M.; Gordon, M.B.; Bolanowski, M.; Labadzhyan, A.; Ur, E.; Molitch, M.; Ludlam, W.H.; Patou, G.; et al. Maintenance of Acromegaly Control in Patients Switching From Injectable Somatostatin Receptor Ligands to Oral Octreotide. *J. Clin. Endocrinol. Metab.* **2020**, *105*, e3785–e3797. [CrossRef] [PubMed]
14. McLaren, D.S.; Murray, R.D. Paltusotine, a Novel Oral Somatostatin Receptor Ligand in the Management of Acromegaly. *J. Clin. Endocrinol. Metab.* **2023**, *108*, e193–e194. [CrossRef]
15. Gadelha, M.R.; Casagrande, A.; Strasburger, C.J.; Bidlingmaier, M.; Snyder, P.J.; Guitelman, M.A.; Boguszewski, C.L.; Buchfelder, M.; Shimon, I.; Raverot, G.; et al. Acromegaly Disease Control Maintained after Switching from Injected Somatostatin Receptor Ligands to Oral Paltusotine. *J. Clin. Endocrinol. Metab.* **2024**, dgae385. [CrossRef]
16. Zhao, J.; Fu, H.; Yu, J.; Hong, W.; Tian, X.; Qi, J.; Sun, S.; Zhao, C.; Wu, C.; Xu, Z.; et al. Prospect of Acromegaly Therapy: Molecular Mechanism of Clinical Drugs Octreotide and Paltusotine. *Nat. Commun.* **2023**, *14*, 962. [CrossRef]
17. Page, M.J.; McKenzie, J.E.; Bossuyt, P.M.; Boutron, I.; Hoffmann, T.C.; Mulrow, C.D.; Shamseer, L.; Tetzlaff, J.M.; Akl, E.A.; Brennan, S.E.; et al. The PRISMA 2020 Statement: An Updated Guideline for Reporting Systematic Reviews. *BMJ* **2021**, *372*, n71. [CrossRef]
18. Sterne, J.A.C.; Savović, J.; Page, M.J.; Elbers, R.G.; Blencowe, N.S.; Boutron, I.; Cates, C.J.; Cheng, H.-Y.; Corbett, M.S.; Eldridge, S.M.; et al. RoB 2: A Revised Tool for Assessing Risk of Bias in Randomised Trials. *BMJ* **2019**, *366*, l4898. [CrossRef]
19. A Study to Evaluate the Safety and Efficacy of Paltusotine for the Treatment of Acromegaly (ACROBAT Evolve). Available online: https://clinicaltrials.gov/study/NCT03792555?a=3 (accessed on 15 June 2024).
20. Martin, S.; Bender, R.H.; Krasner, A.; Marmon, T.; Monahan, M.; Nelson, L. Development and Evaluation of the Acromegaly Symptom Diary. *J. Patient Rep. Outcomes* **2023**, *7*, 15. [CrossRef]
21. A Study to Evaluate the Long-Term Safety and Efficacy of Paltusotine for the Treatment of Acromegaly (ACROBAT Advance). Available online: https://clinicaltrials.gov/study/NCT04261712 (accessed on 15 June 2024).
22. A Study to Evaluate the Safety and Efficacy of Paltusotine for the Treatment of Acromegaly (PATHFNDR-2). Available online: https://clinicaltrials.gov/study/NCT05192382 (accessed on 15 June 2024).
23. Zhao, J.; Wang, S.; Markison, S.; Kim, S.H.; Han, S.; Chen, M.; Kusnetzow, A.K.; Rico-Bautista, E.; Johns, M.; Luo, R.; et al. Discovery of Paltusotine (CRN00808), a Potent, Selective, and Orally Bioavailable Non-Peptide SST2 Agonist. *ACS Med. Chem. Lett.* **2023**, *14*, 66–74. [CrossRef]
24. Madan, A.; Markison, S.; Betz, S.F.; Krasner, A.; Luo, R.; Jochelson, T.; Lickliter, J.; Struthers, R.S. Paltusotine, a Novel Oral Once-Daily Nonpeptide SST2 Receptor Agonist, Suppresses GH and IGF-1 in Healthy Volunteers. *Pituitary* **2022**, *25*, 328–339. [CrossRef] [PubMed]
25. Biller, B.M.K.; Casagrande, A.; Elenkova, A.; Boguszewski, C.L.; Jallad, R.; Hu, B. 12535 Efficacy and Safety of Once-Daily Oral Paltusotine in Medically Untreated Patients with Acromegaly: Results from the Phase 3, Randomized, Placebo-Controlled Pathfndr-2 Study. *J. Endocr. Soc.* **2024**, *8*, bvae163.1201. [CrossRef]
26. Efficacy and Safety of Octreotide (MYCAPSSATM [Formerly OctreolinTM]) for Acromegaly. Available online: https://clinicaltrials.gov/study/NCT01412424 (accessed on 15 June 2024).
27. Efficacy and Safety of Octreotide Capsules (MYCAPSSA) in Acromegaly. Available online: https://clinicaltrials.gov/study/NCT03252353 (accessed on 15 June 2024).
28. Samson, S.L.; Nachtigall, L.B.; Fleseriu, M.; Jensterle, M.; Manning, P.J.; Elenkova, A.; Molitch, M.E.; Ludlam, W.H.; Patou, G.; Haviv, A.; et al. Durable Biochemical Response and Safety with Oral Octreotide Capsules in Acromegaly. *Eur. J. Endocrinol.* **2022**, *187*, 733–741. [CrossRef]

29. Fleseriu, M.; Dreval, A.; Bondar, I.; Vagapova, G.; Macut, D.; Pokramovich, Y.G.; Molitch, M.E.; Leonova, N.; Raverot, G.; Grineva, E.; et al. Maintenance of Response to Oral Octreotide Compared with Injectable Somatostatin Receptor Ligands in Patients with Acromegaly: A Phase 3, Multicentre, Randomised Controlled Trial. *Lancet Diabetes Endocrinol.* **2022**, *10*, 102–111. [CrossRef]
30. Comparison of Oral Octreotide Capsules to Injectable Somatostatin Analogs in Acromegaly. Available online: https://clinicaltrials.gov/study/NCT02685709 (accessed on 15 June 2024).
31. Fleseriu, M.; Molitch, M.; Dreval, A.; Pokramovich, Y.; Bondar, I.; Poteshkin, Y.; Macut, D.; Obermayer-Pietsch, B.; Gilgun-Sherki, Y.; Haviv, A.; et al. MPOWERED Trial Open-Label Extension: Long-Term Efficacy and Safety Data for Oral Octreotide Capsules in Acromegaly. *J. Clin. Endocrinol. Metab.* **2023**, *108*, 3214–3222. [CrossRef]
32. Gadelha, M.R.; Gordon, M.B.; Doknic, M.; Mezősi, E.; Tóth, M.; Randeva, H.; Marmon, T.; Jochelson, T.; Luo, R.; Monahan, M.; et al. ACROBAT Edge: Safety and Efficacy of Switching Injected SRLs to Oral Paltusotine in Patients With Acromegaly. *J. Clin. Endocrinol. Metab.* **2023**, *108*, e148–e159. [CrossRef]
33. A Study to Evaluate the Safety and Efficacy of Paltusotine for the Treatment of Acromegaly (ACROBAT Edge). Available online: https://clinicaltrials.gov/study/NCT03789656 (accessed on 1 June 2024).
34. A Study to Evaluate the Safety and Efficacy of Paltusotine for the Treatment of Acromegaly. Available online: https://clinicaltrials.gov/study/NCT04837040 (accessed on 15 June 2024).
35. Maione, L.; Albrici, C.; Grunenwald, S.; Mouly, C.; Cimino, V.; Lecoq, A.-L.; Souberbielle, J.C.; Caron, P.; Chanson, P. IGF-I Variability Over Repeated Measures in Patients With Acromegaly Under Long-Acting Somatostatin Receptor Ligands. *J. Clin. Endocrinol. Metab.* **2022**, *107*, e3644–e3653. [CrossRef]
36. Sisco, J.; Furumalm, M.; Yssing, C.; Okkels, A.; Zavisic, S. Preferences for Different Treatment Options among People Living with Acromegaly in the US. *Curr. Med. Res. Opin.* **2024**, *40*, 657–664. [CrossRef]
37. Betz, S.F.; Markison, S.; Kusnetzow, A.K.; Athanacio, J.D.; Rico-Bautista, E.; Madan, A.; Johns, M.; Zhu, Y.F.; Schonbrunn, A.; Struthers, R.S. Suppression of Growth Hormone and Insulin-Like Growth Factor 1 in Rats After Oral Administration of CRN00808, a Small Molecule, Sst2 Selective Somatostatin Biased Agonist. *Endocr. Rev.* **2018**, *39*, i1–i1417.

MDPI AG
Grosspeteranlage 5
4052 Basel
Switzerland
Tel.: +41 61 683 77 34

Pharmaceutics Editorial Office
E-mail: pharmaceutics@mdpi.com
www.mdpi.com/journal/pharmaceutics

www.ingramcontent.com/pod-product-compliance
Lightning Source LLC
Chambersburg PA
CBHW040824250926
51850CB00007BA/1252
* 9 7 8 3 7 2 5 8 6 9 1 8 3 *